WELCOME TO

LABOR AND DELIVERY

A Bedside Companion to Your Hospital Childbirth Experience

KIMBERLY E. HEATHCOTE, BSN, RN
Labor Nurse

Published by:
Welcome to Labor and Delivery Press, LLC.
New Jersey, USA

ISBN (paperback): 979-8-9943173-0-3
ISBN (hardcover): 979-8-9943173-1-0

Cover design by Sole from Luna Design
Book Formatting by Daiana Morales

Disclaimer:
This book is intended for educational and informational purposes only. It is not a substitute for professional medical advice, diagnosis, or treatment. Always seek the guidance of your healthcare provider or qualified medical professional with any questions regarding medical conditions or treatment.
Clinical practices, policies, and protocols may vary by institution. The perspectives shared in this book reflect the author's professional experience and are not intended to represent any specific hospital, healthcare system, or employer. The author's views are her own and do not reflect the views or policies of any healthcare organization or employer. Nursing is both an art and a science. Care approaches may vary between providers, institutions, and regions.

First Edition
Printed in the United States of America

A Special Dedication to My Labor & Delivery Family

To my L&D staff — **you know who you are.**

Every nurse, midwife, doctor, scrub tech, anesthesia provider, postpartum and NICU nurse, housekeeping staff who quietly care for our spaces and our patients, and even the registration team who greets our families at the door — this chapter of my life belongs to all of you just as much as it belongs to me.

We are a team.
A family built through adrenaline, laughter, tears, relentless shifts, and the sacred moments we witness together.

You have shaped me into the nurse I am today.

In every emergency, every shoulder dystocia, every hemorrhage, every birth that made the room hold its breath — you stood beside me, guided me, supported me, and believed in me.

Everything I know, everything I teach, and everything I pass on to my patients and fellow nurses comes from standing shoulder-to-shoulder with you.

To the seasoned nurses — thank you for carrying the kind of wisdom that can only be learned through years of birth, loss, and everything in between.

To the new nurses — thank you for reminding me what passion looks like, for the questions that made me think deeper, and for the fire you reignite in all of us.

To the midwives and doctors — thank you for trusting me, teaching me, and challenging me to grow.

To the scrub techs — thank you for your incredible support in the OR and beyond. Your preparation, focus, and quiet confidence hold the unit together more than you'll ever know. Nursing could **NOT** do this work without you.

To the NICU and postpartum units — thank you for caring for our babies and families the moment they leave our hands.

To every nurse I have ever taught — you made me a better teacher. You pushed me to explain more clearly, speak more compassionately, and care more intentionally.

To my people:
I could not have written this book without you.
Your fingerprints are on every page.

No matter where I go in this profession, I will carry you with me — **in my practice, in my teaching and endeavors, and in my heart**.

Thank you for helping me become the nurse capable of writing this.

With all my Love and Gratitude,

Kim

Disclaimer

This book is **not** a substitute for the care, expertise, or guidance of the healthcare professionals assigned to you during your hospital stay. It is intended for educational purposes only.

Nursing is both an **art and a science**, and every nurse practices it a little differently. No single way is better or worse — just different. What you'll read here reflects **my practice**, shaped over many years of caring for women and families through one of the most meaningful experiences of their lives.

These are the approaches and insights that have worked for me — the small things that have made labor, birth, and recovery a little less frightening and a lot more empowering. My goal for this book is to make your birthing experience feel **safe, informed, and deeply human,** giving you real bedside wisdom that helps you embrace one of life's most powerful moments.

Use this book as a **supplementary guide and reference**, but always follow the advice and instructions of your professional healthcare provider regarding your individual situation.

We share the same goal: **the best possible outcome for you, your family, and your baby**.

TABLE OF CONTENTS

1

Welcome to Labor and Delivery! Introduction

"In giving birth to our babies, we may find that we give birth to new possibilities within ourselves."

— **Myla and Jon Kabat-Zinn**

Welcome to Labor and Delivery! That is quite literally what I say to my patients — and I mean it every single time. I'm so excited for you. What you're about to do will change your life forever and I feel privileged to be part of one of the most meaningful moments you'll ever experience.

With that said, I know that you may also feel uncertain, maybe even a little afraid of what this process will look like for you. Whether you're a first-time mom or this is your fifth baby, it's completely normal to feel nervous. It's scary for the first-time mom because she doesn't know what to expect and it's scary for the seasoned mom because she does.

But please believe me when I say this: **you are made to do this**. Everything within you was created to be the mother of this baby. You were a mother long before you ever walked through these doors.

The goal of this book is to make your experience a little less intimidating by walking you step-by-step through the childbirth and hospital process, while explaining the reasoning behind what we do as healthcare providers. Read this book **before** you come in for your big day so you feel prepared, confident, and empowered. Then, **bring it with you** to the hospital — you can reference it throughout labor, during questions, and in those moments when you need clarity or reassurance. I wrote this book for you and it is meant to be your ultimate bedside companion.

I truly believe that when you understand **why** things are happening, you can let your guard down, trust the process, and begin to truly appreciate what is about to unfold — one of the greatest experiences of your life.

So come with me — **I'll show you the way.**

A Note From the Author

I realize this book is long. That was never the intention. But the more I thought about you — the patient, the mother, the family — the more information I wanted to give you. I didn't want to leave a single stone unturned. I didn't want anyone to feel unseen or unheard.

Every topic, every explanation, every chapter came from a place of wanting you to feel prepared, informed, and comforted. Some sections you may never need — and that's okay. Visit one chapter or visit them all.

This book is a **toolbox**, a **companion**, a **hand to hold**. Everything inside it is here because I care about you. I care about your birth experience. I care about the questions you don't know to ask. I care about the moments that scare you, the ones that excite you, and the ones you'll remember for the rest of your life.

You may not need every piece of information in these pages, but I wanted it to be here if you did. Because you deserve to feel supported, informed, and empowered — **every step of the way**.

2

Your Birth Plan and Beyond

"The power of a birth plan isn't the actual plan, it's the process of becoming educated about all your options."

— Plus Sized Birth

A Kinder, Clearer Version

Everyone comes into labor with a vision of how they hope their birth will unfold — and I deeply respect that. **Your wishes matter. Your preferences matter. Your voice matters.**

As your healthcare team, we genuinely want to honor what's important to you and make your experience as close to your hopes as possible.

Birth plans are wonderful tools. They help us understand what matters most — things like delayed cord clamping, staying mobile, avoiding unnecessary interventions, or wanting a low-intervention birth. Sharing those wishes helps us care for you in a way that aligns with your values.

But sometimes, labor takes unexpected turns. And in those moments, **safety becomes the priority** — your safety and your baby's. If a request doesn't align with what's medically safe in that moment, we'll explain why, talk through your options, and help you make the best decision with the information we have.

You never lose your voice in the process.

You always have the right to ask questions.
You always have the right to say yes or no.
You always deserve to understand the risks, benefits, and alternatives.

Empowered decisions aren't about sticking rigidly to a plan — they're about feeling **informed, supported, and respected**, no matter how your birth unfolds.

Our goal will always be the same as yours:
a healthy mom, a healthy baby, and a birth experience that leaves you feeling seen, heard, and cared for.

Nurse's Tip: Questions to Ask When Creating Your Birth Plan

When you sit down to write your birth plan, keep these questions in mind:

- What aspects of birth are most important to me? (comfort, mobility, partner involvement, environment)
- How do I feel about pain management options – both medical and natural?
- What are my preferences for immediate newborn care? (delayed cord clamping, skin-to-skin, feeding)
- Who do I want to be present and what role will they play?

- If unexpected circumstances arise, how flexible am I willing to be?
- What questions can I ask my care team to better understand the risks and benefits of each decision?

Remember: A birth plan is not a contract — it's a **conversation**. The best outcomes happen when you and your care team work together, guided by **trust, safety, and respect.**

You Are Beautiful Here: A Love Letter to the Laboring Body

Before anything else, know this — **you are powerful, worthy, and never need to apologize for your body.**

Your Body, Your Beauty: Embracing Yourself in Pregnancy and Beyond

Pregnancy and birth change your body in ways that are powerful, unexpected, and often humbling. You'll see and feel shifts that remind you every day that your body is doing sacred work — creating life.

But for many women, being in a hospital gown under bright lights, surrounded by strangers and medical equipment, can make them feel vulnerable and exposed.

I see this every day — women apologizing for how they look, covering themselves up, or saying "I'm sorry" before we even begin an exam. Let me say this clearly:

You have nothing to be sorry for.

The Hospital Is a Place of Care, Not Judgment

In Labor and Delivery, we don't see imperfections — we see strength, anatomy, and purpose. Every mark, curve, and change tells a story about your pregnancy and how your body has worked to bring your baby this far.

When I walk into your room, I don't see your stretch marks or swollen ankles — **I see a woman doing the hardest, bravest thing imaginable.** (Granted, I *am* taking note of those swollen ankles to be sure they don't mean anything else — but that's what nurses do. We look out for you, not down on you.)

We know you may feel exposed but we treat every part of you with dignity, respect, and compassion. We see beauty in the process — not in perfection. Your body is doing something extraordinary and our goal is to make you feel safe and supported through every step.

Why You Shouldn't Feel Self-Conscious

Pregnancy and birth are not "pretty" by society's standards — they're **real**. They're raw, powerful, and filled with moments of both strength and surrender. There will be fluids, noises, and positions you never imagined yourself in — and that's okay. **That's labor.**

You might worry about your appearance, how your body looks on the table, or if your provider will think something about you. I promise you — **we don't.**

We are focused on your:

- Safety
- Comfort
- Progress

- Strength
- And how your baby is doing

Not your size, shape, or scars.

> **Nurse's Tip**
>
> Try to let go of self-consciousness and allow yourself to be cared for.
> Your nurses and providers have seen every kind of body – every shape, every story.
> You deserve to be here exactly as you are, without apology or embarrassment.

Celebrating the Body That Carried You Here

Your body has grown organs, increased blood volume shifted and stretched in ways most people never think about. And it will continue to serve you through birth, recovery, and motherhood.

Take a deep breath and thank your body for what it's doing right now — even if you're scared or uncomfortable. That simple gratitude can shift your mindset from shame to pride.

You don't need to look a certain way to be beautiful.
You don't need to be perfect to be powerful.
You already are.

Your body is not just a vessel — **it's the home where your baby began,** and that alone makes it sacred.

3

Let's Get the Party Started!

"It's not my birthday party, I'm just invited to it!"

– Kim Heathcote

When you first arrive in Labor and Delivery — whether it's for a scheduled induction, spontaneous labor, or a planned cesarean section — you're going to be greeted by several people. Registration will check your ID and insurance, the nurses will get you settled, help you change into a gown, and maybe ask for a urine specimen if your facility requires it. Then we'll sit you up in bed and place the monitors on your belly to check on your baby.

At this point, you might feel like you've just pulled into the pit lane at the Indy 500 — a lot is happening all at once! Take a deep breath. This is normal. We'll connect you to fetal monitors, check your blood pressure and temperature, draw admission labs, and start an IV.

I want you to be aware of **any** information we take from you.
Your blood pressure? You should know it.
Your temperature? We should tell you it.
This is **your** information — you have a right to it.

If your facility offers portable monitors, ask for them! Mobility during labor is key — it helps your baby move down into the pelvis during contractions, reduces the risk of blood clots, and serves as both a distraction and a natural coping mechanism for pain.

It's not my practice to connect you to IV fluids unless medically indicated. I want you to have the freedom to move around, use the birthing ball, and feel less restricted. And if your plan includes an epidural, I'll encourage you to stay active while you can.

The Q&A Session

Next comes what I like to call the **questions and answers** portion of our time together. I need to know everything about your medical history. Don't leave anything out. Tell me about your allergies, past and current medical conditions, medications, and even any recreational or illicit drug use.

This information helps me care for you safely and make the best decisions for your baby. Think of talking to me like you're talking to your pastor, priest, or chaplain — I'm not here to judge you. What you do outside these hospital walls isn't my concern; **my concern is you and your baby.**

For example, if you withhold that you're taking opioids and I give you a medication called **Nubain**, it could send you into immediate withdrawal. I've seen this happen before and my heart broke watching that patient suffer. Even conditions like hypertension or asthma affect which medications we can safely use in Labor and Delivery. So please — be honest and forthcoming.

Spill your guts like no one is listening. And if you have nothing to offer, God bless you — because you are few and far between!

Paperwork and Consents

Most hospitals will have a few forms for you to sign, including a general consent that allows us to perform standard care for a laboring patient. Have your provider explain what each form means and take a moment to read before you sign.

Know your rights, including policies about **drug testing**. Not all facilities do this routinely anymore, but some still do — and a positive test can lead to a social services consultation.

You'll also likely be asked to sign a **blood transfusion consent**. I don't want to alarm you, but it's important to understand that this could become medically necessary. Postpartum hemorrhage (PPH) remains one of the leading causes of maternal morbidity and mortality worldwide, affecting roughly **14 million women** each year and resulting in **70,000 deaths** (Weller et al., 2025).

I'll discuss this more in a later chapter but know that transfusions are only given when absolutely indicated — blood is precious and never offered lightly.

Your Initial Assessment

Once the paperwork is done, your nurse will complete a head-to-toe assessment. We'll listen to your heart and lungs, check for swelling, and note any wounds or rashes that could affect your care.

In Labor and Delivery, we pay close attention to signs of **preeclampsia and HELLP syndrome** — such as:

- Headaches
- Blurred or double vision
- Epigastric pain (right under your breasts)
- Abnormal swelling

You might notice your nurse checking your reflexes or tapping on your knees. We're not just "messing around" — we're assessing for **hyperreflexia** or **clonus**, which help us understand how your nervous system and blood pressure are responding to pregnancy.

Getting Ready for the Next Step

Once you're settled in and we've completed your admission work, the real fun begins! What happens next depends on why you came in — induction, scheduled cesarean, or spontaneous labor.

In the next sections throughout the book, I'll walk you through what to expect for each of these situations so you can visualize the process and feel confident about what's ahead.

Nurse's Tip: What to Keep in Mind at the Start of Your Experience

Bring your comfort items.

Hospital rooms can feel sterile, but a familiar blanket, pillow, playlist, or essential oil (if allowed) can make a big difference. Comfort calms the nervous system – and calm helps labor progress.

Communicate early and often.

If you're anxious, in pain, or unsure about what's happening – speak up. Your nurse can't help with what they don't know. There's no such thing as over-communicating in Labor and Delivery.

Stay hydrated.

Even if you're limited to clear fluids, sip water or ice chips as permitted. Dehydration can slow contractions and worsen fatigue.

Know your partner's role.

Back rubs? Ice chips? Distraction? Quiet presence? A little guidance goes a long way for support people.

Embrace flexibility.

Labor is unpredictable – sometimes we zig when we expected to zag. Staying open to changes reduces stress and keeps the focus on safety.

Protect your peace.

This is **your** birth space. Lights, visitors, volume, music – you get to choose. I encourage your partner to be close by. And by close, I mean sitting right next to you. If your partner needs to move or I need them to shift, trust me – I'll guide them.

Eat when we say you can.

If we give the green light – **eat!** Once you're in active labor or get an epidural, that window may close. Fuel up while you can.

Keep an empty bladder.

A full bladder can increase pain, slow labor, or prevent your uterus from contracting well after delivery. Emptying often helps more than you'd expect.

Sleep when you can.

This also means before you get there!

Labor can take hours or days. Rest early – you'll need the strength. If you need medication to help you relax, tell your nurse.

Tell us if anything feels "off."

Smells, rashes, fluid changes, bleeding, discomfort – don't hesitate. We've seen it all, and early clues help keep you safe.

Remember:

Your nurse is here for you. There's no such thing as a stupid question or an inconvenience. Never hesitate to use your call bell — a dedicated nurse will *never* be bothered by your needs.

And if they are? They're in the wrong profession.

We got you.

4

Understanding the Language of Labor and Delivery

"However much we know about birth in general,
we know nothing about a particular birth.
We must let it unfold with its own uniqueness."

– Elizabeth Noble

Before we dive into the details of Labor and Delivery, I want to lay the foundation and help you get familiar with the language, phrases or practices you'll hear or experience during your hospital stay. Terms like cervical dilation, effacement, station, or even procedures like foley catheter placement and membrane rupture can sound intimidating — especially when you're hearing them for the first time in the middle of labor.

This section is designed to help you understand those words and phrases so that nothing your nurse or provider says feels like a mystery. When you know what terms like "checking your cervix" or "pain management options" actually mean, you'll feel more confident and part of the conversation.

Labor and Delivery comes with its own vocabulary and each word tells an important part of your story. My goal here is to make sure you understand not just what's happening to your body, but why — turning medical jargon into meaningful information that helps you feel calm, informed, and in control.

Knowledge turns uncertainty into confidence — and that's exactly what I want for you.

KEY TERMS

Admission & Assessment

Cervical Dilation: Opening of the cervix, measured 0–10 cm.

Effacement: Thinning and softening of the cervix (0–100%).

Station: Baby's head position relative to the pelvis (-3 to +3).

Presentation: The part of the baby entering the birth canal first (head, breech, transverse, or shoulder).

Engagement: When baby's head settles into the pelvis ("lightening").

Membrane Status: Whether the amniotic sac (your water) is intact, ruptured, or artificially broken (AROM).

Blood Work: Routine lab tests done on admission usually includes:

CBC (Complete Blood Count): Checks red/white blood cells, hemoglobin/hematocrit & platelets. All important information for baseline, starting numbers.

CMP (Comprehensive Metabolic Panel): Evaluates organ and electrolyte function.

Type & Screen: Identifies blood type and antibody compatibility in case transfusion is needed.

PCR (Protein/Creatinine Ratio): Often ordered if we suspect Pre-eclampsia or HELLP syndrome.

These first steps help your team plan safe, individualized care for you and your baby.

Monitoring & Baby's Well-Being

US (Ultrasound Transducer): Tracks baby's heart rate externally.

TOCO (Tocodynamometer): Measures contraction frequency and duration.

Fetal Scalp Electrode (FSE): Internal monitor that measures the baby's heart rate directly.

Intrauterine Pressure Catheter (IUPC): Internal monitor that measures contraction strength.

Variability: Beat-to-beat changes in baby's heart rate — a good sign.

Accelerations: Heart rate increases that show baby is well oxygenated.

Decelerations: Temporary heart rate drops; sometimes normal, sometimes need action.

Labor Process & Interventions

Contractions: Uterine muscle tightening that opens the cervix and pushes baby down.

Stages of Labor:

- **1st Stage** - Latent Phase 1: Early contractions, 0–6 cm. Active Phase 2: 6–10 cm

- **2nd Stage** – Pushing and Birth of your beautiful baby
- **3rd Stage** – Delivery of the Placenta

Induction or IOL (Induction of Labor): Starting labor using medication, amniotomy (breaking your water), or mechanical methods.

Augmentation: Strengthening or speeding up labor that has already begun.

Epidural: Regional anesthesia injected into the spine for pain relief.

Peanut Ball: A peanut-shaped cushion that helps open the pelvis and promote descent while in bed.

Foley/Straight Catheter: Tube inserted to drain urine, placed often during c-sections or after epidural placement.

TOLAC: "Trial of Labor After Cesarean" — attempting vaginal birth after a prior C-section. Successful completion of a **TOLAC** is a **VBAC** – "Vaginal Birth after Cesarean".

C-Section (Cesarean Section): Surgical delivery of the baby through the abdomen and uterus.

Every intervention has one goal — a safe delivery for you and your baby.

Medical Conditions & Complications

Preterm Labor: Labor that begins before 37 weeks of pregnancy.

Gestational Diabetes: High blood sugar that develops during pregnancy; managed with diet, monitoring, or medication.

Pre-eclampsia: High blood pressure with signs of organ involvement (like protein in the urine).

Eclampsia: Seizures resulting from severe pre-eclampsia — treated as a medical emergency.

HELLP Syndrome: A severe variant of pre-eclampsia with Hemolysis, Elevated Liver Enzymes, Low Platelets.

Polyhydramnios: Too much amniotic fluid.

Oligohydramnios: Too little amniotic fluid.

Placenta Previa: Placenta covers the cervix, increasing risk for bleeding.

Vasa Previa: Fetal blood vessels cross the cervix — requires immediate C-section if ruptured.

Placenta Accreta: Placenta grows too deeply into the uterine wall.

Shoulder Dystocia: When baby's shoulder gets stuck after the head is delivered — requires skilled maneuvers by the team.

Uterine Rupture: Rare but serious tear of the uterus, usually along a prior scar.

Postpartum Hemorrhage (PPH): Excessive bleeding after birth, often from uterine atony or retained tissue.

Cholestasis of Pregnancy: Liver condition causing severe itching and increased bile acids; monitored closely near term.

Group B Strep (GBS): Common bacteria tested for late in pregnancy; treated with IV antibiotics in labor if positive.

These conditions are closely monitored — early recognition and skilled response keep you and baby safe.

Delivery & Postpartum

Crowning: When the baby's head becomes visible during pushing.

Golden Hour: The first hour after birth — quiet bonding time with uninterrupted skin-to-skin and breastfeeding initiation.

Colostrum: The thick, golden "first milk" rich in antibodies that nourishes and protects your newborn.

Fundus: The top of your uterus — we check to ensure it's firm and contracted.

Lochia: Normal vaginal discharge after delivery (blood, mucus, tissue).

Perineal Care: Cleaning and soothing of the vaginal and perineal area after birth.

Skin-to-Skin: Baby placed directly on your chest to stabilize temperature, heart rate, and bonding. This can happen with your partner as well!

Apgar Score: A quick newborn assessment at 1 and 5 minutes after birth.

The work of birth doesn't end when your baby arrives — it shifts into recovery, bonding, and healing.

Understanding this language will make the conversations you have with your healthcare team feel a lot less like a foreign language — and a lot more like a shared experience.

5

“Necessary Evils: The Things We Do That Don’t Always Feel Good”

“The tough parts are temporary — the safety they give you isn’t.”

Vital Monitoring & Constant Observation

One thing you’ll quickly notice after being admitted is that we keep a very close eye on you — sometimes it feels like we’re checking something every five minutes. That’s not because we don’t trust your body; it’s because our job is to catch the subtle changes before they become big problems. We will absolutely honor your privacy whenever you want it and avoid unnecessary interventions whenever it’s safe to do so. Just know that when our eyes are on you, it’s never about control—it’s about keeping both you and your baby safe.

Why Constant Monitoring Matters

Your body is going through one of the most intense physiological events it will ever experience — your heart rate, blood pressure, oxygen level, temperature, and respiratory rate can all shift quickly depending on what stage of labor you're in, what medications you've received, or how your baby is tolerating the process.

Regular checks help us detect things like:

- Early signs of pre-eclampsia or postpartum hypertension
- Reactions to medications (Pitocin, magnesium sulfate, epidural anesthesia)
- Changes in blood loss that could signal hemorrhage
- Drops in oxygen if you're breathing fast or anxious
- Fever or infection after your water breaks

It's not meant to interrupt your experience — **it's meant to protect it.**

What We Monitor

Blood Pressure (BP):
The intervals in which we take your blood pressure will depend on your situation. Trust me — we will only bother you as much as we have to in order to keep you safe.

Heart Rate & Oxygen Saturation:
Via a pulse oximeter on your finger and only if indicated.

Temperature:
Every 1–4 hours, especially if your membranes are ruptured (to watch for infection).

Respirations:
Especially important if you're on magnesium or have an epidural.

Pain Score:
We'll keep asking — not to annoy you, but to help us adjust interventions if needed. If you don't want to be asked, just tell us.

Bringing up your pain can elevate it — I get that. Just communicate with us and we will do what we can to accommodate you.

For moms on continuous fetal monitoring, we're watching **two lives at once** — your numbers and your baby's heart tracing.

Blood Pressure Cuffs

Yes, it squeezes. Yes, it's annoying — especially when it goes off every 5 minutes. But that cuff tells us how your body is handling labor, medication, or blood loss.

Nurse's Insight:

I know it's repetitive, but every reading gives us data that could save your life if your pressure spikes suddenly or, conversely, goes down. **Knowing is the power!**

Nurse's Tip: I know the cords, wires, and beeping monitors can make you feel like you're in a sci-fi movie. You're not. You're safe - and we're simply keeping tabs on your incredible body while it does the hardest work it's ever done.

If the cords get tangled or feel overwhelming, ask us to reposition them. You deserve comfort and connection even while being monitored.

Again, being constantly checked can feel invasive, I get it - like you can't move or rest without someone touching you or a machine beeping. Please know we don't take that lightly. Every

> number we record has a purpose, and every alarm is a reminder that we're watching closely so you can focus on the most important thing: **bringing your baby safely into the world.**

Blood Draws & Lab Work

When you arrive on Labor and Delivery, one of the first things we do is draw your blood. I know — not the best way to start your birthing adventure — but these labs give us a snapshot of your health and help us plan your care safely.

What We're Checking

CBC (Complete Blood Count):
Tells us your red blood cell level (how much oxygen you can carry), white blood cell count (infection or stress), platelets (how well you'll clot), and includes your **hemoglobin and hematocrit**, which show how much oxygen your blood can deliver and help us assess for anemia or blood loss.

Type & Screen:
Determines your blood type and checks for antibodies. If you were ever to need a transfusion, we already know exactly what's compatible — no delay, no guesswork.

CMP (Comprehensive Metabolic Panel):
Checks blood sugar, kidney and liver function as well as electrolytes. This is especially important if you have pre-eclampsia, HELLP, or are on magnesium sulfate.

PCR or Infection Panels:
Sometimes ordered to rule out pre-eclampsia/HELLP syndrome or infections that could affect you or your baby.

Additional Tests:
Depending on your history, we may check coagulation studies (PT/INR, fibrinogen) or other labs to prepare for a higher-risk birth.

Why It Matters

Your blood work helps us make decisions before they ever become emergencies. For example:

- If your platelets are low, we know to hold off on an epidural until it's safe.
- If your hemoglobin is low, we'll keep an eye out for postpartum bleeding and make sure a transfusion can happen quickly if needed.
- If your blood type shows you're Rh-negative, we'll plan for RhoGAM to protect future pregnancies.

In other words, **these numbers tell us your story behind the scenes.**

Compassion Note: I know this part isn't fun. It's often your first real "hospital" moment, and it can set the tone for your experience. My promise to you? We'll explain everything before we do it and if something hurts more than it should, say so. Labor is about teamwork — and that includes the little things like a blood draw.

IV Access

An IV (intravenous) line will be the next task we complete when you arrive for labor, induction, or certain procedures. It's simply a small, flexible plastic catheter that allows us to give you fluids, medications, or anesthesia quickly and safely.

We usually place it in your hand or forearm, depending on where your veins are most visible and easy to access. In my practice, I try to avoid placing IVs in the antecubital area — that's the bend of your arm. During labor, you'll be moving that arm constantly — holding your belly, pushing, adjusting your position, or cradling your baby after birth. Every time you bend your arm, it can temporarily kink the IV line, blocking the flow of fluids or medications your body needs.

The process only takes a few minutes, and once it's in, you'll be able to move your arm normally.

What It Feels Like

You'll feel a quick pinch or sting when the needle first goes in — kind of like getting your blood drawn. The difference is that once the IV is in place, the needle is removed, leaving only the soft plastic tubing behind.

You might notice a little soreness or tightness at the site for a few minutes, but that usually fades quickly.

Your IV might be connected to fluids or we may simply "saline lock" it — meaning it's capped off and ready to use if needed later. We'll secure it with clear tape so you can move freely without worrying about pulling it out.

Also, keep in mind that in some situations, your care team may need to place a second IV line, especially if you're at risk for postpartum hemorrhage (PPH) or other complications. Having two IVs allows us to give fluids and medications in the one site and potentially blood products in the other quickly if needed.

And trust me — it's much easier to start a second IV **before** an emergency happens, while your blood volume and veins are still stable. Trying to place one during a heavy bleed is far more difficult for both you and your care team.

It's a precaution we take to keep you safe — not because anything is wrong but because we're planning ahead.

Nurse's Tip

- If you're nervous about needles, look away and take slow, deep breaths – it really does help.
- Some moms feel like they are going to pass out. Consider breathing in a small alcohol swab – moms tell me it works.
- Let your nurse know if you've ever had trouble with IVs before (small veins, previous bruising, etc.). Often times we can do a ultrasound guided placement for difficult access.
- If your IV site burns, swells, or feels painful after placement, tell your nurse right away – it might need to be adjusted.
- Hydrating before you come in (if allowed) can make your veins easier to find! So drink up the day before so that your urine is a pale yellow, similar to straw color.
- If you're right-handed, ask for the IV in your left arm so your dominant arm stays free.
- If the sight of the IV makes you uncomfortable, ask for netting so you don't have to see it.

The IV may seem small, but it's one of the most important safety tools we use – it gives us quick access to fluids or medications if you or your baby needs them.

Compassion Note: Some women hate needles and refuse IVs or second lines. That's okay — it's your body. But understand the risks: during emergencies, IV access saves lives. Starting one in a crisis is significantly harder. My goal is to prepare you — not pressure you.

Foley Catheter

A foley catheter is a thin, flexible tube inserted into your bladder to drain urine. In labor and delivery, you might need one if you're on magnesium sulfate, have an epidural, get a C-section, or are otherwise unable to get up to use the bathroom safely. It helps your care team monitor urine output — an important indicator of how your body is handling labor and medications.

What It Feels Like

Most patients describe mild discomfort as the catheter is inserted, like a brief burning or pressure. Once it's in place, you generally don't feel much, although having a tube in your bladder can feel unusual at first.

The catheter has a small balloon at the tip which is inflated to keep it in place — you may feel gentle pressure as it's inflated, but it shouldn't be painful.

You'll be able to move and change positions, though your mobility may be somewhat limited depending on other interventions.

Who Needs a Foley Catheter (and Why)

- **You choose (or need) an epidural.** Once you get an epidural, you may lose the urge and ability to empty your bladder. A full bladder can block the baby's descent and make contractions less effective.
- **You're having a C-section.** While current literature is challenging this need, most surgical births require a foley and it has always been

my practice to place one. It keeps your bladder empty so the surgeon has a clear field and reduces injury risk. It also helps monitor urine output in recovery and the color of the urine can be an indicator of possible bladder injury during surgery.

- **You have pre-eclampsia or are on magnesium sulfate.** If we are concerned about your urine output relating to having this condition, we need accurate measurements of your fluid balance. The foley is essential for this.
- **You're critically ill or high-risk.** Your safety may require limited mobility.
- **You've just delivered and can't void.** Swelling or anesthesia can temporarily make it hard to urinate. Having a full bladder can increase your risk of postpartum hemorrhage.

> **Nurse's Tip:** If you feel burning, tugging, or discomfort, let your nurse know. Also – always keep the drainage bag **below** bladder level to prevent backflow.

Straight Catheterization (In-and-Out Cath)

Sometimes, instead of a foley catheter that stays in place, we'll insert a straight catheter — exactly what it sounds like. It goes in once, drains your bladder, and comes right back out.

We sometimes use this method for:

- Collecting a sterile urine sample
- Emptying your bladder after an epidural
- Helping you void after delivery if swelling or ability prevents it

You'll feel a brief burning or pressure, but once the urine drains, most patients feel **immediate relief.**

Nurse's Tip: A little stinging the first time you urinate afterward is normal. Persistent burning? Tell us – we can help.

Monitoring Your Output

Your urine output tells us how your body is responding to fluids, medications, stress, and labor. It's one of the earliest indicators that something might be off.

Two ways we measure:

- **Foley catheter:** continuous drainage into a clear bag
- **"Hat" in the toilet:** a basin that collects urine for measurement

Nurse's Tip: Always tell your nurse when you void – even if it seems routine.

Compassion Note: Measuring your pee isn't glamorous — but it helps keep you safe.

The Importance of SCDs (Sequential Compression Devices)

There may be certain medical conditions or procedures that put you at higher risk for blood clots and we ask that you wear SCDs. You may notice your nurse rolling in a pair of strange-looking sleeves that wrap around your lower legs and make a soft "whoosh" sound every few seconds. They're called Sequential Compression Devices (SCDs).

They can feel awkward but they're one of the most important tools we use to keep you safe during the labor process or after delivery.

SCDs gently squeeze your calves in a rhythm that mimics walking. They help push blood back toward your heart, preventing blood clots from forming while you're lying in bed.

After having a baby — especially if you had a C-section, epidural, magnesium infusion, or any period of prolonged bedrest — your blood naturally becomes "stickier" as your body works to stop bleeding. Combine that with being less mobile, and you've got the perfect recipe for a **deep vein thrombosis (DVT)** — which we absolutely want to avoid.

So when we say, **"keep your SCDs on," please do!** I know they're warm, noisy, and not the height of comfort, but they're quietly protecting you from something far more dangerous.

> **Nurse's Tip:** If you're sweating or your legs feel itchy under the sleeves, tell your nurse – we can take them off for short breaks or help adjust them for comfort. Once you're up and walking, you won't need them anymore – **movement is the best natural clot prevention there is.**

Compassion Note: Nothing about antepartum and postpartum care feels particulary glamorous. You've got cords, cuffs, IVs, and buzzing leg wraps. But every one of them has a purpose — and SCDs are among the quiet protectors that save lives. Wear them proudly — they're part of your healing team.

Incentive Spirometer: Breathe Like You Mean It

You might notice a small plastic device appear on your bedside table that looks like something out of a science fair project — that's your incentive spirometer. It's not the most glamorous tool, but it's one of the simplest ways to keep your lungs healthy after delivery or during a condition that requires them.

Not everyone gets one of these — **you are the chosen few.**

You'll use it by inhaling through a mouthpiece to make a little ball rise inside the chamber. Sounds silly, I know — but here's why it matters:

- After a C-section or long labor, you're at risk for shallow breathing. Pain, anesthesia, and lying flat can make you take smaller breaths, which allows fluid to collect in your lungs and increases the risk for pneumonia or atelectasis.
- If you've been on magnesium sulfate, your respiratory system is a little slower than usual. The incentive spirometer helps you take deep, intentional breaths to re-expand your lungs.
- If you've had a long epidural or limited mobility, deep breathing helps counteract the effects of being in bed — just like SCDs help your legs, the spirometer helps your lungs.

> **Nurse's Tip:** Try using your spirometer every hour while awake, especially after surgery or while on medications that make you sleepy. Take **10 slow, deep breaths**, hold for a two or three seconds, and exhale gently. It's normal to cough afterward – that's your lungs clearing themselves, not a sign of trouble.

Compassion Note: I know it's the last thing you want to do when you're sore, tired, and balancing a new baby on your chest. But those few extra deep breaths help keep your oxygen up, your lungs clear, and your recovery smooth. **Think of it as one small act of self-care that makes a big difference.**

Alarms and Monitor Beeps

Those beeping machines drive everyone crazy — patients, families, and nurses alike. But each alarm has meaning: low oxygen, IV occlusion, fetal heart rate dips, blood pressure readings that need attention.

Compassion Note: The noise might be irritating, but it's how we know you and baby are safe. Trust me — **if I'm not running, it's nothing to panic about.**

Repositioning – A Lot

We're constantly adjusting you: side to side, upright, tilt, knees in, knees out — and sometimes into what feels like *Olympic-level yoga poses.*

We do it to help baby move down, improve oxygen flow, and get a better fetal heart rate pattern.

> **Nurse's Tip:** Each move has a purpose, even if it feels random. Think of it as **labor choreography** – and yes, **you're the star.**

Nurse's Action: If you find yourself in the same position for too long, ask your nurse to help you move. Changing positions during labor isn't just about comfort — it's physiologically important. Movement creates progress and even small adjustments can make a big difference in how smoothly labor unfolds.

6

What's Going On Down There?

"The check is quick — the info is priceless."

Cervical Assessment: Presentation, Dilation, Effacement & Station

At initial assessment and as your labor progresses, one of the biggest questions on everyone's mind—yours, your partner's, and your care team's—is what exactly is happening "down there." Before we can talk about pushing, pain management, or how close you are to meeting your baby, we first need to understand what your starting place is. That's where a cervical assessment comes in.

This chapter will walk you through the key terms and concepts we use to describe labor progress, so when your nurse or provider gives you an update, it actually makes sense. Think of this as your quick guide to what we're evaluating and why it matters — so you can follow along with confidence, feel informed, and understand how beautifully your body is doing the work it was made to do.

Presentation

"Presentation" refers to which part of your baby is coming down first — ideally, the head, which we call a cephalic or vertex presentation. Sometimes, babies present breech (bottom or feet first) or shoulder first, which can affect your delivery plan and often lead to a cesarean section.

It's important to know your baby's position when you arrive at the hospital. When your provider checks you and says, "I feel a head," that's great — but don't hesitate to ask for confirmation. With that said, do me a favor and request that they use the beauty of modern imaging — a quick bedside ultrasound. It's painless, fast, and ensures we're working with the safest and most accurate information. Trust me, breech deliveries are not fun for anyone and it's always better to know before labor is in full swing.

Cervical Dilation, Effacement & Station

These are the three big measures of labor progress — the language every nurse and provider uses to describe how close you are to meeting your baby:

Dilation: How open your cervix is — measured from 0 to 10 centimeters.

Effacement: How thin and stretchy your cervix has become — expressed as a percentage (0–100%).

Station: How far your baby's head has descended into your pelvis, measured from –3 (high) to +3 (crowning).

Back in the day, we used to say "+4 is on the floor" — meaning the baby has made their debut!

> **Nurse's Tip:** Progress isn't always linear – sometimes the cervix takes its time before making big moves. Patience and positioning go a long way.

Engagement

Engagement happens when your baby's head "drops" into your pelvis and stays there — a reassuring sign that your body is gearing up for delivery.

In some cases, however, the baby's head doesn't fully engage because the pelvis and the baby's head don't fit together well — what we call cephalopelvic disproportion (CPD). This can happen even when contractions are strong and measured perfectly by Montevideo units (MVUs), but the cervix isn't changing.

That's because the baby's head isn't making enough contact with the cervix to help it dilate. Sometimes, the baby will even "tell" us they're uncomfortable — their fetal heart rate tracing might show signs of distress, prompting us to step in and reposition, reassess, or intervene to help labor progress safely.

Every cervical exam tells part of your story — how your body and your baby are working together. It's not just a number; it's a snapshot of teamwork in progress.

Cervical Exams: What to Expect

Getting your cervix checked isn't anyone's favorite part of labor, but it's an important one. Think of it as similar to a Pap smear — uncomfortable, yes, but bearable. We'll always ask for your permission before we begin, explain what we're doing, and do our best to make the experience as quick and gentle as possible.

Once you give consent, your provider or nurse will gently separate your labia and insert two gloved fingers into your vagina to feel for your cervix. If your water has already broken, those gloves must be sterile to reduce infection risk.

You'll feel pressure, not necessarily pain, as we locate your cervix. If your baby has started to descend into the pelvis, this is often straightforward. But if your baby is still high, your cervix may be positioned more posterior (toward your back), and yes — it can feel like we're "trying to pick your nose through your vagina." We're sorry — we really don't mean it!

Sometimes, we may ask you to raise your hips using your fists or place an upside-down bedpan under your bottom to help us reach your cervix. If your IV is in your hand, be mindful not to bend or pull it — you don't want to go through that again!

You're encouraged to hold your partner's hand or even your nurse's hand if you need support. It helps distract from the discomfort and gives you something to squeeze (until our fingers turn blue — and yes, we're okay with that).

How We Measure Dilation

Once we locate your cervix, we'll estimate how open it is — this is where our "appraisal skills" come in. Each nurse or provider may measure slightly differently based on experience and hand size, so small differences are completely normal.

Think of it like a house appraisal: one expert might say it's worth $200,000, another might say $205,000. Both are close enough to show progress

— and that's what matters most. We're not looking for perfection; we're looking for change over time.

If we can fit one finger, you're about 1 centimeter dilated.
Two fingers — about 2 centimeters.
Beyond that, the stretch between our fingers helps us estimate further — what I jokingly call my "exaggerated peace sign" is roughly 6 to 7 centimeters for me (and I have short fingers!). So yes — someone else with longer or wider fingers might give you a slightly different number and that's okay.

Here's a quick visual to help you picture what dilation looks like:

Cervical Dilation	Approximate Size
1 cm	About the width of a Cheerio
3 cm	About the width of a quarter
5 cm	About the width of a ping pong ball
10 cm	Fully dilated - about the size of a bagel or the top of a coffee mug and we can no longer feel cervix

Effacement and Station: The Other Half of the Story

While we're checking dilation, we're also assessing two other important things: effacement and station.

Effacement refers to how thin or soft your cervix has become. A cervix that's still firm feels like the tip of your nose, while one that's soft and ready feels more like your lips. Effacement is what allows dilation to happen — the thinner and softer your cervix becomes, the easier it can open.

This is especially important during inductions or augmentations of labor. If your cervix is still thick and firm, starting Pitocin too soon is like "hitting your head against a wall" — it'll hurt, but it won't make progress. Instead, your provider may start with a cervical ripening medication or device to help your cervix prepare before labor stimulation begins.

Station tells us how far down your baby's head is in your pelvis — measured in centimeters above or below the ischial spines (the bony points of your pelvis). A –3 station means baby's still floating high; 0 station means baby's engaged at the pelvis; and +3 means baby's practically here.

More In-depth Understanding of Effacement and Station at a Glance

Labor progress isn't just about how open your cervix is — it's also about how thin it's becoming (effacement) and how low your baby has moved (station). Here's a quick guide to help you picture it:

Effacement (Thinning of the Cervix)

Effacement describes how thick or thin your cervix is as it prepares for delivery. Think of your cervix like a turtleneck sweater — it starts thick and long, then gradually shortens and softens to make way for your baby.

Effacement	Description	What It Feels Like
0% Effaced	Cervix is thick and long (like the tip of your nose).	Firm, not ready to open.
50% Effaced	Cervix is halfway thinned out.	Softer, starting to stretch.
100% Effaced	Cervix is completely thinned and ready for dilation.	Soft like your lips – the "green light" for delivery.

Effacement allows dilation to happen — the thinner your cervix, the easier it is for it to open.

Station (Baby's Descent into the Pelvis)

Station tells us where your baby's head is in relation to your pelvis — specifically, the ischial spines.

Station	What It Means	Visual Reference
-3	Baby is high in the pelvis ("floating").	Still "dancing" above the doorway.
-2 to -1	Baby is moving down, but not yet engaged.	You're making progress!
0	Baby's head is at the ischial spines – "engaged."	Officially in the pelvis.
+1 to +2	Baby's head is lower, visible during pushing.	The finish line is near!
+3	Baby is crowning – it's go time!	You're about to meet your baby.

Nurse's Tip: Effacement, dilation, and station all work together like a team.

Effacement softens and shortens the cervix.
Dilation opens it.
Station tells us how far your baby has traveled.

Progress in one usually helps the others along – it's your body and your baby working together in perfect sync.

Remember: no two labors look exactly the same. Whether it's slow and steady or fast and furious, progress is still progress. Trust your body – it knows the way.

Frequency of Cervical Checks

Every provider has their own approach when it comes to how often they check your cervix. Some take a hands-off approach and only perform exams when there's a clear reason — for example, if you request pain medication, your baby's heart rate shows something on the monitor, or you start feeling pressure that suggests you're close to pushing.

Others prefer to check at the beginning of their shift and then at regular intervals to track your progress over time. Neither style is wrong; it just depends on your provider's practice and your specific situation.

Once your membranes rupture (your water breaks), things change. Even though our exams are done using sterile technique, every check slightly increases your risk of infection because the protective "bag of water" around your baby is no longer there. For that reason, we only check when it's medically necessary — not just out of curiosity.

> **Nurse's Tip:** If you ever wonder why your provider isn't checking as often (or why they suddenly want to check now), just ask! There's always a reason behind it, and we're happy to explain. The fewer unnecessary checks we do, the safer it is for both you and your baby.

When We Decide to Check

We don't check your cervix just because we can and again, it's usually provider preference — every exam has a reason behind it. Our goal is to gather the information we need while keeping both you and your baby safe.

Here are a few of the most common reasons we decide it's time for another check:

Changes in Contractions:

If your contractions suddenly become stronger, closer together, or take on a new pattern, we may check to see whether your cervix is responding and making progress.

You Request Pain Relief:

Before giving pain medication or calling anesthesia for an epidural, we often perform a check to see how far along you are. It helps guide whether it's the right time and what type of medication will work best.

You Feel Pressure or the Urge to Push:

That deep, unmistakable "I need to push" sensation often means baby is much lower. We'll check to confirm if you're fully dilated and ready — or if we need to help you breathe through the urge a bit longer.

Changes in the Baby's Heart Rate:

If your baby's heart rate tracing shows dips or accelerations that we want to understand better, a cervical check can help us identify whether baby's position or descent is playing a role.

After a Long Period Without Progress:

Sometimes, we re-check after a few hours to see how your cervix is responding to contractions, induction medications, or position changes.

Remember: every check should serve a purpose. The fewer unnecessary exams we do, the safer and calmer your experience will be.

The Reality of Progress

A not-so-fun fact: getting from 0 to 6 centimeters is often the hardest and slowest part of labor. In early or induced labors, this stage can take hours — even days. Some providers don't consider "active labor" to start until 6 centimeters, so please don't get discouraged.

Once you hit that point, textbook labor progress is about 1 to 2 centimeters per hour — but every body and every baby have their own rhythm. If things slow down, we'll help figure out why and make adjustments safely.

Nurse's Tips:

- Cervical exams are not a competition – they're just one part of your overall progress.
- You can always ask how far effaced or what station you are – these details help paint the full picture.
- Breathe deeply, hold someone's hand, and remember – every centimeter means you're getting closer.
- Try to relax as much as possible during checks. The more you tighten up, the harder it is for us to feel your cervix.

I often tell my patients, "Go to your happy place" – the beach, the mountains, Disney World, or lately, their own bed (and honestly, that sounds perfect). Wherever that place is for you – go there.

Each check brings a little more information and a lot more anticipation. Your body is doing exactly what it was designed to do.

Nurse's Note: Cervical Swelling & Benadryl

Sometimes, during a long or intense labor, the cervix can become a little swollen — especially if you've been pushing before you're fully dilated or if your body is working really hard against a contraction pattern that isn't quite ready yet. A swollen cervix can slow progress and make it harder for your baby to move down.

One tool we sometimes use is **Benadryl**, not for sleep, but because it can help reduce inflammation and allow the cervix to relax. A calmer, less swollen cervix can open more effectively and make your labor more comfortable and productive.

While this recommendation is based on anecdotal experience rather than research-based evidence, your nurse or provider may suggest it to help your body return to a more efficient rhythm.

When You Might Decline a Cervical Check

Just because cervical exams are routine in labor doesn't mean they're mandatory. You always have the right to say yes or no to any part of your care — and that includes vaginal exams.

There are moments when it's absolutely appropriate to decline or delay a check. Your comfort, safety, and trust matter as much as your progress.

Reasons You Might Decline

You're not ready emotionally or physically.
Labor is vulnerable and sometimes you just need more time to breathe, reposition, or mentally prepare. That's okay — tell your nurse.

There's no medical reason at that moment.
If everything looks stable — your contractions are consistent, baby's heart rate is reassuring — it may be perfectly fine to wait.

You're ruptured and want to limit infection risk.
Once your water has broken, minimizing checks helps protect your baby. Declining a non-essential exam is sometimes the best evidence-based choice.

How to Communicate Your Preference

You don't have to make a speech or defend your decision. A simple statement works:

- "Can we hold off for now?"
- "I'd rather wait until there's a reason."
- "I'd like to know what the check is for before I agree."

Any good nurse or provider should respect that. Those are signs of an engaged, informed patient — exactly the kind of collaboration we want.

> **Nurse's Tip:** Ask:
>
> "What information will this exam give you and how will it change the plan?"
>
> If the answer isn't clear or medically necessary, it's okay to delay.
>
> Remember: This is your body, your birth, and your experience. We're here to guide and protect you – not to take control away from you.

What to Expect Emotionally During Exams

Let's be honest — being checked is one of the most vulnerable moments of your hospital stay. You're exposed, anxious, and already working through pain, pressure, and anticipation. It's okay to feel uncomfortable, shy, or even emotional. Most women do.

As nurses, we understand that this isn't just a physical exam — it's an emotional one too. We know you're letting us into your most private space and that takes a lot of trust. Whether it's your first baby or your fifth, it's never routine for you.

If you've ever experienced trauma, anxiety, or fear related to medical or intimate exams, please tell your nurse quietly. We can take extra care — explaining each step before it happens, adjusting positions, or minimizing how often we check. You deserve to feel safe, respected, and in control.

Nurse's Tip:

- Ask your nurse to talk you through the exam before and during.
- Request that only essential staff remain in the room.
- Use your support person – hold their hand, make eye contact, breathe with them.

You are strong, you are safe, and you have every right to feel comfortable during your care. Your nurse is there not only to assess your progress – but to protect your peace.

For Support Persons: Protecting Her Privacy and Comfort During Exams

As a partner, friend, or loved one, your presence means more than you realize. During labor — especially moments like exams or procedures — your calm, protection, and reassurance can make all the difference.

Here's how you can help her feel safe, respected, and supported:

1. Be Her Anchor

Stay by her side, hold her hand, maintain eye contact.
A gentle "You're okay, I've got you" can ground her when she feels vulnerable.

2. Help Protect Her Privacy

If extra staff enter the room, it's okay to ask:
"Does everyone here need to be present right now?"
You are her advocate, not her barrier.

3. Mirror the Energy She Needs

If she needs calm — soften your voice.
If she needs motivation — encourage her.
Your emotional tone sets the temperature of the room.

4. Respect the Medical Space

Stay close but out of the sterile field.
Your awareness helps us care safely while keeping her centered.

5. Ask Questions — Kindly

"What can I do to support her through this?"
We love when partners are engaged. It makes everything smoother and more connected.

> **Nurse's Tip:**
> You are her mirror.
> If you stay steady, she feels steady.
> If you stay calm, she can breathe.
>
> Your presence can turn a vulnerable moment into one of connection.

Partner Reflection: "What She Feels When You Stay Present"

She might not say it out loud — not in the middle of contractions, not when the room gets busy — but she *feels* you.

She feels your hand, your words, your steady presence.
She feels the way you look at her like she is strong and capable.
When she doubts herself, your quiet *"you can do this"* becomes the rope she holds onto.

You don't have to fix anything or say the perfect thing.
Just stay. Stay grounded. Stay kind. Stay hers.

Long after the monitors are off and the birth story settles into memory, she will remember how you loved her through it. Your presence becomes part of that memory forever.

7

All Things Fluid

"Every drop has a purpose. Trust the process."

Let's be honest — Labor and Delivery comes with fluids. Lots of them. Some you expect, some you don't, and some will have you looking at me like, "Is that normal?" (Spoiler: it usually is.)

Whether it's a little bloody show, a gush of amniotic fluid, or the constant "Did I just pee myself?" mystery, this chapter is your guide to everything that can leak, drip, or gush during labor. Fluids are one of your body's biggest ways of communicating what's happening as you progress. So instead of feeling confused or embarrassed, I want you to feel prepared. Consider this your no-judgment, tell-it-like-it-is breakdown of all the fluid-related surprises you might encounter on your way to meeting your baby.

Bloody Show

One of the earliest signs that your body may be preparing for labor is something called the bloody show — a mix of mucus and a small amount of blood that comes from your cervix.

Your cervix is a highly vascular structure, meaning it has many tiny blood vessels. As it begins to soften, thin, and dilate, those vessels can break slightly, allowing small streaks of blood to mix with the normal cervical mucus. The result is what you might notice as a pink, red, or brown-tinged discharge on your underwear, tissue, or pad.

This is perfectly normal and can happen in a few situations:

- As your body naturally prepares for labor.
- After a cervical exam, when the cervix is gently stretched.
- Following sexual intercourse during late pregnancy.

> **Nurse's Tip:** Don't panic if you see a little mucus and blood – it usually just means your cervix is getting ready for the main event.

When to Call Your Nurse or Provider

While light spotting or mucus with blood is common, **heavy bleeding is not.**

Contact your nurse or provider immediately if you notice:

- A sudden gush or steady stream of bright red blood.
- Large clots or tissue-like material.
- Bleeding accompanied by pain, dizziness, or weakness.

Those could signal something more serious and may need immediate attention.

Your body has a beautiful way of signaling when it's getting close to labor. The bloody show is one of its gentle reminders that things are progressing — but your care team is always there to make sure it's progressing safely.

Rupture of Membranes (ROM) / Artificial ROM (AROM)

(a.k.a. "Water Breaking")

Your baby spends nine months surrounded by a thin, strong amniotic sac filled with amniotic fluid — which, fun fact, is basically baby urine! This warm fluid cushions and protects your baby, helps maintain temperature, and allows them to move and grow comfortably.

Sometimes, your water breaks naturally, and other times, your provider will intentionally break it (called an artificial rupture of membranes or AROM) to help labor progress.

When this happens, you may feel a **small trickle**, a **huge gush**, or it might just feel like you accidentally peed yourself. Everyone's experience is different.

Often, the baby's head acts like a **cork in a wine bottle**, blocking the cervix and holding fluid back. When you move or shift positions, the "cork" moves too, and you may feel another gush.

It's completely normal to continue leaking fluid until your baby is delivered — after all, they're still in there **urinating and floating around** in what's left!

What We Look For: Color and Consistency

Once your water breaks, one of the first things your nurse will check is the color and consistency of the amniotic fluid. This fluid can tell us a lot about what's happening with your baby:

Clear or Slightly Cloudy

This is what we love to see! Normal amniotic fluid is usually:

- Clear or pale straw-colored

- Mild, sweet smell
- Sometimes a little cloudy with white flecks (vernix + skin cells)

Totally normal.

Yellow or Green (Meconium-Stained Fluid)

If the fluid is yellow, green, or brownish, it means your baby has passed **meconium** — their first bowel movement — before birth. This can happen for several reasons, including being past your due date or if the baby has had a temporary stress episode in utero.

While meconium in the fluid doesn't always mean there's a problem, it tells us we need to monitor your baby's heart rate closely.

Meconium Aspiration Syndrome (MAS)

If a baby inhales meconium-stained amniotic fluid, it can:

- Block the airways
- Irritate lung tissue
- Cause airway trapping
- Lead to infection or pneumonia

Most of the time, if meconium is present, the delivery team is ready and waiting. After birth, a neonatologist will assess your baby right away.

- If baby cries and breathes well → **no extra intervention needed.**
- If baby shows distress → airway suction, oxygen, or breathing support may be needed.

Pink or Red-Tinged

A light tint usually means a small amount of cervical bleeding — part of the normal bloody show. We'll keep an eye on it, but it's usually expected during labor.

Dark Brown or Foul-Smelling

This can indicate **old blood** or **infection (chorioamnionitis)**. In these cases, we act quickly to evaluate you and your baby. You might be started on antibiotics and delivery may be expedited for safety.

> **Nurse's Tip:** When your water breaks, note the:
>
> - Time
> - Color
> - Smell
>
> Don't be embarrassed – we've heard it ALL. The more accurate you are, the safer you and your baby are.
>
> Even if you're not sure whether your water broke, come to Labor & Delivery triage to be checked. We have special tests that can confirm it quickly.
>
> As a nurse, I like to have the **fetal heart rate volume up** so I can hear how your baby reacts when you are AROM'ed. This can tell me a lot about what's going on inside.

Amniotic fluid tells a story — one that helps your team understand what your baby might be experiencing before they even arrive.

Testing to See if Your Baby's "Swimming Days" Are Over"

Here are the ways we check if your membranes have ruptured:

1. Speculum Exam

Your provider will perform a sterile speculum exam (just like a Pap smear) to look for fluid pooling in the vagina. If fluid is seen trickling from your cervix, that's often enough to confirm your water has broken.

2. Nitrazine (pH) Test

We use pH-sensitive paper that turns **blue** when exposed to amniotic fluid. Vaginal fluid is acidic; amniotic fluid is more alkaline. Quick and useful.

3. Ferning Test

A small sample of fluid is placed on a microscope slide and allowed to dry. Amniotic fluid forms a distinct **fern-like pattern** under the microscope. This, by the way, is the most definitive test.

4. AmniSure or ROM-Plus Test

A rapid diagnostic test that detects specific proteins only found in amniotic fluid.

✔ Fast

✔ Accurate

✔ Doesn't usually require a speculum exam

8

Riding the Waves: Understanding Your Contractions

"The power and intensity of your contractions cannot be stronger than you, because it is you."

– Unknown

Let's talk about contractions—the part of labor everyone loves to fear but is actually your body doing exactly what it was built to do. Contractions are the powerhouse behind getting your baby into the world, the tightening and releasing that opens your cervix and moves your little one down with every wave. I know they can be intense, overwhelming, and sometimes take your breath away, but they are also your progress. They're the rhythm of labor, the steady drumbeat moving you closer to meeting your baby. And I promise, once you understand what's happening and how to work with them instead of fighting them, the whole experience feels a lot less scary and a lot more empowering. Contractions aren't the enemy—they're the engine.

Contractions

Contractions are the tightening and relaxing of your uterine muscle that help open your cervix and push your baby down. The tightening begins at the top of your uterus and radiates downward, guiding your baby deeper into the pelvis with each wave.

They typically last 40–100 seconds and gradually become closer together — every 1 to 3 minutes — as you approach delivery. In early labor, contractions may feel like mild menstrual cramps or pressure in your back. As labor progresses, they grow stronger, longer, and more intense.

But here's the truth I always tell my patients: **Contractions alone don't necessarily mean labor.**

You can have contractions all day long, but if your cervix isn't changing — opening, thinning, or moving the baby down — then you're not yet in true labor. This is one of the most frustrating things for women in triage. You may feel like you're working hard, timing contractions, and still get sent home. I know how discouraging that can be, but those are likely Braxton Hicks contractions — your uterus practicing for the big day.

Don't lose faith. Your body is still doing important work, even if you're not quite there yet.

What Real Labor Contractions Feel Like

Real contractions don't feel like period cramps — that's what everyone *thinks*, but it's only the beginning.

True labor contractions feel like a wave that builds, peaks, and melts away… and then keeps coming back again and again with a rhythm your body has no control over.

Most people describe them as:

1. **A deep tightening that starts in your back and wraps around your belly**

It's not a surface pain — it's a deep, internal squeeze, almost like someone is wringing your uterus out like a towel from the inside.

2. **Pressure in your pelvis that increases with each contraction**

As baby moves down, the pressure becomes heavier —
like a bowling ball sitting low in your hips.

3. **You cannot talk through real contractions**

Braxton Hicks = you can still carry a conversation.
Real labor = at the peak, talking becomes impossible — your breath shifts and your focus narrows.

4. **Each wave takes your full attention**

The contraction builds like this:

- starts slowly
- rises and intensifies
- peaks for a few seconds
- fades away
- gives you a break

That predictable "build–peak–release" pattern is the hallmark of true labor.

5. **They come closer and closer together**

If the contractions are getting:

- longer
- stronger
- closer together

…that's the real deal.

6. They don't stop with rest, baths, or hydration

Braxton Hicks calm down when you sit, rest, or drink water.
True contractions laugh in the face of water bottles and warm showers — they keep going.

7. **The pain has a PURPOSE**

This is the part I always tell my patients:

Labor pain isn't random pain.
It's productive pain.
Every contraction is pulling your cervix up and open, moving your baby down, and preparing you to push.

When moms understand that, they cope differently.

Nurse's Tip

If the contraction makes you stop, breathe, close your eyes, or brace your body – it's likely real labor.

If you can:

- walk
- talk
- joke
- scroll your phone
- clean your house

...then we're probably not in the "real" stage yet.

How to Cope

Here's what I tell my patients: **ride your contractions like a wave.**

Every contraction builds, peaks, and fades — just like an ocean swell. When you feel it rising, take a deep breath in through your nose, out through your mouth, slow and steady. Focus on breathing through the peak, knowing it will always come back down.

Don't hyperventilate.

Quick, shallow breathing increases anxiety and can make the pain worse. Keep your breaths calm and controlled — one at a time.

Sometimes, the best way to get through a contraction is to not be present for it. Let your mind drift somewhere else. Zone out. Go to your happy place — wherever that may be. The beach, the mountains, your own cozy bed. The more you focus on the pain, the more power it has. The more you let go, the more your body can do what it already knows how to do.

I know it's counterintuitive to relax during a contraction, but that is exactly what your body needs you to do. Your uterus is working hard to open your cervix, and when you tense up, clench your muscles, or hold your breath, you're actually fighting against that natural process.

When you soften your shoulders, unclench your jaw, breathe slowly, and let your body melt into the contraction, you allow your uterus to do its job more efficiently. Think of it like opening a door—if you pull against it, it sticks, but if you release and lean with it, it opens much more easily.

Plus, holding your breath affects the amount of oxygen your baby receives. During a contraction, your uterus temporarily tightens and reduces blood flow to the placenta—that's normal and expected. But if you also hold your breath or tense up, you're limiting the oxygen your baby gets at the exact moment they need it most.

By breathing slowly and steadily through your contractions, you help keep oxygen moving to your baby and support them through each wave. Think of it as working as a team: your uterus squeezes, you breathe, and together you help your baby handle the journey. Breathing isn't just for comfort—it's part of keeping both you and your baby protected, calm, and supported during labor.

Your breath, your mindset, and your ability to let go become powerful tools in helping labor progress. Relaxation isn't weakness—it's cooperation with your own body's strength.

REMEMBER THIS:

You can do anything for 60 seconds.

That's the average length of a contraction. It's temporary. It passes. And each one brings you closer to your baby.

Focus on something outside of your body — a sound, an object, a voice — and trust your body to take over. These contractions are not happening to you; they're happening for you.

Every contraction is progress. Every breath is strength. Every moment brings you closer to the incredible moment when you'll meet your baby.

You are in control of your reaction, your breath, and your mindset. Believe in yourself— because I believe in you. You were made to do this.

Pain Management

Every labor is unique — and so is every woman's experience of pain. Some women feel it deep in their lower back as it radiates forward. Others describe it as strong menstrual cramps or pressure that builds and spreads through the pelvis. The further you progress, the more you'll feel that pain low in your vagina and rectum.

And not to sound heartless — but if you're in pain, **I'm happy for you.** It means your body is doing exactly what it's supposed to do. Labor is meant to be intense — it's a sign of progress, not punishment and it is the only time I'm kinda okay with someone being in pain. It means we are getting somewhere.

That said, no one gets a medal for suffering through pain, and there are plenty of options to help you stay comfortable and in control. My goal is for you to look back on this experience with pride and maybe even a smile — not to feel like you survived something miserable or traumatic. You deserve a birth that feels supported, not one that feels like you were dragged through hell. I'm here to help make sure of that.

Breathing Techniques

The simplest and one of the most powerful tools you have.
In through your nose, out through your mouth — slowly.
Breathe with purpose.
Focusing on your breath keeps oxygen flowing to your baby and keeps your body from tightening up against the pain.

Hydrotherapy

If your hospital allows it, slipping into a warm tub or shower can work wonders.
Warm water relaxes your muscles, eases back pain, and can even help you progress faster by helping you stay calm.

Massage and Counter-Pressure

Think of this like redirecting your pain sensors. When someone presses on your lower back, applies firm counter-pressure to your hips, or rubs your shoulders, your brain focuses on that touch instead of the contractions.

Some patients even bring **old-fashioned hair combs** to squeeze during contractions — the discomfort in your hand tricks your brain into paying less attention to what's happening in your abdomen. It sounds silly, but many swear by it!

Medications

Most hospitals have their go-to pain-relief medications — mild narcotics or "labor cocktails." These take the edge off, but they won't take the pain away completely, so don't expect total relief.

These medications can make you drowsy or groggy and you may even find yourself dozing off between contractions. Because the medicine crosses the placenta, your baby feels some of the effects too — we'll see this reflected in their heart rate tracing, which may look a little "sleepy" afterward. This is expected and not dangerous, but for that reason, we often time medications carefully so your baby isn't affected right before delivery.

If you're close to pushing, your provider may hold off and offer other comfort methods to protect your baby from potential breathing issues at birth.

Distraction Techniques

Labor is as mental as it is physical.
Listen to music, sway, breathe rhythmically, focus on a mantra, or talk with your partner or nurse.

These methods help release endorphins — your body's natural painkillers — and give you a sense of control when everything else feels out of your hands.

Epidural

An epidural is a form of pain relief given through a small catheter placed in your lower back that numbs you from the waist down. It continuously delivers medication throughout your labor, keeping pain signals from reaching your brain. You'll still feel pressure but not sharp pain.

I dedicate an entire chapter to epidurals later on, but know this: **it's a safe and effective option for most women and it doesn't make you weak.** Choosing comfort doesn't make your birth less meaningful — it just makes it more manageable.

Compassion Note: There's no "right" way to labor. Whether you breathe through every contraction or ask for pain relief at 2 cm, it's your experience — and your body. My job isn't to judge you; it's to support you.

Laughing Gas (Nitrous Oxide)

This one surprises a lot of patients — **yes, we still use laughing gas in Labor and Delivery!** Nitrous oxide is a mild inhaled pain relief option that helps take the edge off contractions and anxiety. You'll hold a small mask yourself and breathe it in during contractions. It works fast and wears off within seconds once you stop breathing it in — so you're always in control.

One of the facilities that I have worked for incorporated it into use by our unit but has since discontinued due to COVID and never got it back.

It won't make you "loopy" or numb like an epidural, but it can help you relax and feel less tense between contractions. Many moms say it takes that overwhelming edge off enough to help them focus on their breathing and stay calm.

Nurse's Insight: I'll be honest — I've never been a huge fan of nitrous. In my practice, many patients expect it to do more than it actually does. After a few good breaths, most end up asking for another form of pain management because the relief just isn't strong enough for active labor pain.

That doesn't mean it doesn't have value — for some, it takes the edge off enough to help them breathe and refocus. But I always tell my patients to think of nitrous as a tool for relaxation, not total pain control. It's a great bridge if you're waiting for an epidural or want something light that you control yourself but it's rarely the final answer for significant pain.

> **Nurse's Tip:** Because nitrous doesn't affect your baby and clears quickly from your system, it's a great option if you want a lighter, flexible form of pain relief – or if you're waiting for your epidural and need a little help getting through those early contractions.

Pudendal Block: What It Is and When We Use It

A pudendal block is a lesser-known but very effective type of pain relief used during labor — especially during the pushing stage or right before delivery. It's not an epidural and it doesn't numb your entire body. Instead, it targets the pudendal nerves, which provide sensation to the vagina, the perineum, and the area where you will feel the most burning and stretching as the baby crowns.

Think of it as numbing just the exit.

When We Use a Pudendal Block

We typically use a pudendal block when:

- the baby is about to be born
- you don't have an epidural
- you need quick, local relief
- we anticipate you may need stitches after birth
- the pressure and burning during crowning are intense
- an episiotomy or instrumental delivery (vacuum/forceps) may happen

It works fast and is a great option for moms who want to stay fully mobile but need some help with the final stretch of labor.

How It's Given

Your provider will:

- Place two fingers inside your vagina
- Use a small needle to inject numbing medication (usually lidocaine)
- Target the pudendal nerve on each side of your pelvis

The entire process takes less than a minute per side, and the relief is almost immediate.

What It Feels Like

You may feel:

- pressure from the provider's fingers
- a quick pinch or burn (like a dental numbing shot)
- a warm, slightly tingly sensation as the medication spreads

Once it kicks in — usually within 1–2 minutes — the perineal area feels significantly more comfortable. You will still feel pressure, but not the sharp burning as the baby crowns.

How Long It Lasts

A pudendal block typically lasts:

That depends on your provider. It depends on the type and how much of the medication they used.

Generally, long enough to get through the pushing and immediate postpartum repairs.

Benefits

- fast relief
- preserves your ability to push
- does not affect the baby
- keeps you fully awake and mobile
- reduces pain with crowning and stitching
- great alternative for moms without an epidural
- minimal medication compared to systemic options

Nurse's Reassurance

If you're nearing the end of labor and the pressure becomes overwhelming, a pudendal block can be a game changer. It doesn't take away your ability to push or the sensation of your baby being born — it simply makes those intense moments more manageable.

And if you need stitches afterward, the block keeps you comfortable, so you don't feel every suture.

You're still in control.
You're still fully present.
You're just more comfortable — **and that matters.**

Just make sure you have a conversation with your provider before you arrive to see if they even offer that option. Many do not.

Position Changes and Movement

Even small movements can make a huge difference.
Rolling from side to side, sitting upright, getting on hands and knees, or using tools like the peanut ball can help relieve pressure and encourage your baby to descend.

Gravity is your friend — so if your provider allows it, use it.

> **Nurse's Tip:** Even if you have an epidural, side-lying with a peanut ball can help open the pelvis and shorten labor.

Aromatherapy and Environment

Creating a calm, soothing space can lower stress hormones and reduce how intensely you feel pain. Lavender, peppermint, or citrus oils can be grounding (if your hospital permits them). Dim lighting, quiet voices, and your favorite playlist help your body relax — and a relaxed body labors more efficiently.

Mind-Body Techniques

Guided imagery, mindfulness, meditation, or prayer can help you stay centered through contractions. Some women visualize waves, light, or even opening flower petals to help their minds work with their bodies rather than fighting against them.

Support and Touch

Don't underestimate the power of touch and presence. A steady hand to hold, a nurse whispering "You're doing great," or your partner's gentle voice — all help you feel safe and capable.

That emotional safety is one of the best pain management tools there is.

Compassion Note: Labor pain is primal and purposeful, but you don't have to walk through it alone. The right support team makes all the difference.

Heat and Cold Therapy

A warm compress on your lower back or abdomen can ease muscle tension. A cool washcloth on your neck or forehead can bring comfort between contractions — especially during transition when you may feel flushed or overheated.

Partner Power

If you have a partner or support person, give them a role. Have them time contractions, offer massages, help you change positions, or simply keep you laughing. Labor isn't just physical — **it's emotional endurance**, and connection helps keep your energy grounded.

Compassion Note: Your birth story may start slowly, but it's still yours — and it's still powerful. When you look back, you won't remember how long it took. You'll remember the moment it all shifted and your baby finally arrived.

The Partner's Role During Contractions

When contractions hit, it can be overwhelming — not just for the person laboring, but for the partner too. You may find yourself wanting to help but not knowing exactly how. Here's the truth: **you don't need to have all the answers.** You just need to be there — steady, calm, and connected.

Your energy becomes her anchor.

Help Her Breathe

When a contraction begins, help guide her breathing if she starts to lose focus. Try quiet, calm reminders:

- "In through your nose… out through your mouth."
- "Breathe slow — you've got this."

If she starts breathing too fast, model slow breathing yourself — she'll naturally follow your rhythm.

Sometimes, all it takes is your presence and a few steady breaths to help her regain control.

Provide Physical Support

Offer your hand, your shoulder, or your chest to lean into during contractions.

Use counterpressure on her lower back or hips if she's having back labor — ask the nurse or doula to show you how.

Gently massage her shoulders or lower back between contractions if she finds it soothing.

If she prefers silence, just stay close — quiet presence can be more powerful than words.

Offer Encouragement

Your words matter. Keep them short, sincere, and focused on what she's doing right.

- "You're doing amazing."
- "That was a big one — you handled it beautifully."
- "You're getting closer."

Avoid phrases like "Just relax" or "Calm down." Even with the best intentions, they can feel dismissive in the moment.

Instead, focus on strength, progress, and teamwork.

Stay Steady

You might feel nervous or emotional watching her in pain — that's completely normal. The best thing you can do is stay steady and calm. When you breathe slowly, speak softly, and move with purpose, you create an energy that helps her feel safe.

If you need a moment to collect yourself, quietly step out for a deep breath, then come back in ready to be her anchor again.

> **Nurse's Tip:** You don't have to fix the pain – you just have to hold space for it.
> She'll remember how you looked at her, how you spoke to her, and how you never left.
> **Your presence is one of the strongest tools she has.**

Personal Experience Tip from Your Nurse

In my own labor, in addition to having my favorite old soul play list blasting in my ears, I had my husband play with my hair. It relaxed me so much in early labor — the soft, repetitive motion helped my whole body unclench.

But the moment labor shifted into *real-deal, deep-focus intensity*, I gently shooed him away. I needed to be in my own zone, with no outside influence, no talking, no touching… just me, my breath, and the work my body was doing.

And guess what?

That's okay.
You're allowed to change what you need at any moment.
Support doesn't always mean being physically close — sometimes it means loving you from a few steps away.

Your preferences may shift throughout labor. Let them. Your birth space should always match what your body and mind need *in that moment.*

Labor Is Teamwork

She's doing the physical work, but **you're doing the emotional heavy lifting** — grounding her, protecting her peace, and reminding her she's not alone.

9

Your Epidural — What to Expect, What It Feels Like, and Why It's Okay to Want One

"Pain is not a measure of love or bravery. An epidural doesn't change your strength—it changes your experience."

– Kim Heathcote

For many women, the idea of an epidural can feel both comforting and intimidating. You've probably heard stories from friends, TikTok, or random strangers who love to share their birth experiences. But here's the truth:

Epidurals are one of the safest, most effective pain relief options in modern childbirth. Choosing one is NOT a failure. It does NOT mean you "couldn't handle it." It simply means you chose comfort and calm—and that is strength, not weakness.

Let's walk through everything you need to know.

How Common Are Epidurals?

You are not alone if you're considering one.

About 80% of laboring women in the developed countries receive an epidural (Xu et al., 2023).

That means the majority of moms choose this option. Epidurals are widely available, highly effective, and have been used safely for decades.

So if you're even thinking about it — you're already in the same boat as most women giving birth today.

What an Epidural Actually Is

An epidural is a form of pain relief that:

- numbs the nerves that carry pain signals from your uterus
- allows you to stay awake and alert
- lets you rest or even sleep during labor
- still allows you to feel pressure (so you know when to push)

It is **not** a shot into your spine.
It is **not** a needle that stays in your back.
It is **not** a full-body numbness that takes over everything.

The needle is only used to place a very thin, flexible catheter (tube) that delivers medication.
The needle comes out immediately afterward.
The catheter stays in place — soft, bendy, and taped.

Epidural ≠ C-Section Risk

In my experience:

Epidurals do NOT increase your risk of needing a C-section.
They also do NOT slow labor significantly when managed appropriately.

These are old myths. Your L&D nurses and anesthesiologists follow evidence-based protocols to keep things safe and balanced.

Nurse's Note: Do Epidurals Slow Down Labor?

I know that there is a long-standing myth that epidurals slow labor — but in my experience at the bedside, that isn't always true. In fact, my anesthesiologist "boyfriend" — whom I lovingly used to refer to as *"my magical injection guy"* — became famous on our unit for how quickly many patients delivered after he placed their epidural.

Once their pain eased and their body relaxed, their cervix often did the same. I witnessed this over and over again: a patient finally gets comfortable, takes a deep breath... and suddenly their labor *moves forward,* not backward.

While every labor is different, and every body responds uniquely, I can honestly say that I have seen far more epidurals **help patients progress** than slow them down. When pain decreases and tension releases, the body can often work more efficiently — and sometimes, surprisingly quickly.

So if an epidural is part of your plan, please know:
It doesn't automatically slow labor.
In many cases, it can actually help your body do exactly what it needs to do.

You deserve comfort *and* progress — and yes, you can absolutely have both.

You Are NOT a Failure for Wanting One

Please read that again.

Pain relief is not failure.
Motherhood does not come with a medal for suffering.
You do not have to "prove" anything to anyone.

Some women labor beautifully with epidurals.
Some labor beautifully without them.

Both are equally strong.
Both are equally valid.

There is **no "right way"** to give birth — only the way that feels right for you.

Why We Give You Fluids Before an Epidural (The Bolus)

Before your epidural, your nurse will start giving you a fluid bolus — basically a big, fast dose of IV fluids.

Why?

Because:

- an epidural can temporarily lower your blood pressure
- more IV fluid = more blood volume
- more volume = steadier blood pressure during the procedure
- steady blood pressure = steady oxygen and blood flow to the baby

This is standard, safe, preventative care.
It's one of the reasons epidurals are so safe today.

What the Epidural Feels Like

Let's break it down step-by-step in a real, honest way.

1. Getting into position

You'll sit on the edge of the bed and curve forward like a "angry cat" or gentle "cooked shrimp." Chin to chest, relax shoulder down.

Your nurse will help hold you steady, especially during contractions.

2. Cleaning the area

Cold.
Wet.

Scratchy.
Sterile.

Then what feels like a shower curtain on your back. This is the drape.

This is all to reduce infection risk.

3. The numbing medicine

You'll feel a quick pinch and burn. It's like a bee sting. This is what is described as the worse part — this lasts seconds and the numbing makes the actual epidural placement much more comfortable.

4. The pressure

You may feel:

- pressure
- pushing
- a dull "weird" sensation

Not pain — just awareness that something is happening.

5. A warm, tingling wave

As the medicine starts working, your pain begins to fade. Most women say:

"I can still feel my contractions, but they don't hurt."
"I feel pressure, but not pain."
"I can breathe again."

That's exactly what we want.

Nurse's Tip: Listen Closely to Your Anesthesiologist

Your anesthesiologist will explain a few important **warning signs** to pay attention to when you receive your epidural. These signs help us quickly identify if the medication is going somewhere it *shouldn't* – such as into a blood vessel or too close to the spinal space.

Please take this part seriously and really **listen to what they say**. These symptoms are rare, but if they happen, **we need to know immediately**.

Let us know right away if you notice:

- **A sudden ringing or buzzing in your ears**
- **A metallic taste in your mouth**
- **Numbness or tingling in your face or lips**
- **Severe dizziness or confusion**
- **Feeling extremely weak or like you might pass out**
- **Shortness of breath or difficulty speaking**

These sensations can be signs that the epidural medication entered your bloodstream or was placed incorrectly and catching it early keeps you safe.

Why this matters

Your care team, especially anesthesia, is trained to respond instantly. The faster you alert us, the faster we can stop the medication, correct the issue, and keep you and your baby safe.

The Bottom Line

You are not bothering us – **your voice keeps you safe**.
If something feels off after the epidural, **tell us right away**.
Your anesthesiologist and your nurse are right there with you, watching, listening, and ready to act.

You Will Still Be Able to Push

Epidurals do not take away the ability to push.

You will still:

- feel pressure
- feel the urge
- feel your baby moving down
- feel present and involved

The goal is comfort, not paralysis. And even if you did get too much of a good thing, you have your nurse to help guide you along during the pushing process. Do not worry!

What You Might Feel Afterward

Normal sensations include:

- warm, heavy legs
- numbness that varies by side
- the ability to sleep (which is GOOD!)
- relief so deep you may cry (also normal)

Your nurse checks your level frequently to make sure it's balanced and safe.

Why You May Notice More Interventions After Your Epidural

Once your epidural is in place, you may notice a few extra pieces of equipment or checks happening more often — and that's completely normal.

Because an epidural can temporarily affect your blood pressure and sensation, we keep a closer eye on you and your baby during this time.

You may see:

- a blood pressure cuff cycling more frequently
- a pulse oximeter on your finger
- SCDs (compression boots) to keep blood flowing
- a foley catheter if your numbness prevents emptying your bladder

None of these interventions mean anything is wrong — they're simply part of keeping you safe, comfortable, and well-supported while your epidural does its job.

You're still in control, still doing beautifully, and we're just adding layers of care around you.

Nurse Tip: You may have an epidural ***bolus button*** at your bedside. This allows you to give yourself an extra dose if the continuous medication isn't providing enough relief. Don't worry, you can't overdose yourself. There are programmed parameters. Before using it, always let your anesthesiologist or nurse know so they can guide you and make sure it's safe and effective for you.

Epidural Expectations

It's completely normal to still feel pressure with an epidural — pressure is your body's way of telling us your baby is moving down. Sometimes that pressure can become very strong or intense and that often means it's getting close to baby time. You also may still feel the squeezing and tightening of your uterus. All completely normal.

Epidurals take away the sharp, painful sensation of contractions, but they don't always remove the tightening sensation or deep pressure that comes with your baby descending.

That said, every body is different. Some women feel only mild pressure, and some feel nothing at all — not even the urge to push.

Anatomically, our spines, nerves, and pelvic floors vary, so everyone's epidural experience is unique.

What matters most is that you're comfortable, supported, and reassured that everything you're feeling — whether it's a lot, a little, or nothing — is completely normal. Your nurse and provider will guide you every step of the way.

Epidural Myths – Busted

Myth #1: "The needle stays in my back."
Nope. It comes out immediately. Only a thin tube remains.

Myth #2: "I'll be paralyzed."
Modern epidurals do not enter the spinal cord.

Myth #3: "It hurts to get."
Most women say the contractions hurt far more than the epidural. Some even complain more about the IV insertion.

Myth #4: "It will slow my labor."
Not when managed properly.

Nurse's Wisdom Note

I like to remind my patients of this simple truth: if **80% of laboring women get epidurals**, then ask yourself — do you see **80% of mothers out in the world** walking around with bad backs or paralysis **(Xu et al., 2023)**?
No, you don't.

Epidurals are one of the most common and safest forms of pain relief in labor. Complications are extremely rare, and the overwhelming majority of women have **no long-term issues** at all. So if you're nervous, that's okay — but know that the fear is far greater than the reality. You're safe and you're in good hands.

Nurse's Note: You're Allowed to Be Scared

It's okay to feel nervous.
It's okay to ask questions.
It's okay to pause if you need to.

Your nurse will:

- stay with you
- help position you
- hold you steady
- talk you through each step
- support you emotionally
- advocate for you if you need more reassurance

You are not doing this alone.

Nurse's Heads Up: Don't Wait Too Long to Ask for Your Epidural

There is a common belief that you have to "earn" your epidural or wait until you're almost unable to talk through contractions. That's simply not true and waiting too long can actually make the whole process harder for you.

Here's why:

1. You need to be able to sit still for placement

During the epidural, you'll need to stay curled forward and steady — even during contractions.
If you're already overwhelmed by pain or losing control of your breathing, holding still becomes much harder.

Getting the epidural sooner can make the placement smoother, faster, and safer.

2. You need time for the fluid bolus

Before an epidural, we give you a big dose of IV fluids to protect your blood pressure.
If you wait until you're in severe pain, these extra minutes can feel endless.

Asking earlier gives your body time to prep without rushing.

3. The anesthesiologist may be tied up

At busy hospitals, anesthesia may be in:

- a C-section
- an epidural across the hall
- an emergency procedure

If you ask when you're already at your limit, you may have to wait — and that wait can feel unbearable.
Asking earlier helps avoid this.

4. Epidurals don't work instantly

Even after placement, it takes **10–20 minutes** for full relief.

If you wait until you're exhausted, panicking, or losing control, those minutes feel like hours.
Getting the epidural early enough helps you stay calm and centered.

5. Being comfortable helps labor progress

When you're in extreme pain, your body produces stress hormones that can:

- slow dilation
- tighten your pelvic floor
- make contractions less coordinated
- increase maternal exhaustion

Relaxation helps your body open.

An epidural can support that process — not hinder it.

6. There is NO benefit to "toughing it out" unnecessarily

You don't get a trophy for suffering.
You don't become a better mother by enduring more pain.
And you are not weak for wanting relief.

Asking earlier is smart, not soft.
It's about staying in control, not losing it.

Bottom Line

Ask for your epidural when you need it — **not when you're at your breaking point.**
You don't have to wait until you're crying, shaking, or unable to breathe through contractions.

You are in charge.
Your comfort matters.
And getting ahead of the pain often leads to a smoother, calmer, more positive birth experience.

When an Epidural Feels One-Sided (And What We Do About It)

Sometimes after an epidural, you may notice that one side of your belly or one leg feels more numb than the other. This is surprisingly common and nothing to worry about.

Epidural medication is gravity-driven, which means it tends to flow toward whatever side you're lying on.
If you've been in one position for a while — especially if you're tilted slightly — more medicine may collect on that side and create uneven relief.

The good news?
We can usually fix this quickly.

What Your Nurse Does to Even Out the Epidural

1. Reposition You

This is the biggest fix and works most of the time.

We might:

- switch you to the opposite side
- place a peanut ball between your knees
- tilt you slightly with pillows
- elevate one hip or drop one knee

A small shift can completely change how the medication spreads.

2. "Rock and Roll" Positioning

Sometimes we'll gently help you:

- lie on your right for 20 minutes

- then left for 20 minutes
- then center with a small tilt

This helps the medicine coat your epidural space more evenly.

3. Check the Epidural Catheter

If repositioning isn't enough, anesthesia may:

- pull the catheter back a tiny bit
- adjust it slightly
- give a small extra dose

These micro-adjustments often fix one-sided numbness instantly.

4. Give an Additional Bolus

If baby is tolerating labor and everything looks safe, anesthesia can give a bolus (a small boost) of medication through the catheter to balance your relief.

This is quick and highly effective.

5. Assess Your Progress

Sometimes sensations change because you're getting close to pushing. If the pressure is increasing on one side only, it might actually be baby's position — not epidural imbalance.

Your nurse knows the difference and will explain what's normal and what's not.

Nurse Reassurance:

Uneven epidural relief is **not a failure**, **not dangerous**, and **not unusual**. Most of the time, it's simply gravity doing its job a little too well.

With a few adjustments, we can almost always help the medication spread evenly — and get you back to feeling balanced, comfortable, and in control.

When an Epidural Lowers Your Blood Pressure (and How We Fix It)

One of the normal, expected side effects of an epidural is a temporary drop in your blood pressure. This doesn't happen to everyone, but it's common enough that we prepare for it ahead of time with IV fluids. Still, sometimes your blood pressure dips a little after the medication is placed.

Here's what that means—and why it matters.

Why Blood Pressure Can Drop After an Epidural

Epidurals relax the nerves in your lower body, which can also relax the blood vessels. When blood vessels relax, they open up—and your blood pressure naturally drops.

It doesn't mean anything is wrong with you.
It's simply how your body responds to the medication.

What It Feels Like When Blood Pressure Drops After an Epidural

If your blood pressure dips after an epidural, the sensation can come on **quickly** and may feel unsettling — but it's **common, expected, and very treatable**.

You might feel:

- **Suddenly lightheaded or dizzy**

- **Nauseated** or like you might vomit
- **Warm, flushed, or clammy**
- **Weak or heavy**, like your arms and legs feel hard to move
- **A little "out of it"** or fuzzy-headed
- Occasionally **short of breath** or like it's harder to take a deep breath

Some people describe it as:

"That feeling when you stand up too fast — but stronger."

How It Affects the Baby

Your baby relies on healthy blood flow through the placenta.
So when your blood pressure drops:

This is very common and usually corrects quickly.

Your nurse and anesthesia team watch for this in real time.

What We Do to Fix It – Quickly and Safely

If your blood pressure drops or baby shows they don't like the change, we act fast and confidently. Here's what happens:

1. We reposition you

Often, turning you to your side or adjusting your tilt fixes the issue immediately.
Side-lying improves blood return to your heart and boosts blood flow to the placenta.

2. We give you more IV fluids

Remember the fluid bolus before the epidural? Sometimes you need a little extra.

More fluid = more circulating volume = better blood pressure.

3. We give a small dose of medication (if needed)

If fluids and position changes aren't enough, anesthesia can give you medications, which gently raises your blood pressure back to normal.

These medications:

- work extremely fast
- are safe in labor
- help baby instantly look happier on the monitor

4. We watch the monitor closely

You will NOT be alone during this. Your nurse stays right at your bedside, watching:

- your blood pressure
- how you feel
- your breathing
- and most importantly, your baby's heart rate

Most babies perk up immediately once blood flow improves.

Nurse Reassurance:

This is one of the reasons epidurals are safest in the hospital—you have a whole team monitoring you moment by moment.

A blood pressure dip is:

- common
- expected
- treatable

- usually gone within minutes
- not harmful once corrected

And your nurse will talk you through every step so nothing feels scary or unexpected.

Why Epidurals Can Make You Itch

If you get an epidural and suddenly notice your nose itching like crazy—or your face, chest, or arms—don't worry. Itching is one of the most common and harmless side effects of epidural medication.

Here's why it happens:

1. Some Epidural Medications Contain a Small Amount of Opioid

To make the epidural work well and last longer, anesthesia often mixes a tiny dose of opioid medication (like fentanyl) into the local anesthetic.

Opioids can trigger itch receptors in your skin and brain even though you're not allergic.

It's not a rash.
It's not an allergy.
It's simply a known side effect of that class of medication.

2. Your Body's Histamine Response Gets Triggered

Opioids can release a small amount of histamine, a natural chemical that causes:

- itching
- warmth

- flushing

This is why your face, nose, or neck tend to itch the most.

3. It's More Common When You're Relaxed

Once your pain eases, your nervous system shifts into "rest mode," and your body becomes more aware of little sensations—like itching—that you probably wouldn't even notice during strong contractions.

Is It Dangerous?

No. Epidural-related itching is totally safe and usually mild.

It may feel annoying, but it doesn't mean:

- you're allergic
- something is wrong
- your epidural is misplaced
- the medication is too strong

None of those are true.

What We Can Do to Help

If the itching bothers you, we can:

Give a small medication to counteract the itching
There are safe anti-itch or anti-histamine options that work quickly.

Adjust the epidural dose or medication mixture
Sometimes a simple tweak helps.

Reassure you that it's normal and temporary
The itching usually fades as your body settles into the medication.

Nurse's Note

Itching is one of those quirky little side effects that almost everyone with an epidural experiences at some level. It's harmless, temporary, and easy for us to help with if it becomes bothersome.

You're not having a reaction–your body is just responding to the medication in a very normal way.

Why You Might Not Be Able to Urinate With an Epidural

When you get an epidural, you may notice that you suddenly can't pee on your own—even if your bladder is full. This is very normal and happens for a few important reasons:

1. The Epidural Numbs the Nerves That Tell Your Brain "I Have to Pee"

Your bladder sends signals to your brain through nerves in your lower back. An epidural numbs those nerves, which means:

- You may not feel pressure
- You may not feel fullness
- You may not feel the urge to go at all

So even if your bladder is full… your brain isn't getting the message.

2. The Pelvic Floor Is Relaxed (Sometimes Too Relaxed)

Your pelvic floor muscles normally help "release" urine. With an epidural, those muscles can be so relaxed that they don't coordinate the way they normally do.

It's not that you won't pee—it's that your muscles can't coordinate the process.

3. Your Baby's Head May Be Lowering Into the Pelvis

As your baby moves down, their head can physically compress your urethra—the tube urine comes out of.

This can make it:

- harder to start a stream
- harder to push urine out
- or make urination impossible

This is **SUPER common** in active labor.

4. You're Usually Lying Down

Epidurals often mean:

- you're in bed
- you're side-lying
- or semi-reclined

And your bladder simply doesn't empty well in these positions.
Your body isn't designed to pee lying down.

What Your Nurse Does to Help

✓ Straight catheterization
A tiny catheter is used to empty your bladder as needed. With an epidural, you likely won't feel it at all.

✓ Foley catheter
If your epidural is dense or labor is long, we may place a Foley catheter to continuously drain the bladder.

Regular bladder checks

This prevents overstretching—because a full bladder can slow your baby's descent.

Nurse Reassurance:

Not being able to urinate with an epidural is completely normal and nothing to be embarrassed about. You didn't do anything wrong—your body is simply responding to the medication and the way it changes nerve signals.

Your nurse handles this quietly and professionally while keeping you comfortable and safe. It's just one more part of supporting you through labor.

Why Emptying Your Bladder Helps Labor

Your bladder and your baby share the same space in your pelvis, so what happens to one can affect the other. Keeping your bladder empty during labor can make a noticeable difference in how smoothly things progress.

Here's why:

1. A Full Bladder Takes Up the Space Your Baby Needs

As your baby moves down, they need room to rotate, descend, and line up with your birth canal. A full bladder sits right in front of your baby's head and can act like a little roadblock.

When your bladder is emptied:

- baby has more space
- descent becomes easier
- rotation improves
- pushing becomes more effective

2. A Full Bladder Can Slow Dilation

Your bladder rests right under your uterus. If it's too full, it can press upward and cause:

- more discomfort
- less efficient contractions
- slower cervical dilation

An empty bladder gives your uterus the freedom to work the way it needs to.

3. It Helps Prevent Cervical Swelling

When the baby's head is pushing downward but the bladder is pushing upward, it can create extra pressure on the cervix. This can sometimes contribute to swelling—especially if you're pushing early.

Keeping the bladder empty helps maintain the right kind of pressure.

4. It Keeps Contractions More Effective

Contractions work best when:

- the uterus has room
- pressure is directed downward
- nothing is obstructing baby's path

A full bladder can "absorb" some of that force, making contractions feel stronger but do less work. Emptying it helps each contraction do its job more efficiently.

5. It Makes Pushing MUCH More Comfortable

When you start pushing, a full bladder can make you feel:

- pressure
- burning
- discomfort

- difficulty focusing your push

Once the bladder is emptied, pushing usually feels smoother and easier.

Signs Your Bladder Might Be Full (Even If You Can't Feel It)

- Increasing pressure low in your pelvis
  Not sharp pain—just a heavy, full feeling.
- Contractions suddenly feeling more uncomfortable
  A full bladder can make contractions feel crampier or more intense.
- A bulging feeling when we check your cervix
  Your nurse will notice this during exams.
- Baby seems "higher" than expected
  A full bladder can temporarily block descent.
- A sudden feeling of needing to push too early
  Sometimes fullness mimics the urge to push.
- Your nurse gently suggests a bladder check
  We can often feel it on your lower abdomen
- You haven't emptied your bladder in a while
  With an epidural, you won't get the natural urge—so time matters.

Nurse Reassurance:

A full bladder is totally normal in labor but avoidable—especially with an epidural. Emptying it can make you instantly more comfortable and help your baby come down smoothly. You did nothing wrong. Your body just isn't sending the usual signals right now.

How a Full Bladder Can Affect Postpartum Bleeding (PPH)

After your baby is born, your uterus needs to clamp down firmly to stop bleeding where the placenta was attached. This tightening is what keeps you safe and prevents postpartum hemorrhage (PPH).

But here's something many people don't realize:

A full bladder can actually get in the way of the uterus tightening the way it needs to.

This is why nurses pay close attention to your bladder right after birth.

Why a Full Bladder Increases PPH Risk

1. It Pushes the Uterus Out of Place

When the bladder is full, it sits right in front of the uterus and pushes it upward and to the side. This makes it harder for the uterus to contract firmly.

A "boggy," soft uterus is the biggest risk factor for PPH.

2. It Prevents Good Uterine Contraction

Your uterus is a muscle—and like any muscle, it needs to be able to tighten. If the bladder is taking up too much space:

- contractions become less effective
- bleeding increases
- the uterus struggles to stay firm

Emptying the bladder often makes the uterus firm up immediately.

3. It Can Hide a Soft Uterus

Sometimes, when the uterus is being pushed up and off center by a full bladder, it can feel misleadingly "firm," even though it's not contracting well.

Once the bladder drains, the uterus shifts back into place and the true tone becomes obvious.

4. It Makes Fundal Massage Less Effective

If your bladder is full:

- fundal massage is harder
- the uterus may not respond as well
- it takes longer to stop heavy bleeding

A quick bladder emptying can make massage suddenly more effective.

What We Do to Protect You

Your nurse will often check your bladder soon after birth—especially if:

- your uterus is boggy
- bleeding is heavier than normal
- you had an epidural
- you haven't voided in a while
- your bladder looks full on palpation
- bleeding isn't improving like expected

If needed, we'll:

✓ Straight cath you
✓ Encourage you to attempt the bathroom
✓ Give you time, privacy, and support
✓ Place a foley if medically necessary

You may be surprised how often we see this:

We empty the bladder and the uterus responds instantly—becoming firm, centered, and clamping down the way it should.

It's one of the simplest and most effective interventions for preventing or treating early postpartum bleeding.

Nurse Reassurance:

Needing help to empty your bladder after delivery is normal—especially with an epidural, heavy IV fluids, swelling, or exhaustion.

You didn't cause the bleeding.
You didn't do anything wrong.
Your body is adjusting after doing the biggest job of your life.

Your care team watches this closely so your uterus can contract the way it needs to and keep you safe.

Partner's Note for your Epidural Decision

If your partner is in the room, remind them:

- This is routine
- It's safe
- You are in good hands
- Their job is to help you stay still and breathe
- They are supporting your choice, not judging it

The First Two Hours: Your Sweet Spot of Comfort

The first two hours after your epidural is placed are often the most comfortable you will feel during your entire labor. The medication is fresh, evenly spread, and working at its absolute best.

If you haven't slept yet—**this is your moment.**

Use this window to:

- rest your body
- reset your mind
- recharge your energy

Labor is a marathon, not a sprint, and giving yourself permission to close your eyes now can make all the difference later, especially when it's time to push.

Many moms wake up from this little epidural nap feeling clear, calm, and ready for whatever comes next.

Rest isn't indulgent—it's strategic.

Your body is working hard; let it recover while your epidural does its job.

A Hidden Benefit of an Epidural

One thing many women don't realize is that an epidural can also serve as an extra layer of safety if an unexpected situation arises.

If you need to go to the operating room for a C-section—whether urgently or unexpectedly—your epidural is already in place and ready to be quickly dosed with stronger medication.

This means you can be:

- kept comfortable
- kept awake
- safely numbed
- quickly prepped

Having the epidural catheter already in your back gives the anesthesia team immediate access, allowing them to get you numb safely and much faster.

Most moms never need this benefit, but it's a reassuring part of why epidurals are such a useful tool during labor: **comfort now and a ready plan just in case.**

Epidural Highlights

1. An Epidural Doesn't Affect Your Baby's Apgar Score

Many moms worry the medication will make their baby sleepy.
The great news: epidural medications stay in your epidural space, not the baby's bloodstream.
This means:

- Baby stays alert
- Breastfeeding is not affected
- Apgar scores are not decreased

This is a HUGE reassurance for anxious mamas.

2. You Still Control Your Labor With an Epidural

An epidural doesn't take over your birth — you are still an active participant.

You still:

- choose your positions
- help rotate your baby
- work with your nurse
- push your baby out
- decide your comfort level

You're not "stuck" — we reposition you constantly to help your labor progress beautifully.

3. Pushing With an Epidural Is Absolutely Possible

Some moms worry they won't know how to push. But your body still cues you with:

- pressure
- stretching

- rectal heaviness
- the classic urge-to-push

And if you don't feel the urge?
Your nurse and provider will coach you with every push and teach you exactly how to direct your energy. Once the baby is low enough, majority of woman feel the urge to push. We will get you there!

4. Epidurals Do Not Increase Your Chance of a C-Section

This is one of the most outdated myths in obstetrics.
Modern research shows:

A well-managed epidural does **NOT** raise C-section rates.
In fact, for exhausted moms, it can prevent a C-section by helping the body relax enough to dilate.

5. Epidurals Can Help Lower Stress Hormones

Pain releases adrenaline and cortisol — hormones that can stall labor and make dilation slower.
An epidural brings:

- relaxation
- muscle release
- improved oxygen flow
- decreased maternal stress

A calmer body = a more efficient labor.

6. You Can Still Move (More Than You Think)

Even though you're not walking, we can do:

- side-lying
- hands-and-knees (with support!)

- peanut ball positions
- throne position
- exaggerated side-lying release
- pelvic tilts

These positions help baby move down and rotate — even with an epidural.

7. Epidurals Can Sometimes Be "Lightened"

If you feel too numb or want more pressure so you can push better, anesthesia can adjust it.
Epidurals are customizable, not one-size-fits-all.

8. You Don't Need to Suffer First

Some moms feel they "should" wait as long as possible.
But epidurals are not a reward for suffering.
You don't need to hit a certain pain level for it to "count."

Your comfort is valid the moment you say it is.

9. They Can Help Moms With High Blood Pressure

The relaxation effect of an epidural can sometimes help stabilize or lower blood pressure in moms with:

- preeclampsia
- gestational hypertension
- severe anxiety

It's not a treatment, but it can be a helpful supportive measure.

10. Epidural Placement Is Usually Fast

Most epidurals take:
5 to 10 minutes to place
5–15 minutes thereafter to feel relief

This surprises many moms who expect a long, dramatic procedure.

11. They Don't Rob You of the "Birth Experience"

Many moms actually report the opposite.

With an epidural, you can:

- breathe
- relax
- laugh
- talk
- rest
- enjoy the moment
- stay connected to your partner
- feel present and powerful

You're not less brave — you're more focused, more centered, and more in tune with your birth.

12. You Can Still Feel Your Baby Being Born (Without Pain)

Many women say: "I felt the moment my baby came into the world — but it didn't hurt." That's the beautiful balance an epidural gives you.

> **Nurse's Tip: Understanding Spinal Headaches (Rare but Treatable)**
>
> It's rare, but sometimes a spinal headache can occur after an epidural or spinal.
> This happens when a tiny amount of spinal fluid leaks through the spot where the needle went in, causing a drop in pressure around the brain.

Most women never experience this, but I want you to know what it means – just in case.

What it feels like:

- A very intense headache
- Worse when sitting or standing
- Better when lying completely flat
- Sometimes accompanied by neck stiffness, nausea, or sensitivity to light

What you should do:

Tell your nurse or provider right away. Don't just "tough it out."

There are several treatments we can try:

- Fluids, caffeine, and rest for mild cases
- A blood patch for more severe headaches – a quick procedure done by anesthesia that usually fixes the problem almost immediately

A spinal headache is uncomfortable, but it's not dangerous and it is very treatable.

If you ever feel a headache that gets dramatically better when you lie flat, please let us know.

We've got you and there are effective solutions to get you feeling normal again.

Epidural Recovery: What to Expect After Birth

Once your epidural is turned off, it takes about **two hours** for full feeling and strength to return to your legs. Every body is different — some feel sensations sooner, some take the full two hours — but this window helps us keep you **safe and steady**.

Nurse's Heads Up

Even if you're excited to get up, **please don't try to get out of bed without your nurse.**
Your legs may feel:

- Heavy
- Wobbly
- Numb
- "Not quite yours yet"

That's normal but trying to stand too early can lead to a fall — and falls in postpartum are no joke.

What You Should Do While You Wait

For the next two hours, gently:

- **Lift your legs** one at a time
- **Bend your knees**
- **Wiggle your toes**
- **Shake out your legs**
- **Move your ankles in circles**

These little movements help circulation, help sensation return, and give your muscles a chance to "wake up."

Before You Stand...

Your nurse will always:

- **Assess your strength**
- **Check your balance**
- **Make sure you can safely bear weight**
- **Stay with you during your first walk to the bathroom**

We will never expect you to do this alone — your safety is our priority.

Closing Thoughts: Your Birth, Your Choice

Choosing an epidural isn't about pain or strength—it's about clarity, control, and honoring your own needs in one of the most powerful moments of your life.

Whether you use it to rest, to breathe, to refocus, or simply to meet your baby with calm, your decision is valid and respected.

There is no one "right" way to give birth—there is only your way.

And if an epidural helps you feel safe, supported, and present, then it is the right choice for you.

In labor, strength isn't measured by how much pain you can endure, but by how confidently you make the choices that feel best for your body and your baby.

You are doing an incredible job—and your story continues beautifully from here.

10

Epidural vs. IV Pain Medication

"Pain has choices. You have control."

Understanding your options so you can choose what feels right for you.

Labor pain relief isn't "all or nothing." You have choices, and every option works differently. Here's a simple, honest comparison to help you understand the difference between an epidural and IV pain medication (also called systemic or narcotic pain relief).

Epidural Pain Relief

The most effective form of labor pain control.

What it does:

- Numbs the nerves that carry pain from your uterus
- Dramatically reduces pain while still allowing you to feel pressure
- Helps you relax, rest, and stay calm during labor
- Can be adjusted constantly through a pump

What it feels like:

- Contractions become pressure instead of pain
- Warm, heavy legs
- Sense of relief and the ability to breathe and focus again

Pros:

✓ Most effective pain relief available
✓ Allows deep rest during long labors
✓ Does not enter baby's bloodstream
✓ You remain awake, alert, and fully present
✓ Adjustable, steady comfort

Cons:

- **Requires IV fluids**
- **Restricts walking until cleared**
- **Requires more frequent monitoring** (blood pressure checks, pulse ox, and assessments for how your body is responding)
- **Can cause difficulty urinating on your own**, sometimes requiring a temporary foley or straight cath
- **May cause one-sided numbness** (usually fixable with repositioning or adjustment)
- **Takes a few minutes to place and activate**

IV Pain Medication (Systemic Narcotics)

Helps "take the edge off" without numbing you completely.

Common medications: Morphine, Stadol, Nubain, Fentanyl (small doses)

What it does:

- Helps you relax between contractions
- Reduces the intensity of pain but does not remove it
- Can help early or mid-labor feel more manageable

What it feels like:

- More drowsy
- "Floaty" or slightly disconnected
- Contractions may still hurt, but feel less overwhelming

Pros:

✓ Works quickly
✓ No need to sit still for placement
✓ Does not require an anesthesiologist
✓ Can be used before an epidural
✓ Lets you rest if you're tense or anxious

Cons:

- Can make you sleepy or loopy
- May have to be in bed for a period of time for safety
- Can make you itchy
- Crosses the placenta (baby may feel sleepy temporarily)
- Can't be given too close to delivery
- May not provide enough relief for active labor
- Does not numb pain — only softens it

Side-by-Side Comparison

Feature	Epidural	IV Pain Medications
Pain control	Excellent	Mild to moderate
Effect on baby	None (does not cross placenta)	Yes, can cause temporary sleepiness
Mobility	Limited	Can usually move more freely under supervision of your nurse after an hour or so
Onset time	10–20 minutes	2–15 minutes
Best for	Active labor, long labors, epidural-level relief desired	Early labor, anxiety, quick "take the edge off"
Awareness	Fully awake	Can feel drowsy or "out of it"
Push effectiveness	Very good (pressure remains)	Good, but may feel groggy
Duration	Continuous	Traditional are given every 4 hours in labor

Nurse's Note: You Can Use BOTH

Many moms start with IV pain medication early in labor and later switch to an epidural when their contractions intensify. You don't have to pick one path–your plan can change as labor changes.

There is no failure in changing your mind. There is only choosing the support you need in the moment.

Bottom Line

If you want the strongest pain relief, epidural is best.

If you want a little help early on but want to stay mobile after the initial "be safe in bed" phase, IV meds can be a great option.

If you're unsure—you're allowed to try one, switch to the other, or do both. Most providers will not give the narcotic after the epidural.

Your labor, your comfort, your choice.
And your nurse will guide you every step of the way.

Chart: When IV Pain Meds Make Sense vs. When an Epidural Makes Sense

Category	IV Pain Medication *"Take the edge off"*	Epidural *"Strong, steady relief"*
Best When...	· Early in labor · Contractions painful but manageable · You're anxious & need to relax · You want something quick · You want to stay mobile	· Active labor · Pain is intense or overwhelming · You need to rest or sleep · You're exhausted or losing control · You want reliable, long-lasting comfort
Good If You...	· Want "a little something" without committing · Want short-term relief · Want to take a nap · Want flexibility before deciding on an epidural	· Want the strongest pain relief · Want to stay calm and present · Want steady comfort through labor · Prefer not to feel intense pain at all

Category	IV Pain Medication *"Take the edge off"*	Epidural *"Strong, steady relief"*
Keep in Mind...	• Relief is mild to moderate • May make you sleepy or loopy • Crosses the placenta (baby may feel sleepy temporarily) • Can't be given too close to delivery	• Requires sitting still for placement • Takes ~10–20 minutes to work • Legs may feel warm or heavy • You'll feel pressure, not pain
Perfect For...	• Early labor • Buying time before an epidural • Moms who want mobility • Moms not ready for an epidural yet	• Active labor • Long inductions • Moms who need to rest • Moms who want maximum comfort

Nurse's Tip

You don't have to pick one and stick with it. Many moms choose IV medication first to take the edge off... and then request an epidural once contractions intensify. Your comfort plan can change at any time–and that's completely normal.

11

Hello from the Inside!

"I don't make music for eyes. I make music for ears."

– Adele

There is nothing—I mean nothing—quite like hearing your baby's heartbeat, steady and strong. It's the closest thing to music your body will ever make, and trust me, I've spent plenty of shifts be-bopping along to those little thumps and rhythms.

When we place the monitors on your belly, we're not just listening for safety—we're listening to your baby's own soundtrack.

Electronic fetal monitoring lets us tune in to how your little one is handling labor, how strong your contractions are, and what your uterus is up to behind the scenes.

Think of this chapter as your backstage pass to the concert happening inside your belly.

Electronic Fetal Monitoring (EFM)

Electronic fetal monitoring is the system we use to track your baby's heartbeat and your contractions — it's how we keep tabs on what's happening "on the inside."

When we talk about monitoring in labor, you'll often hear your nurse mention the **"US and TOCO."**

US (Ultrasound Transducer)

This is the round monitor that picks up your baby's heartbeat. It uses gentle sound waves — the same kind used in routine pregnancy ultrasounds — to track:

- how fast your baby's heart is beating
- how it changes with movement
- how it responds to contractions

TOCO (Tocodynamometer)

This is the second round monitor placed near the top of your uterus. It measures your contractions by sensing the tightening of your belly — letting us know:

- how often your contractions occur
- how long they last

Together, the **US and TOCO** create a full picture of how your baby is handling labor and how your body is progressing.
Think of them as two parts of the same conversation:
Your uterus does the talking… and your baby tells us how they're feeling about it.

Types of Fetal Monitoring

1. External Monitoring

These are the stretchy belts placed around your belly — one for the baby's heart rate and one for your contractions.

This is the most common type of monitoring you'll see in Labor and Delivery.

2. Internal Monitoring

Sometimes we need a more accurate reading. In that case, we may use one or both of the following:

Fetal Scalp Electrode (FSE)

A small spiral wire that gently attaches to your baby's scalp to measure their heart rate directly.

Intrauterine Pressure Catheter (IUPC)

A thin tube placed inside the uterus to measure the *actual strength* of your contractions.

Internal monitors are **not used routinely** — only when medically needed.

Reasons might include:

- baby's position
- extra adipose tissue making it hard for the external monitor to pick up a clean signal

a very active baby who keeps "running away" from the monitor
(Mom, did you just drink a Red Bull?)

If You're Planning a Low-Intervention Birth

Check your hospital's policies in advance:

- Some allow **intermittent monitoring**
- Others require **continuous monitoring** for safety

It's always good to know ahead of time what's allowed in your specific facility.

What You Need to Know About Fetal Monitoring

In my experience, patients and their families are often curious about what they're seeing on the monitor.

While your nurse and provider are professionally trained to interpret every rise, drop, and wiggle on that screen, **I still think it's important for you to understand the basics.**

Fetal monitoring is your baby's way of communicating with us — tiny messages like:

- **"I'm doing great!"**
- **"I need a minute to recover."**
- **"Hey, can you help me out here?"**

In the next section, I'll break down what these patterns mean so you can feel:

- informed
- reassured
- empowered
- and part of the conversation

The Top and Bottom Lines on the Monitor

The **top line** on the fetal monitor is created by the **US (ultrasound transducer)** — this line shows your baby's heart rate. It rises and falls with every beat, giving us a picture of how your baby is responding to labor.

The **bottom line** comes from the **TOCO (tocodynamometer)** — this one tracks your contractions, showing when they start, peak, and fade.

When we look at **both lines together**, we can see how your baby's heart rate responds to each contraction. That relationship tells us how well your baby is tolerating labor and helps guide every decision we make.

Think of it like a conversation — the bottom line (your uterus) speaks, and the top line (your baby) answers. When both are in sync, we know things are going beautifully.

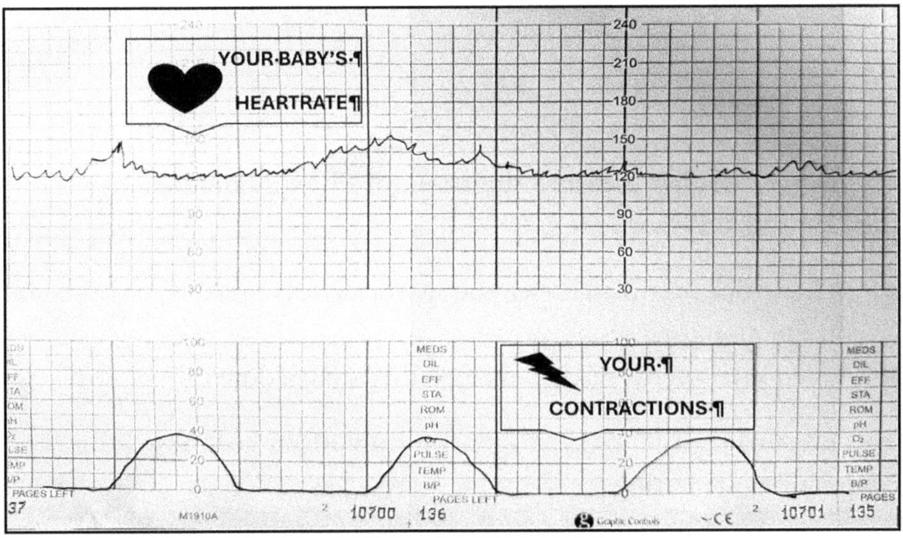

US (Ultrasound Transducer)

The US, or ultrasound transducer, is the round monitor placed on your belly that tracks your baby's heartbeat during labor. It works by sending out gentle sound waves (the same kind used in regular pregnancy ultrasounds) that bounce off your baby's heart. The returning echoes are translated into a signal that shows your baby's heart rate pattern on the top line of the fetal monitor strip.

Think of it as your baby's microphone — it lets us "listen in" to how they're doing inside the womb.

The TOCO: Tracking Your Contractions

Alongside monitoring your baby's heart rate, we also keep an eye on your contractions using a monitor called a **tocodynamometer**, or simply **TOCO** (pronounced *toe-co*).

The TOCO is the second round disc you'll see on your belly, usually placed near the top (the **fundus** — that's where contractions start). It measures the tightening and relaxing of your uterine muscle — the rise and fall you feel with each wave.

How It Works

The TOCO **doesn't measure the strength** of your contractions — just their **timing and frequency**.

- When your uterus tightens, the sensor detects pressure and the line on the monitor rises.
- When your uterus relaxes, the line drops back down.

This gives us a visual pattern showing **how often and how long** your contractions are lasting.

Think of it like a weather radar: it doesn't feel the storm, but it shows us when it's rolling in and when it's passing.

Fetal Scalp Electrode (FSE)

Sometimes, it's difficult for the external ultrasound monitor to pick up your baby's heartbeat clearly — especially if your baby is moving a lot, is in a tricky position, or if you have extra soft tissue between the monitor and your uterus. In these cases, we may use an internal fetal monitor called a **fetal scalp electrode (FSE).**

The FSE is a tiny, spiral-shaped wire that gently attaches to the top layer of your baby's scalp after your water has broken. It gives us a very accurate, beat-by-beat reading of your baby's heart rate, even during strong contractions or active labor.

You can think of it as your baby's personal EKG.

How It Feels and What to Expect

You won't feel the electrode being placed, other than the exam itself—your cervix is already dilated, and your baby's head is close enough for us to reach. The wire is extremely thin and flexible, and once it's secured, only a small portion comes out and connects to the fetal monitor.

Most moms don't even realize it's there after placement.

> **Nurse's Tip:** The FSE doesn't hurt your baby. It's placed carefully to attach only to the top layer of skin – like twisting a strand of hair. It can leave a small red mark or scratch on your baby's scalp after birth, which heals quickly.

Why We Use It

We place an FSE when:

- External monitoring can't pick up a consistent heart rate.
- The baby's tracing looks suspicious and we need more detail.
- The mother's heart rate is being mistaken for the baby's.
- There's a lot of movement or adipose tissue interfering with the signal.

The fetal scalp electrode is just another way for us to "hear" your baby's heartbeat more clearly when the outside world gets too noisy.

Intrauterine Pressure Catheter (IUPC)`

Sometimes during labor, we need a more accurate way to measure your contractions than what the external monitor can provide. That's when we use an **Intrauterine Pressure Catheter (IUPC)** — a small, flexible tube that sits just inside your uterus next to your baby after your water has broken.

The IUPC measures:

- the **exact strength** of your contractions
- how long they last
- how often they come
- how well your uterus relaxes between them

While the external TOCO only senses pressure from the outside, the IUPC gives us a **true numeric reading** (in millimeters of mercury) and helps us determine whether contractions are strong enough to make cervical change.

What to Expect

Placement is quick and usually painless — most women describe it as pressure during a routine cervical exam. Once it's placed, only a small tube runs along your leg and connects to the monitor. You can still move, breathe, and rest comfortably.

> **Nurse's Tip:** If you hear us mention **"Montevideo units,"** that's just our way of calculating the total strength of contractions over 10 minutes.

Why We Use It

An IUPC might be used when:

- Labor is induced or augmented with Pitocin.

- The cervix isn't changing and we need to assess contraction strength.
- External monitoring isn't clear enough.
- We need to evaluate resting tone between contractions.

What We're Looking For

Your nurse will monitor:

- **Frequency** – how often contractions begin
- **Duration** – how long they last
- **Resting tone** – how well the uterus relaxes in between

Ideally, contractions are:

- every **2–3 minutes**
- lasting **60–90 seconds**
- with a **full relaxation** between each one

> **Nurse's Tip:** If you're on Pitocin, you'll see us watching the monitor closely – not because we don't trust your body, but because we're making sure your contractions stay safe and effective because we are controlling them.

Your contractions are your body's natural communication — and the TOCO helps us see the conversation happening between you and your baby in real time.

The IUPC is like a translator, helping us understand exactly how your contractions are performing so we can support your labor safely and effectively.

Fetal Heart Rate (FHR)

Your baby's heart rate normally ranges between **110 and 160 beats per minute**. This tells us how well your baby is tolerating labor and how effectively oxygen is being delivered.

When your uterus contracts, it temporarily reduces blood flow — and therefore oxygen — to your baby. The way your baby's heart rate responds gives us important clues about how they're coping.

Variability

Variability refers to how much your baby's heart rate changes from beat to beat. Think of it as your baby's **energy level.**

A baby with **good variability** is:

- well-oxygenated
- active
- showing gentle, natural fluctuations

That's exactly what we want to see.

When variability decreases, it can mean your baby is resting, or it could signal that they're not getting quite enough oxygen. That's why we watch it closely throughout labor.

Decelerations

Decelerations are temporary dips in your baby's heart rate during labor that we see on the monitor.

Some are **completely normal** — especially when the head is being squeezed by contractions (their first workout!).

Others can signal that your baby may need a little help — maybe a position change, extra oxygen, or IV fluids for you.

We monitor the **pattern, depth, and timing** of each deceleration to decide what interventions are needed.

> **Nurse's Tip:** If your nurse suddenly asks you to roll to your side, hands and knees, or switch positions, don't panic. We're just helping your baby get more oxygen and relief from the pressure. It's teamwork in action.

Electronic fetal monitoring is our window into your baby's well-being. It's how we listen to their story — one heartbeat at a time.

What Your Baby's Heartbeat Tells Us

Your baby has their own way of communicating during labor — and we listen through the monitor. Each pattern we see tells us a little about how your baby is handling contractions, oxygen flow, and the overall stress of birth.

There are **three main categories** we use to describe what we're seeing:

Category I / Reassuring (Normal) Patterns

This is exactly what we LOVE to see.

Your baby's heart rate:

- stays between **110–160 bpm**
- has **moderate variability**
- may show **accelerations** (little mountains!)

Accelerations are wonderful signs of a healthy baby reacting to movement, stimulation, or contractions.

When we see this pattern, we smile. It means your baby is thriving and tolerating labor beautifully.

Category II / Non-Reassuring (Concerning but Recoverable) Patterns

Sometimes babies show signs that they're getting a little tired or need more oxygen.

This might include:

- **Minimal variability**
  (this can happen after pain medication or during sleep cycles)
- **Occasional decelerations**
  (A heart rate that is below your baby's baseline for a period of time)

These patterns don't always mean something is wrong — they simply signal that we need to watch more closely.

Your care team may:

- Reposition you
- Give you oxygen
- Adjust IV fluids
- Stop or lower Pitocin
- Encourage deep breathing

Most of the time, these fix things quickly — your baby just needed a little extra help.

Nurse Tip: If your baby has a persistent heart rate above 160, it may indicate that *you* have a fever. Your nurse should be taking your temperature just to make sure.

Category III/Concerning Patterns

These are rare but important.

We may see:

- **Absent variability** (a very flat line)
- **Repetitive, deep decelerations**
- A consistently **low heart rate** that doesn't recover

If we see this:

- Your nurse and provider will act quickly
- You may be repositioned
- We may prepare for urgent delivery

Every action taken is to keep you and your baby safe.

Nurse's Tip: Try not to let the sound or changes of the monitor alarm you. We're trained to interpret every squiggle and beat in real time – and we're always one step ahead.

Your baby's heart rate tells us their story — when they're calm, when they're active, and when they need a little extra love. Every beat is a message, and we're listening closely the whole way through.

When the Monitor Gets It Wrong

Electronic fetal monitors are amazing tools — but they're not perfect. Sometimes the tracing on the screen looks alarming, when in reality, nothing is wrong at all. The monitor gives us data, but it doesn't always tell the whole story.

Why It Happens

There are several reasons the monitor might show irregular or "concerning" patterns that don't reflect what's truly happening:

- **Baby movement:** If your baby wiggles, flips, or kicks, the heart rate sensor can lose contact, creating sudden dips or gaps in the tracing.
- **Maternal movement:** Sitting up, rolling over, or walking around can shift the monitor bands just enough to distort the reading.
- **Monitor placement:** Every belly is different! The baby's position (and a little extra padding or amniotic fluid) can make it hard for the monitor to get a consistent signal.
- **Twin pregnancies:** Two heartbeats in close proximity can sometimes "cross signals," making the monitor think something's off when it's not.

What Nurses Do When That Happens

When the tracing looks strange, the first thing we do is go to you — *not* the screen.

We may:

- check monitor placement
- listen directly to your baby with a handheld Doppler or get an ultrasound for better placement
- reposition you for a better signal

Most of the time, that's all it takes to get things back on track.

Sometimes, what looks like a dramatic deceleration is really just the monitor picking up your pulse or the movement of the belt. We can usually tell the difference within seconds.

> **Nurse's Tip:** If your nurse seems calm while the tracing looks messy, that's your clue everything is fine. We've seen every pattern imaginable – and we can tell when it's a true concern versus a monitor hiccup.

Trust the Team, Not the Screen

It's easy to get caught up in the sounds of the monitor — the whooshing heartbeat, the alarms, the beeps. But remember: **the screen is just a tool.** *We* are the interpreters.

We combine what we see on the monitor with what we see in you:

- your breathing
- your contractions
- your color
- your instincts as a mother

When technology and human care work together, that's where the magic happens — because no monitor will ever replace a nurse's intuition.

Normal and Abnormal Fetal Heart Fluctuations

During labor, your baby's heart rate will naturally go up and down — these fluctuations are normal and show us how your baby is responding to contractions, movement, and the birth process itself.

Babies are resilient, and their heart patterns change often as they adjust to what's happening inside your uterus.

Sometimes the monitor may show a dip or variation that *looks* unusual to you — but to us, it's part of what we expect and know how to interpret. It could be a normal response to head compression or rapid descent through the birth canal.

In other words, it means your baby is getting closer to making their grand entrance.

Rest assured, we're trained to recognize which changes are normal reactions and which ones need attention.

Nurse Reassurance:
Please don't panic if you hear us mention "decelerations" or see extra people step into your room. Let us decide what's concerning and what's not — that's our job.

I always tell my patients, **"Do I look nervous or concerned?"** When they answer no, I smile and say, **"Good — because you shouldn't be either."**

Your nurse's demeanor is your best indicator of how things are going. If I'm calm, it's because I know you and your baby are safe, and we have everything under control.

So take a deep breath, match my energy, and let that reassurance carry you through.

You focus on your breathing and your baby — I'll focus on everything else.

We are highly trained professionals who specialize in reading these patterns, and our goal is always the same:
to keep you and your baby safe.

Let us carry that worry for you — your job is to focus on the moment you've been waiting for.

What We See When We're Looking at Contractions

When your nurse glances up at the monitor, we're not just staring at squiggly lines — we're reading your body's story in real time.

Every contraction tells us something about how you and your baby are handling labor.

We're looking for:

- patterns
- rhythms
- spacing
- how strong each wave seems

What the Boxes on the Contraction Monitor Mean

When you look at the fetal monitor strip, you'll notice a grid of tiny boxes behind the lines. These boxes aren't random — they help us measure time and contraction frequency.

Here's the simple way to understand them:

Each small box = 10 seconds

You'll see lots of little squares across the strip.
Each one represents **10 seconds** of time.

So:

- **6 small boxes = 1 minute**
- **30 small boxes = 5 minutes**

This helps your nurse and provider measure exactly how often your contractions are coming.

⏱ Each darker vertical line = 1 minute

Every minute is marked by a darker or thicker line.
These are our landmarks for timing contractions accurately.

1

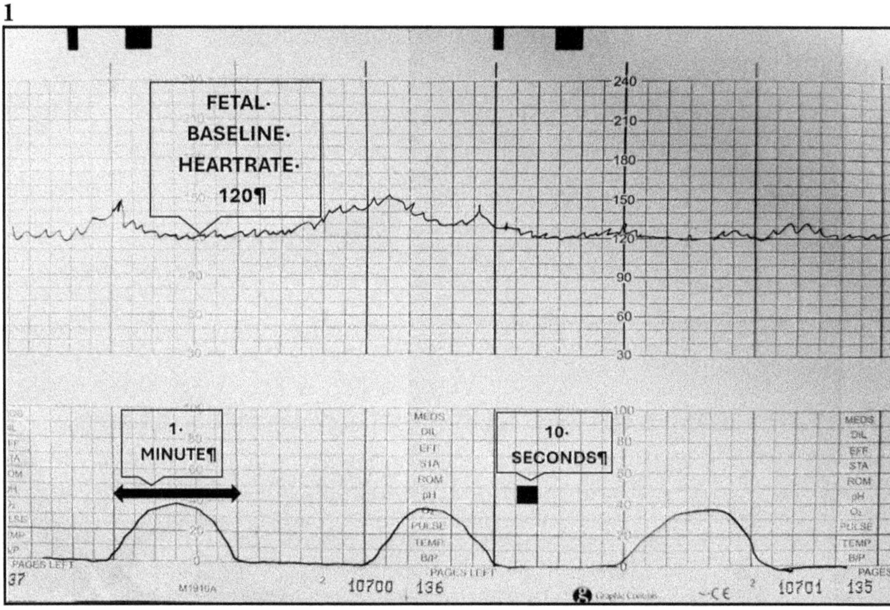

How We Count Contractions

When we talk about contractions, we describe them in **frequency** — how many you have in a 10-minute window.

It's **NOT:**

- how long they last
- how intense they feel

- how far apart you think they are
- from the **end** of one to the end of the next

It **IS:**

From the start of one contraction to the start of the next.
That's the official way labor contractions are counted.

We Also Look At:

- **How often your contractions are coming**

Are they every 5 minutes? Every 2 minutes? Back-to-back?
This tells us where you might be in labor and whether things are moving along safely and comfortably.

- **How long each contraction lasts**

A typical contraction lasts **60–100 seconds**.
This helps us understand how coordinated your uterus is as it works to open your cervix.

- **How strong they are (to the best the monitor can tell)**

External monitors don't measure true intensity, but they show us whether contractions are building or spacing out.
If you have an **IUPC**, we can measure strength more accurately.

- **Whether your uterus is getting a full rest in between**

This is **huge**.
Your body and your baby need time to recover after each wave.
If contractions are too close together (tachysystole), we may need to help your uterus take a break.

- **How your baby responds to each wave**

Every contraction temporarily reduces blood flow to the placenta. That's normal — but it's also why your nurse keeps such a close eye on baby's heartbeat during and after each contraction.
We want to make sure your baby is tolerating labor beautifully.

Nurse's Tip: Don't Hold Your Breath

During contractions, remember to **breathe**. The contraction itself already temporarily reduces blood flow and oxygen to your baby – that's normal and expected. But when you hold your breath on top of that, it can make that reduction more pronounced.

Steady, intentional breathing helps:

- Keep oxygen moving to your baby
- Reduce tension in your body
- Make contractions more manageable

So when the wave builds, **exhale**, don't brace. Your breath is one of your strongest tools in labor.

Why This Matters to You

Understanding what we're looking at helps you feel **empowered** instead of overwhelmed.
The monitor isn't just a machine — it's a window into how you and your baby are doing, moment by moment.

And remember:

You don't have to read the monitor.
That's our job.
Your job is to breathe, relax, and work with your body.
Our job is to protect you, guide you, and make sure everything we see is safe, healthy, and reassuring.

What Is Tachysystole?

Your uterus is designed to contract, then rest — over and over — giving your baby time to recover and get oxygen between each contraction. **Tachysystole** means your uterus is contracting **too often**.

Clinically, it's defined as:

- **More than 5 contractions in 10 minutes**, averaged over 30 minutes.

But here's the simple version:
Your uterus isn't getting enough rest time between contractions and neither is your baby.

This can happen:

- on its own (natural labor)
- with **Pitocin**
- with cervical ripening methods like **Cytotec, Cervidil, or the balloon**
- or a combination of these

The good news?
We can fix it — and we act fast.

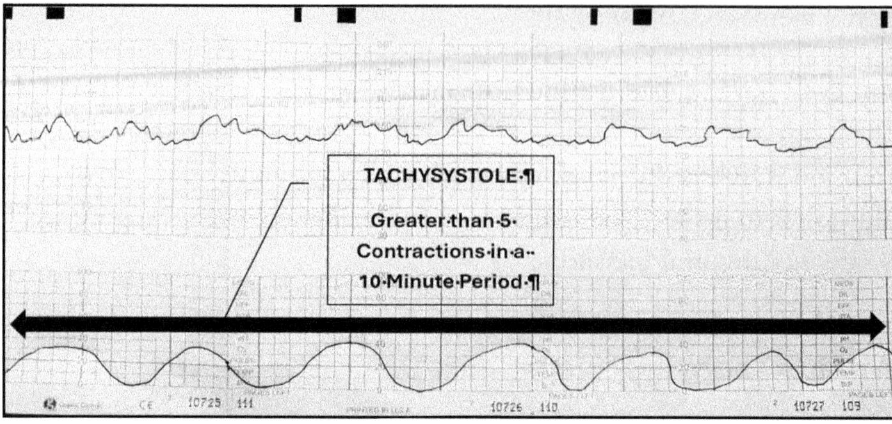

Why Tachysystole Matters

Between contractions, your placenta sends oxygen and nutrients to your baby. When contractions are too close together:

- Baby doesn't get as much time to recover
- You may feel overwhelmed and unable to breathe through the pattern
- Baby's heart rate may show signs that they're stressed by the rapid pace

Tachysystole isn't dangerous when caught early — and that's exactly why we monitor you so closely.

What We Do When We See Tachysystole

What we do depends on whether you're being induced/augmented or you're laboring naturally.

If You're on Pitocin (Oxytocin)

Pitocin is wonderful for helping labor progress, but it can also make contractions come too strong or too fast.
If we see tachysystole, we step in right away:

We turn the Pitocin down
We may decrease your dose to give your uterus more rest time.

Or we shut it off temporarily
This allows your body to reset and gives your baby the break they need.

We reposition you and give fluids
Sometimes a simple position change or extra hydration helps regulate contraction spacing.

Our goal is always the same:
safe, steady contractions — **not nonstop ones.**

If Tachysystole Happens With Cervical Ripening

Even before Pitocin starts, certain induction methods can occasionally make your uterus contract too often. When that happens, we respond quickly to keep both you and your baby safe and comfortable.

Balloon (Foley or Cook Balloon)

A balloon works mechanically, not with medication — but the pressure on your cervix can still trigger frequent contractions.
If we see tachysystole:

- We adjust your position
- We may deflate or remove the balloon
  Relieving that pressure usually calms the uterus down right away.

Cervidil (Dinoprostone)

Cervidil gently releases medication over several hours but if contractions become too close together:

- We remove the Cervidil insert
- Repositioning and fluids can also help
  Because Cervidil can be taken out quickly, it's one of the easiest ways to stop tachysystole fast.

Cytotec (Misoprostol)

Cytotec is effective for softening the cervix but it can sometimes overstimulate the uterus. If we see tachysystole:

- We hold your next dose
- We reposition you and give IV fluids
- We may give **a tocolytic** to help your uterus relax
  Cytotec can't be "removed," so we manage the effects with supportive care and medications until the pattern slows down.

In Natural Labor (No Pitocin)

Even without medication, your uterus can sometimes take off on its own.
If contractions become too frequent and baby doesn't like the pattern, we act quickly to help both of you.

We may give you a tocolytic.
This will help the uterus relax.
It slows the contraction pattern, giving your baby time to recover and get the oxygen they need.

We use it when:

- your contractions are too close together
- you're feeling overwhelmed and can't catch your breath

- baby's heart rate shows us they're not tolerating the pattern well
- or all the above

It works fast and safely and it often makes a world of difference in how you feel.

Why This Matters

You might think strong, frequent contractions mean faster progress — but that's not always true.

Your uterus, like any muscle, needs rest to work effectively.
Your baby needs those breaks even more.

When contractions are too fast:

- you become more uncomfortable
- your cervix may not actually open faster
- baby may show signs of stress because of lack of blood supply and oxygen
- labor can become less efficient

With the right adjustments — turning Pitocin down, changing positions, giving fluids, or using Terbutaline — you and your baby get the balanced rhythm you both need.

> **Nurses's Tip: What to Expect With Terbutaline, a known Tocolytic**
>
> Terbutaline works fast to relax your uterus, but it can also cause your heart rate to speed up for a short time.

This is completely expected and usually lasts only a few minutes.

You might feel:

- a little shaky
- warm or flushed
- your heart beating faster (tachycardia)
- slightly anxious or jittery

These effects fade quickly and we stay right with you while it happens.
The goal is simply to give your baby more oxygen and give your uterus the break it needs.

The Bottom Line

Tachysystole sounds scary, but it's something we are trained to recognize instantly and treat quickly.
You are never going through it without us watching, guiding, and adjusting your plan in real time.

When the Monitor Doesn't Match the Pain

If I had a dollar for the number of patients that have said to me, "these contractions really hurt but don't show strong on the monitor"....

The strength of your contractions can only be measured accurately with an internal monitor (an intrauterine pressure catheter), not from the external TOCO on your belly.

The TOCO only senses **pressure changes**, not **intensity** — so don't ever feel like you shouldn't be in pain just because the contractions on the screen look small.

Every woman feels contractions differently depending on her baby's position, uterine tone, and individual pain threshold.
Some of the strongest contractions barely register on the monitor, while others look huge but feel mild.

I remember being monitored with my first, pre-term, and I was contracting away and didn't feel a thing.

What matters most is what your body feels — not what the line shows.

Trust your body — not the paper.
You're the one doing the work and your experience tells us more than any machine ever could.

When We Measure Contractions Internally

Sometimes, we need a more accurate picture of how strong your contractions really are — especially if labor isn't progressing as expected or if we're adjusting medications like Pitocin. In these cases, your provider may place an internal uterine pressure catheter (IUPC).

An IUPC is a thin, flexible tube that goes just inside your uterus, past the cervix, and sits alongside your baby.
It measures the exact strength and frequency of your contractions in millimeters of mercury (mmHg).

Unlike the external TOCO, which only senses movement, the IUPC tells us precisely:

- how powerful each contraction is
- whether your uterus is resting properly in between
- if your contractions are strong enough to cause cervical change

Nurse's Tip: If you have an IUPC, you might notice your nurse or provider talking about "Montevideo units."
That's just a fancy way of calculating the overall power of your contractions – not something you need to worry about.

The IUPC isn't used for every patient – only when it's truly needed.
But when we do use it, it helps us make sure your uterus is working effectively, your labor is progressing safely, and your baby is getting all the rest and oxygen they need in between those powerful waves.

When We Use Both: FSE + IUPC

Sometimes, both the fetal scalp electrode (FSE) and intrauterine pressure catheter (IUPC) are used at the same time — and there's a good reason for that.

When labor becomes more complex, we want to know two things with absolute accuracy:

How your baby is responding
→ That's what the FSE shows us.

How strong and frequent your contractions are
→ That's what the IUPC measures.

Using them together gives us the clearest picture possible of what's happening between you and your baby — a real-time dialogue between the uterus and the fetal heart.

> **Nurse's Tip:** If you hear your nurse say, "We're going to put both internal monitors in," don't panic.
> It doesn't mean something terrible is happening – it just means we want the most accurate information to guide your care safely and effectively.
>
> Think of it like tuning both sides of a conversation –
> one tells us what your uterus is doing,
> the other tells us how your baby is handling it.
> Together, they help us make the best decisions for you and your little one.

When We Give Baby Back Their Pool Water (Amnioinfusion)

One of the coolest things about an IUPC is that it doesn't just measure contractions — **it also gives us a way to help your baby if they need a little extra "cushion."**

This is done through something called an **amnioinfusion**, where we gently infuse warm sterile fluid through the catheter and back into the uterus.

Think of it as adding a little extra padding around your baby.

We use this technique when:

- the amniotic fluid is low
- baby is having **variable decelerations** from cord compression

With more fluid around them:

- the cord is less likely to get squeezed
- baby can move and "float" more comfortably
- the heart rate pattern often improves

It's safe, effective, and honestly one of the most satisfying interventions because babies usually respond beautifully.

Sometimes just giving them that extra little float helps the whole room breathe easier.

> **Nurse's Tip:** Remember – **what goes in must come out.**
> If we're giving extra fluid through an amnioinfusion, that fluid will leak back out of your vagina.
>
> Don't be surprised if you feel more leaking or see your pad getting wetter.
>
> It's normal, expected, and a good sign that everything is flowing the way it should.
>
> You're not peeing yourself.
> Nothing is wrong.
> Just let it leak!

Comfort, Mobility, and What You Can Still Do

Even with internal monitors like the FSE and IUPC in place, you're not confined to the bed. While movement will be more limited (since the monitors are connected by thin wires), you can still change positions, roll from side to side, sit up, or use a peanut ball or birthing bar to help labor progress. Your nurse will help you move safely while keeping the monitors secure and the tracings clear.

> **Nurse's Tip:** Don't feel embarrassed about needing help to shift, use the restroom, or get comfortable – that's what we're here for. Labor is intimate, vulnerable, and powerful all at once, and your comfort matters.
>
> You'll still be able to rest, breathe, and focus on your labor. Internal monitors simply help us take better care of you – they don't take away your power or your birth experience.
>
> Even with a few extra wires, *you're still in charge.* You call the shots and we'll make sure you stay safe, comfortable, and cared for every step of the way.

Staying Calm During Fetal Heart Rate Interventions

Few moments in labor feel more stressful than when the baby's heart rate changes and the room suddenly gets busy. You might see more nurses walk in, hear alarms from the monitor, or notice your provider at your bedside — and your first instinct may be to panic.

Please remember: **This happens often and it rarely means something is seriously wrong.** It simply means your baby is communicating and we're responding.

What's Happening

During contractions, your uterus tightens and briefly limits blood flow (and oxygen) to the baby — this is completely normal. But sometimes, your baby's heart rate may dip a little more than we like or take longer to recover. That's when you'll see us act quickly.

Our goal is always the same: **to help your baby get more oxygen.**

That's why you might see us:

- Reposition you (side-lying or hands-and-knees)
- Give you oxygen (at some institutions)
- Stop or decrease your Pitocin
- Bolus your IV fluids
- Ask you to take slow, deep breaths

Each of these steps is designed to improve blood flow and calm your baby's heart rate pattern.

> **Nurse's Tip:** If you see your nurse move with purpose but stay calm – that's your sign to breathe. We do this every day and we know what to do. You may hear medical terms like "deceleration," "late decel," or "minimal variability." These are just ways we describe what we're seeing on the monitor so the whole team can communicate clearly.

How to Stay Calm

You have more control than you think. Try these grounding techniques while we work:

- Focus on your breath. Inhale through your nose, exhale slowly through your mouth.

- Listen to your nurse's voice. We'll guide you through every step.
- Hold your partner's hand. Let them be your anchor while we take care of your baby.
- Trust the process. Most heart rate changes correct themselves within a few minutes after interventions.

What It Means

Not every change in the fetal heart rate means distress — babies experience natural fluctuations during labor just like adults do when they move, sleep, or react to stress. We monitor these patterns so closely because we can catch even the smallest shifts and correct them before they become a problem.

Remember:
A busy moment in your room means **your team is working** — not that your baby is in danger.
Our calm means your baby is still okay and we're making sure it stays that way.

Why Staying Calm Matters for You and Your Baby

When you feel afraid or panicked, your body releases stress hormones like adrenaline and cortisol — the same ones that activate your "fight or flight" response. While that reaction is useful in danger, during labor it can actually work against you and your baby.

These hormones can:

- constrict blood vessels
- reduce blood flow and oxygen to the uterus and baby
- speed up your heart rate
- make your breathing shallow

- cause your muscles (including the uterus) to tighten

This can make contractions **less effective**, slow labor, and sometimes make your baby briefly show signs of stress on the monitor.

That's why calm, controlled breathing is powerful.
It helps keep oxygen flowing, keeps your uterus working efficiently, and helps your baby stay steady and well-oxygenated.

> **Nurse's Tip:** When you feel fear creeping in, look for your anchor – your nurse, your partner, your breath. Focus on one of those until your body settles.
> A calm mind creates a calm body, and a calm body helps your baby stay safe, strong, and well-oxygenated.
>
> You set the tone for your baby's first environment – your heartbeat, your breath, your strength. The more peace you create for yourself, the more peace your baby feels inside of you.

The Partner's Role During Fetal Heart Rate Changes

When the room suddenly fills with activity — nurses moving quickly, monitors beeping, voices getting serious — it's natural to feel your heart race too. But during these moments, your presence can be one of the most powerful forms of support your partner has.

What You Can Do

Stay calm. Your partner will mirror your energy. If you stay steady and composed, she's more likely to stay grounded too.

Hold her hand or speak softly. Say things like, "You're doing great," or "They've got you and the baby — everything's okay." A gentle, confident tone helps her focus on your voice instead of the flurry around her.

Step aside if asked, but don't leave. Sometimes, the team needs space to work. You might be asked to move a few feet back but stay in the room if possible — your partner will still feel your presence.

Listen, don't panic. When nurses use medical terms or call out numbers, remember it's just how we communicate quickly. It doesn't automatically mean there's an emergency.

What Not to Do

Don't interrupt or ask rapid-fire questions in the moment. It can distract the team. Instead, wait until things settle, and we'll explain everything.

Don't assume the worst — 9 times out of 10, these heart rate dips correct quickly with simple interventions like changing positions or giving fluids.

Why Your Calm Matters

Your partner is vulnerable — she's in pain, emotional, and focused on her baby. When you stay calm, breathe with her, and keep your eyes locked on hers, you become her anchor. She'll remember your steady presence long after the monitors are turned off.

> **Nurse's Tip:** If you're unsure what's happening, look at your nurse. If she's calm, you can be too. We'll always tell you when there's a true emergency – and we'll make sure you understand what's going on as soon as we can.

> In moments of uncertainty, your steadiness becomes strength. You don't have to fix anything – just love, reassure, and breathe beside her. That's the kind of support she'll never forget.

After the Scare: Processing What Just Happened

Once the lights dim again, the monitors quiet down, and your nurse's voice softens back to normal, you might finally have a moment to breathe — and that's when the emotions hit. Even when everything turns out perfectly fine, those few minutes can feel like hours. It's okay to feel shaken, scared, or even tearful afterward.

Give Yourself Permission to Feel

Labor is raw, intense, and deeply personal. Watching your baby's heart rate change or seeing your care team move quickly can trigger fear — even if nothing serious happened. Allow yourself to feel whatever comes up: relief, exhaustion, gratitude, even frustration. All of it is valid.

Talk About It

Ask your nurse or provider to explain exactly what happened. We love when parents want to understand — we'll walk you through the heart rate tracing, what we saw, and what we did to fix it. That understanding can bring peace and closure to an overwhelming moment.

If you're still processing it later — days or weeks after birth — that's normal too. Birth stories are powerful and sometimes we need time to make sense of them.

Nurse's Tip: Don't carry fear from one moment into the rest of your labor. Once your baby's heart rate stabilizes and we're smiling again, that's your cue to let the fear go and step back into the moment. You're safe, your baby's safe, and you're doing exactly what you need to do.

Labor isn't just about physical strength – it's about emotional resilience. The way you and your partner weather those intense moments together becomes part of your birth story, one that ends with the sweetest sound of all – your baby's heartbeat, steady and strong.

12

How You Arrive: The Many Paths to Labor and Delivery

"It's not the destination, it's the journey."

– Ralph Waldo Emerson

No two birth stories start the same way. Some moms arrive cool and calm, suitcase in hand, ready to check in like it's a hotel. Others come flying down the hallway gripping the wheelchair rails, praying we don't hit a bump.

However you get here, you're in the right place.

Now that we've laid the foundation for what to expect during your stay, let's walk through the most common ways patients come through our doors — whether it's planned, spontaneous, or somewhere in between — and what happens next for each.

Triage: The Gateway to Labor and Delivery

Triage is often the very first stop on your journey — kind of like the "front desk" of Labor and Delivery, except instead of handing you a hotel key, we're deciding whether it's time to have a baby or time to go home and rest.

You might find yourself in triage if:

- you think your water broke
- you're contracting
- you haven't felt the baby move as much
- something just feels "off"

And let me say this up front — **please never feel bad about coming in.** You're not overreacting. You're not being dramatic. You're not wasting anyone's time.

You're being a mom — protecting your baby before they're even here.

You'd be surprised how many patients apologize for showing up:

"I didn't want to bother anyone."
"I wasn't sure if it was time."

Please hear me when I say — "you are never a bother". That's literally what we're here for.

What Happens in Triage

When you come to triage, think of it as your first safety checkpoint. We're going to:

✓ get you settled into a triage room
✓ monitor your baby's heart rate
✓ track your contractions
✓ ask questions about what's been going on
✓ focus our assessment on whatever concern brought you in

Depending on the situation, we may also:

- check your cervix
- collect a urine sample
- do a swab if you think your water broke
- check your blood pressure
- draw blood if we're screening for preeclampsia or infection

Sometimes, after monitoring, we find your contractions are early or irregular, and your cervix isn't changing yet. That's what we call **false labor** (prodromal labor).

It's frustrating — especially when you were sure *this was it* — but if your body isn't quite ready, we'll send you home to rest, eat, and let things develop.

If you **are** in active labor or your water is broken, we'll admit you, bring you to a birthing room and begin the real work.

Nurse's Tip: Pack Your Patience

Triage can be busy, especially at night when it feels like every mom in the county suddenly goes into labor.

We'll get to you as fast as we can – and once you're in a room, you'll be well on your way to meeting your baby.

Compassion Note: I know it's nerve-wracking to be hooked up to monitors, waiting for answers. But this part of the process is how we make sure both you and your baby are safe before moving forward.

Every labor story starts here — with reassurance, information, and a team ready to take care of you.

Nurse's Insight: When to Head to Triage

Don't wait or second-guess yourself — if something feels off, trust your instincts. Here are some good reasons to come in for evaluation:

- Regular contractions that are growing stronger, closer together, or more uncomfortable. You cannot walk or talk through them.
- A gush or continuous trickle of fluid (it could be that your water broke)
- Vaginal bleeding that's more than spotting
- Decreased fetal movement or a change in your baby's usual pattern — after 28 weeks, if baby does not move 10 times in two hours, drink or eat something sweet, and wait for movement. If there is no movement or you are unsure, call or come in.
- Severe abdominal pain or intense pressure
- Headache, blurred vision/visual disturbances, or swelling of the face or hands (possible signs of high blood pressure)
- Fever, chills, or flu-like symptoms during pregnancy
- **Any gut feeling that something isn't right — you know your body best**

Remember: It's always better to come in and be told everything is okay than to stay home and wonder. You are *never* an inconvenience.

What's Your Labor Path?

"Birth is a mystery. Words are not enough." – Marie O'Connor

Induction of Labor: When We Give Nature a Nudge

For some women, labor begins all on its own — but for others, we need to help things along a little. That's what we call **induction of labor (IOL)** — using medication or other methods to encourage your body to begin the process when it hasn't started naturally.

If you're scheduled for an induction, it's totally normal to feel a mix of excitement and anxiety. You've had this date circled on your calendar for weeks — you know when it's happening but that also gives you plenty of time to think about it (and overthink it). The night before an induction, sleep usually doesn't happen. Your bag's packed, your nerves are high, and your mind is racing with everything from baby names to epidurals.

Compassion Note: It's okay to feel nervous — even when it's planned. Most moms tell me that the anticipation is worse than the actual process. Once you're here, surrounded by your team, the fear starts to fade and the focus shifts to excitement.

Why We Induce

There are many reasons your provider might recommend starting labor rather than waiting for it to happen on its own:

- You're past your due date (usually 41 weeks for first time moms, 39 weeks for elective seasoned moms).
- You have high blood pressure or pre-eclampsia.
- You have gestational diabetes or other health conditions.
- There are concerns about your baby's growth or well-being.

Sometimes, it's just because your body — or your baby — needs a little encouragement to get moving.

How Induction Happens

There's no one-size-fits-all approach. The method depends on your body's readiness — especially the condition of your cervix (whether it's soft, thin, or still firm).

Here are the most common methods:

Cervical Ripening Agents

Medications like **Cytotec (misoprostol)** or **Cervidil (dinoprostone)** that soften and thin your cervix to prepare it for dilation.

Mechanical Methods

A **Foley balloon** or **Cook catheter** inserted into the cervix to gently stretch it open.

Amniotomy

Artificially breaking your water (if it's safe and your cervix is favorable).

Pitocin (Oxytocin)

A synthetic version of your body's own contraction hormone, given through your IV to start or strengthen contractions.

Each method can be used alone or in combination, depending on how your body responds. Sometimes, things move quickly. Other times, it's a slow process — and that's okay.

> **Nurse's Tip:** Inductions are a marathon, not a sprint. Bring your charger, snacks, and patience. Sometimes we start in the evening and don't meet your baby until the next day – or the day after that. Progress takes time and that's normal.

A Word About Expectations

Inductions don't always go as planned — and that's not failure. Sometimes, your cervix just isn't ready yet and we may need to pause, let your body rest, or even try again another day. What matters most is keeping both you and your baby safe.

Compassion Note: No matter how your labor begins — naturally or with our help — it's still *your* labor. There's no wrong way to bring your baby into the world.

Methods of Cervical Ripening: What to Expect

Before labor can progress, your cervix has to get soft, thin, and ready to open — that's where cervical ripening comes in. The method your provider chooses depends on how "ripe" your cervix already is.

Here's a breakdown of what's used and what it feels like:

Medication-Based Ripening

Cytotec (Misoprostol) and **Cervidil (Dinoprostone)** are medications designed to soften and thin the cervix.

How It's Given

- **Cytotec:** a small pill placed near the cervix, swallowed, or placed buccally in the cheek
- **Cervidil:** a thin strip inserted vaginally close to the cervix and left in place for several hours. Moms describe this as feeling a little scratchy during insertion.

What It Feels Like

Usually mild cramping or period-like pain that builds gradually. Some women barely feel anything at first; others feel stronger contractions as their body begins responding.

Some women, most often moms that have had babies before, can go into *rip-roaring labor* as a result — everyone responds differently.

What Happens Next

You'll be monitored for contractions and baby's heart rate.
If your cervix starts to change, we move forward with other steps like **Pitocin** or **breaking your water.**

> **Nurse's Tip:** If you feel pressure or mild cramps, that's actually a good sign – your body's responding! Try to relax, breathe, and rest while you can.

Mechanical Methods

A Foley balloon or Cook catheter is a small tube with one or two balloons at the end that's gently inserted into the cervix and inflated with sterile water to apply pressure and help it open. This method can be used with medications as well.

What it feels like: Insertion can feel like a strong cervical check — uncomfortable but usually quick. Once the balloon is in, you'll feel pressure low in your pelvis or back, like period cramps. Don't be alarmed if you find this uncomfortable or painful. Many women do. In fact, some ask for pain management as a result and that is o-kay. And then there are some patients walk around with it in place and don't even know it's there. Everyone is different. Contractions will be more uncomfortable with the balloon in place. Also be prepared for that.

How long it stays: Usually **6–12 hours** or until it falls out on its own, which often means you've reached around **3–4 cm dilated.**

Compassion Note: You might feel like things are slow at first — and that's okay. Cervical ripening is the foundation for a smoother labor, not wasted time. Think of it as warming up before the marathon.

Amniotomy (Breaking Your Water)

If your cervix is ready and your baby is low enough in the pelvis, your provider may use a small hook-like instrument to break your water.

What it feels like:

A quick gush of warm fluid — surprising but not painful. You'll probably continue to leak fluid until delivery.

Why it helps:

1. Stronger, More Effective Contractions
When the amniotic sac is broken, your body releases more **prostaglandins**, hormones that help contractions become stronger, longer, and more coordinated.

2. Better Pressure on the Cervix
Without the fluid cushion, your baby's head presses more directly against the cervix. That steady pressure helps the cervix **thin and open more efficiently**.

3. Improved Labor Feedback Loop
Pressure on the cervix sends signals to your brain to release more **oxytocin**, which strengthens contractions — a natural positive feedback cycle.

4. Helps Baby Settle Lower
Breaking the water often allows the baby to **descend deeper into the pelvis**, which can help labor progress, especially if things have slowed.

Nurse's Tip: Whenever my provider breaks your water, I make it a point to be right at your bedside. If your baby doesn't like the change, I'm already there to respond immediately. I also keep the fetal heart monitor volume turned up just enough so I can "hear" what your baby has to say – if your little one needs to tell me something, I want to listen.

Important Things to Know

- Once your water is broken, labor usually needs to **keep moving forward**
- It can make contractions feel **stronger or more intense**
- It's a **deliberate decision**, not a routine step — and it should always be discussed with you first

Why Babies Sometimes React When the Water Breaks:

When your provider breaks your water, your baby suddenly loses that warm, cushiony environment they've been floating in. The quick change in pressure and space can shift the umbilical cord or cause the baby to move, which sometimes shows up as a brief heart-rate dip on the monitor. Most of the time, your baby quickly adjusts, but that's why your nurse stays close — to listen, watch, and respond if needed.

Compassion Note: Even when things look intense on the monitor, remember — your nurse is right there, reading every beat and ready to act. Your baby's just adjusting to a brand-new world that's about to get even bigger.

Word to the Wise: If an epidural is part of your birth plan and you're already feeling uncomfortable, it's perfectly reasonable to ask your provider whether breaking your water can wait until after your epidural is placed.

Here's why: Once your water breaks, contractions often get **much stronger, very quickly** — what might feel like a 3 on the pain scale can jump to a 7 in no time. I never want you to be caught off guard or in unnecessary pain, especially if your intention is to have an epidural for comfort.

Advocate for yourself, ask questions, and let us support you in the timing that feels right for you.

Pitocin (Oxytocin)

Sometimes, once your cervix is ready, we'll start Pitocin to create or strengthen contractions. Our goal is to get them to be **2–3 minutes apart** and for your uterus to **palpate moderate.**

What it feels like:

Contractions will become more regular and intense. Don't be surprised if they come faster than natural labor — we adjust your dose carefully to balance comfort and progress.

> **Nurse's Tip:** Don't hesitate to ask for breaks or adjustments – you *have a say* in your induction process and we will discuss pros and cons of your particular situation. We'll titrate your Pitocin based on how you and your baby respond. I dedicate a whole chapter to Pitocin because I want you to become friends with it.

Know Your Options: Induction Methods at a Glance

Method	How It Works	Pros	Cons
Cytotec (Misoprostol)	Small tablet placed near cervix or taken orally/ buccally to soften and open it.	· Works well when cervix is not ready · May start contractions naturally	· Can't be removed once given · May cause too-frequent contractions · Requires close monitoring
Cervidil (Dinoprostone)	Thin strip placed in vagina that releases medication over several hours.	· Gentle ripening · Can be removed if not tolerated · May help labor start naturally	· Slower to work (up to 12 hours) · May cause mild cramping without progress
Foley Balloon / Cook Catheter	Balloon gently inflated inside cervix to apply pressure and stretch it open.	· Works quickly for many · No medication if used standalone · Low risk of overstimulation	· Insertion can be uncomfortable · Causes pressure or cramping · May fall out early
Pitocin/ (Oxytocin)	IV medication that mimics natural labor hormone to trigger contractions.	· Can start, stop, or adjust easily · Provides controlled, measurable progress · Works quickly once cervix is ready	· Can cause strong, frequent contractions · Requires continuous monitoring · May lead to fatigue or earlier pain relief needs

> **Nurse's Tip:** Your body – and your baby – will guide us in choosing the best method. The goal isn't to rush labor, but to help it happen safely, effectively, and at the right pace for you.

Compassion Note: No two inductions feel the same. Be patient with yourself — progress isn't always fast, but it's always moving toward one incredible moment: meeting your baby.

Coping During Induction: The Waiting Game

If you're being induced, you're signing up for one of the hardest parts of labor — the **hurry up and wait.**
There's nothing instant about an induction.

Some women progress within a few hours; for others, it's a marathon that takes days. The pace depends on your body, your baby, and how your cervix decides to cooperate (or not).

It can be frustrating — you're at the hospital, you're hooked to monitors, but nothing seems to be happening yet.

Trust me, **it is.**
Your body is quietly doing the work of softening, stretching, and getting ready for what's next.

Compassion Note: Inductions can test your patience, but remember — this is still labor, even if it's not happening at lightning speed. You're doing exactly what you need to do. Slow progress is still progress.

Nurse's Note

Bring a simple board game to play with your support person while you're waiting in early labor or during induction. My husband and I love **checkers** – it's easy, almost mindless, and a perfect distraction when the hours feel slow.

Keeping your mind engaged on something light can help the time pass, lower stress, and make those early hours feel a little less like waiting and a little more like being together.

Mind-Body Tips for the Long Wait

Sleep whenever you can.
You'll thank me and yourself later when it's time to push.

Eat before you're told you can't.
Once your cervix starts changing or if you get an epidural, you may be NPO or clear fluids only.

Bring comfort items.
Your pillow, blanket from home, sound machine, or soft lighting can make the room feel calm and cozy.

Move if allowed.
Use the birthing ball, sway, stretch, or walk the halls if your monitors are wireless.

Distract yourself.
Shows, music, games, scrolling — anything that keeps you from staring at the monitor.

Nurse's Tip: Don't obsess over your contraction pattern or dilation number. We'll tell you when it matters. Stay relaxed, hydrated, and calm — tension slows progress.

Understanding the Stages: Early Labor vs. Active Labor

Before we talk about how to manage labor, it helps to know what kind of labor you're actually in. Every birth journey begins in early labor and transitions into active labor — but they feel very different.

Labor Stages at a Glance

Stage	What's Happening	Cervical Dilation	Contractions	What You'll Feel/ Do
Early Labor	Your cervix is softening and thinning, starting to open. Your body is warming up for the main event.	**0–6 cm**	Irregular, 30–45 sec long, 5–10 min apart	You can usually talk through them. Walk, rest, hydrate, and breathe. This phase can last hours or even days.
Active Labor	Your cervix is actively dilating and the baby begins to descend. This is when things get serious.	**6–10 cm**	Strong, 45–90 sec long, 2–4 min apart	Breathing through contractions becomes harder. You'll need focus, support, and pain relief – natural or medical.

Nurse's Tip: You'll know you're moving into active labor when contractions demand your full attention – you can't talk, joke, or scroll between them anymore. That's your cue that baby's on the way and it's time to head in or let your nurse know things are changing fast. Part of active labor includes the transition period.

Compassion Note: It's not a race — every body has its own rhythm. Some labor slowly and steady; others move from zero to baby in hours. What matters most is progress and safety, not speed.

When Induction Turns Into Active Labor

After hours (and sometimes days) of slow, steady progress, your body eventually decides it's ready. The ripening is done, your cervix is opening, and those early contractions shift into **the real deal**.

This is when everything becomes more intense — and your nurse may say:

"Okay, we're getting somewhere now!"

Your contractions will become:

- stronger
- longer
- closer together

You might begin needing to breathe deeply through each one, squeeze your partner's hand, or focus inward as your labor becomes active and powerful.

How We Know You've Transitioned

Your cervix is dilating beyond 6 centimeters and thinning rapidly.
Your contractions are regular, usually every 2–4 minutes, lasting 60–90 seconds.
You may feel pelvic pressure, back pain, or the urge to bear down.
Your baby's heart rate stays steady, showing they're tolerating labor well.

> **Nurse's Tip:** There's also an emotional shift that tells us you're in active labor. The laughter fades, the small talk stops, and you start closing your eyes and breathing with purpose. That's your body focusing - and it's a beautiful thing to witness.

What to Expect Next

Once you've hit active labor, your nurse will:

- Reassess your pain management plan — whether that means an epidural, IV medication, or continued natural coping.
- Adjust Pitocin levels if you're on it, to keep contractions productive but safe.
- Keep a close eye on fetal heart tones and your comfort.
- Encourage you to change positions if possible, to keep your baby descending.

Compassion Note: This is the turning point where all your patience pays off. The waiting, the softening, the endless cervical checks — they've all led to this. You're in it now and every wave brings you closer to the moment you'll finally meet your baby.

Active Labor

Whether your labor began on its own or we gave things a little nudge with an induction, the great news is this: your body is responding exactly as it should for childbirth. Do you believe that out of all the brilliant minds and research out there, no one knows exactly what causes labor to begin naturally? The truth is, we don't. Labor is the result of many systems lining up — hormonal, inflammatory, mechanical, fetal, and maternal — all coming together when the time is right.

Some women are lucky enough, that they just show up in labor by themselves. I'm always in awe of patients who come in full-blown, rip-roaring labor. I had to be induced with all three of my babies, so I know what it's like when your body doesn't "understand the assignment." Some women's bodies just get it — they start the process all on their own, perfectly timed, like nature's clockwork.

So What Happens When You Walk In Already in Active Labor?

Us nurses — we move quickly.

- First things first, we'll check your cervix.
- If you want an epidural, tell us right away. We'll need to draw blood to check your platelets to make sure it's safe.
- We'll start an IV and get fluids running to maintain your volume and blood pressure.

The admission process happens at lightning speed — charting, questions, consents — all at once, while we keep our focus on you and your baby.

We want to meet your needs, but sometimes your baby dictates the timing. And yes, we know you're in pain — and we want to get you comfortable as soon as possible.

Pain Management Considerations

- **If you're planning to use IV pain medication:**
  For your safety, you may need to stay in bed for a while. Narcotics can make you dizzy or lightheaded and I'd rather have you safe than slipping out of bed.
- **If you're planning a non-medicated birth:**
  I might be starting your IV while you're standing, swaying, or leaning over the bed — whatever position feels right to you. I'll ask only the questions I have to ask and keep unnecessary charting for later. When you're in that kind of pain, you need presence, not paperwork.

> **Nurse's Tip:** If you find yourself with a nurse who's too focused on the computer instead of you, it's okay to speak up – kindly but directly. This is your moment. You have every right to ask for care that feels focused, calm, and compassionate.
>
> At my facility, we don't put strict limits on when you can get an epidural. If you can sit safely and hold still, it can be done. In the meantime, your best tools are your breath, your nurse, and your belief that you were made for this.

Compassion Note: Through it all, remember — this is your story, your birth, your moment. The nurse by your side should be the one who honors that and helps create the experience you deserve.

When Labor Needs a Little Boost – Understanding Labor Augmentation

Sometimes, even when labor starts on its own, it doesn't always keep up the momentum. You may have made great progress early on — contractions strong and regular — and then suddenly, things just... stall.

That's when we talk about **augmentation of labor** or giving your body a gentle push to get things moving again.

What Augmentation Means

Augmentation simply means **enhancing labor that's already started.** Your uterus is contracting, but maybe not often or strong enough to keep making cervical change.

It's not failure.
It's not your fault.
It's just a little help to get back into rhythm.

How We Help Things Along

Here's how we support your labor:

Pitocin (Oxytocin)
Given through your IV and adjusted slowly until contractions become regular and effective. The dose can go up, down, or stop depending on how you and baby respond.

Amniotomy (Breaking Your Water)
If your membranes are intact, your provider may rupture them to help the baby's head apply more pressure on your cervix and encourage dilation. (Page back to my tips regarding this!)

Position Changes & Movement
Upright positions, leaning, squatting, birthing balls, side-lying — all help your baby rotate and descend.

Pain Management Options
If exhaustion, tension, or anxiety are slowing labor, an epidural or IV medication can relax your body and help labor progress more efficiently.

> **Nurse's Tip:** Think of augmentation as teamwork – your uterus is the drummer and Pitocin is just helping it find its beat again. You're still doing the work; we're just helping the rhythm stay steady.

Augmentation is Just Induction - Midway

If you're reading this after our section on Induction of Labor, you might notice some similarities — and that's on purpose!

Augmentation = Induction… but AFTER labor has already started.

We use the *same tools*, the *same medications*, and the *same strategies* — we're just joining your body mid-process instead of starting from step one.

If you want the deeper explanations again, just flip back to the Induction section — everything aligns perfectly.

What You Might Feel

Once augmentation begins, contractions may feel stronger or closer together. You might notice less rest time in between — which can be tough, especially if you've been laboring for hours already. That's why communication matters: **tell your nurse what you're feeling.** We can adjust doses, change positions, or help you breathe through the intensity.

Compassion Note: Needing help to progress does *not* mean you're doing anything wrong. Labor is unpredictable — sometimes it just needs a little encouragement. What matters most is the end goal: **a safe delivery and a healthy mom and baby.**

Reasons for Augmentation: Why Labor Sometimes Needs a Boost

Labor isn't always a straight line — sometimes it slows down or stalls, and we have to help it find its rhythm again.
Here are the most common reasons your nurse or provider may suggest augmentation of labor:

1. Uterine Fatigue

Your uterus is a muscle — and like any muscle, it can tire out. After hours of contractions, it might start losing strength or pattern, which makes progress slow or stop.

Pitocin helps re-establish a strong, consistent rhythm.

2. Epidural Effect

Epidurals are wonderful for pain relief, but the relaxation they bring can sometimes slow contractions.
When your body relaxes completely, your uterus might "take a break" too.

A small dose of Pitocin can balance that relaxation with steady progress.

> **Nurse's Tip:** For some woman, you might notice your contractions spacing out after your epidural, don't worry – we can safely encourage them to return without compromising your comfort.

Word to the Wise:
In my practice, I don't often see epidurals slowing labor or stopping contractions — that's a common fear, but it's not usually the reality. If

you're getting uncomfortable, don't be afraid to ask for the epidural or another form of pain management.

Your uterus will keep doing its job or we will help it! You deserve to be as comfortable as you want to be while it does.

3. Fetal Position

If your baby is:

- sunny-side up
- not well-aligned
- tilted in the pelvis

...progress can stall.

Often, changing your position can help baby rotate:

- Hands-and-knees
- Side-lying with pillow support
- Peanut ball
- Throne or upright positions

If baby still doesn't rotate, Pitocin or breaking your water may be needed to increase pressure and aid rotation.

4. Dehydration or Exhaustion

Labor takes *energy*.

If you've been going for hours without enough fluids or rest, your contractions can weaken.
IV fluids or light nourishment (if allowed) can help — but sometimes Pitocin provides the boost your uterus needs to keep labor moving.

5. Ruptured Membranes Without Progress

If your water breaks but contractions:

- don't start
- start and then fizzle
- aren't strong enough to make cervical change

...we need to help things along.
Once membranes rupture, the risk of infection slowly rises over time.

Pitocin or another method may be started to safely initiate or strengthen contractions.

Compassion Note: Needing help to keep labor progressing doesn't mean your body is failing — it means your care team is working *with* your body to get you and your baby safely to the finish line.

13

Pitocin Is Not a Bad Word!

"When your uterus needs a motivational speech."

For many women, the word *Pitocin* sparks instant anxiety. Maybe you've heard stories of contractions coming on too strong, too fast, or too painfully. Maybe you've read posts online warning you to "avoid it at all costs." I understand that fear — I've seen it in countless patients' eyes as they ask:

"Do I *have* to get Pitocin?"

Here's the truth: **Pitocin isn't the enemy of natural birth.**
When used safely, carefully, and with constant monitoring, it's one of our best allies in helping you and your baby have a healthy, successful delivery.

Like any tool, it's all about **how, when, and why** we use it.

What Pitocin Really Is

Pitocin is the synthetic version of **oxytocin**, the same hormone your body naturally produces to cause contractions and create that powerful bond between you and your baby after birth.

Think of it as **a gentle reinforcement** of what your body is already trying to do — not a replacement for it.

> **Nurse's Tip:** You already have oxytocin flowing through your veins. Pitocin simply gives your uterus a little encouragement when it needs a boost.

When We Use Pitocin during Labor

We use Pitocin in two main scenarios:

Induction of Labor

When we help your body start labor that hasn't begun on its own because:

- You're past your due date (usually beyond 41 weeks)
- You have high blood pressure or pre-eclampsia
- You have gestational diabetes
- There are concerns about your baby's growth or well-being
- Your water broke but contractions haven't started

Augmentation of Labor

When labor begins naturally but slows down or stalls.

- Contractions space out or weaken
- The cervix stops dilating
- You're exhausted and need help regaining momentum

Compassion Note: Needing Pitocin doesn't mean you're failing.
It means your body just needs **a little teamwork** to get the job done.

How It Works

Pitocin is given through your IV and **carefully titrated** (adjusted) by your nurse.

We start at a **low dose** and increase it *slowly*, watching how your body and baby respond every step of the way.

Our goal is to **mimic the pattern of natural labor**:

✓ steady
✓ coordinated
✓ effective

...contractions that open your cervix **without stressing your baby**.

> **Nurse's Tip:** Think of Pitocin like a **dimmer switch**, not an on/off button.
> We raise the light gently – never flip it to full brightness all at once.

Safety and Monitoring

Because Pitocin affects your uterus and your baby, you'll be on **continuous monitoring** during use.

Two belts track you and your baby:

US (Ultrasound Transducer)

Monitors your baby's heartbeat.

TOCO (Tocodynamometer)

Tracks the timing and spacing of your contractions.

If readings are unclear or baby keeps wiggling away, we may place internal monitors:

- **Fetal Scalp Electrode (FSE)**
- **Intrauterine Pressure Catheter (IUPC)**

These give us a clearer picture.

My Role as Your Nurse

I watch the screen…
…but more importantly —

I watch YOU.

Your:

- comfort
- breathing
- body language
- facial expressions

…tell me just as much as the monitor does.

Pitocin Management: You're Still in Control

Even though we're the ones administering Pitocin, **you still have a voice** in how it's managed. Pitocin isn't a one-size-fits-all medication — every woman responds differently, and your comfort and preferences matter.

If you ever feel like your contractions are getting too intense, or you want to slow things down, **tell us.**
We can:

adjust the dosage
hold steady
or even turn it off entirely

Likewise, if you're ready for things to move a little faster, we can increase it — always in **small, careful increments**, and always with **your consent** and **our provider's order**.

Nurse's Tip

Our goal with Pitocin is simple:

Steady, effective contractions –
not a nonstop marathon.

We aim for:

- contractions every **2–3 minutes**
- your uterus to feel **moderately firm** when we palpate it

That tells us your body is responding the way we want it to.

What we *don't* want is **tachysystole** (too many contractions, too close together), because that can stress both you and your baby. So, we'll adjust the Pitocin up or down to keep things **safe, controlled, and productive.**

Here's a Pitocin Visual

Think of Pitocin like the **volume knob on a radio** —
we can turn it up or down...

...but **you** get to decide which level feels right.

We'll always explain the **risks and benefits** before making any change. Some women planning an unmedicated birth prefer **slower, gentler** progress rather than fast intensity — and that's completely valid. We honor your plan as long as it's safe for you and your baby.

Pitocin & Pain: Why Induced Labor Can Feel Different

Pitocin is an amazing medication for helping labor progress, but it can change how your body experiences contractions — and that's why some people feel that induced labor is more intense.

Natural Labor: Your Body Builds Up Slowly

During natural labor, your body increases contraction strength **gradually**. Because the intensity rises in small steps, your brain has time to adjust. Your pain threshold adapts little by little and many people tolerate this slow, natural climb surprisingly well.

Induced Labor: Your Body Didn't Start the Process

When we use Pitocin, **your uterus responds faster than your brain does.** Your contraction pattern may strengthen more quickly than your body can naturally "catch up," which can make the pain feel more sudden or overwhelming.

It's not that Pitocin creates "worse pain" — it's that your nervous system didn't get the warm-up it usually gets in natural labor.

The Good News: We Start Low and Go Slow

We begin Pitocin at **very low doses** and increase it **gradually.**
This gives:

- your uterus time to respond,
- your pain threshold time to adjust,
- and you time to stay in control of the process.

Remember: *You Are in Control*

If you need to pause, slow down, reposition, breathe, or request an epidural, you absolutely can.
Your comfort matters just as much as your progress.

And we are right beside you—supporting, monitoring, and adjusting every step of the way.

Compassion Note: You are the center of your care.
Even when medication is involved, your comfort, consent, and instincts lead the way. We're here to **guide**, not rush.

Pitocin Myths vs. Facts

There's a lot of confusion (and anxiety) about Pitocin. Let's clear up some of the biggest misconceptions so you can make informed choices with confidence.

Myth	Fact
"Pitocin makes labor unnaturally painful."	Pitocin can make contractions stronger and closer together, but pain perception varies. With good coaching, position changes, and pain relief options, many women tolerate it well.
"If I get Pitocin, I'll definitely need an epidural."	Not necessarily. Some women labor comfortably without an epidural on Pitocin, especially when doses are increased slowly. Pain management is always your choice.

Myth	Fact
"Pitocin means I'll end up with a C-section."	False. Pitocin is actually used to **avoid C-sections** by restarting stalled labors. Careful monitoring keeps you and your baby safe.
"Once Pitocin starts, I can't stop it."	You're always in control. We can turn Pitocin **down or off** at any time if contractions are too strong, too frequent, or if you just need a break. Just have a discussion with your provider.
"Pitocin is dangerous for my baby."	Pitocin is one of the **most commonly used and well-studied medications** in obstetrics. When monitored properly, it's very safe. Nurses watch both you and your baby closely throughout.

Nurse's Tip

Don't let Pitocin scare you – let it work **with** you.
Labor is a team effort between **your body, your care team, and your baby**.
We'll adjust every step together.

Compassion Note

Every birth plan looks different and that's okay.
Whether your contractions start naturally or with a little help, the goal is the same: **a safe delivery and a healthy mom and baby.**

When Pitocin Isn't Working

Every uterus is different. Sometimes, despite good contractions, the cervix just doesn't budge.
When that happens, we pause and reassess:

Check your baby's position.
Sometimes the baby's head is tilted or facing the wrong way, keeping pressure off your cervix.
Position changes or a peanut ball can help rotate them.

Evaluate contraction strength.
With an IUPC, we measure exactly how strong your contractions are — not just how they look on the TOCO.

Hydrate and rest.
Dehydration and fatigue can make the uterus sluggish. Fluids, food (if allowed), or even a nap can help.

Reassess progress.
Your provider may perform a cervical check to understand why dilation has paused — baby's position, cervix shape, or pelvic factors may all play a role.

Reset and Restart
We call this a **Pit break**, but really, it's your body's intermission.

After resting:

Your contractions may return on their own
Or when we restart Pitocin, your body responds better
Progress resumes without being forced

It's not about pushing your uterus — it's about **finding the rhythm** that works for you and your baby.

Nurse's Tip
Labor isn't a math equation.
If Pitocin has been running for hours without much progress, it doesn't mean it failed –
it means **we listen to your body and change the plan**, not force it.

Nurse's Note: How Tums Can Help Strengthen Contractions

You might be surprised to hear your nurse suggest **Tums** when your contractions aren't quite strong enough — but there's real physiology behind it.

Tums is **calcium carbonate** and calcium is a key ingredient your uterus uses to contract.
Every time your uterus tightens, it's pulling calcium into the muscle cells to create that contraction.

So when contractions are:

- too weak
- too irregular
- or not quite effective enough

a small dose of calcium from Tums can sometimes give your uterus a little extra boost to help those contractions become more coordinated and productive.

This is especially true if you're on **Pitocin**, because Pitocin works by opening the calcium channels in your uterine muscle.
More available calcium → more efficient contractions.

It's not a magic trick and it doesn't replace medication — but it's a simple, safe tool we sometimes use to support the contraction pattern your body is already trying to create.

In short: *Tums can help "fuel" your uterus by providing extra calcium, making contractions a little stronger and more effective.*

When a Change in Plan Is Needed

If your cervix remains unchanged despite strong, regular contractions and baby's position looks good, your provider may start talking about a

C-section. This doesn't mean you "couldn't labor" — it means your team is making the safest call for you and your baby.

Compassion Note: I know how disappointing it can be when labor doesn't go as planned, especially when you've worked so hard. But remember — your strength doesn't depend on **how** you deliver, only that you did everything you could to bring your baby safely into the world.

A Nurse's Perspective

In my years at the bedside, I've seen Pitocin bring countless babies into the world and also save countless lives. I've also seen fear hold women back from understanding what it really is: **a tool, not a punishment**. The difference isn't in the medication — it's in:

- how it's used
- how it's explained
- and how closely it's watched

My job isn't just to hang the bag and push a button.
It's to **guide you, advocate for you, and make sure Pitocin serves *you* — not the other way around.**

Closing Thoughts: From Fear to Empowerment

You don't have to fear Pitocin. You just need to understand it.
When used carefully and collaboratively, it's one of the most effective ways to help your body do what it's already trying to do — bring your baby into the world safely.

You are the author of your story, not the medication in your IV.
Whether your contractions begin naturally or with a little help, your strength, your courage, and your love make this birth **your own**.

14

TRANSITION: The Hardest Part Before the Best Moment

"It is when we are in transition that we are most completely alive."

– William Bridges

Transition is the most powerful, intense, emotionally charged phase of labor — and also the shortest. It is the moment when your body shifts from opening your cervix to bringing your baby down. Transition is often described as the "breaking point," but the truth is far more empowering: it's the moment right before everything changes.

When women reach transition, they often say the same things, look the same way, and behave in the same patterns — not because they're failing, but because their body is doing exactly what it's supposed to do. **Transition is not a sign that something is wrong. It's a sign that you are so close to meeting your baby.**

Below is everything you need to know about this incredible part of labor.

What Transition Really Is (Clinically Speaking)

Transition is the final phase of the first stage of labor. It typically occurs between:

- **7 cm and 10 cm dilation**
- As the cervix completes its final thinning and opening
- As baby descends deeper into the pelvis
- As hormones surge rapidly

During transition, the uterus becomes incredibly efficient and powerful. Contractions often:

- come closer together
- last longer
- peak stronger
- and feel overwhelmingly intense

This is not a sign of distress — it is the hallmark of a body doing its greatest work.

What It Feels Like

Every mother describes it differently, but common themes include:

- **Overwhelming pressure**
  Deep, heavy, rectal pressure as baby descends.
- **Very strong contractions**
  More intense than earlier phases.
- **Shaking or trembling**
  Hormonal surges mimic cold chills.
- **Nausea or vomiting**
  Adrenaline often causes sudden queasiness.

- **Feeling hot or cold suddenly**
  Temperature swings are completely normal.
- **Feeling emotional or panicked**
  Crying, yelling, or withdrawing are all signs you're in transition.
- **Feeling the urge to push**
  Sometimes before you're fully dilated.

Transition feels like a storm — intense, consuming, but short-lived.

Why Women Say "I Can't Do This Anymore"

This phrase is so common in transition that nurses often smile knowingly when we hear it, because it tells us everything we need to know:

You're close.
Your body is shifting.
You're almost at 10 cm.

This phrase is not a sign of weakness — it's a sign that your hormones are peaking exactly as they should.
You are not quitting. You are transitioning.

The Hormone Surge: Nature's Design

During transition, your body releases a massive wave of:

- **Adrenaline**
- **Oxytocin**
- **Endorphins**

This surge makes your contractions stronger and your urge to push more intense. It also increases emotional sensitivity — which means even tiny sensations or noises can feel overwhelming.

But here's the beautiful part:

This is your body preparing you to push.
This is your body mobilizing strength you didn't know you had.
This is the final gateway before birth.

What Nurses See During Transition

As nurses, we watch for signs that tell us a mother is entering this phase — even before she says a word:

- shaking legs
- difficulty focusing
- saying **"I need something for the pain"**
- sudden irritability or fear
- loud vocalizations
- vomiting
- sweating
- gripping the bed rails or partner
- asking for help repeatedly
- withdrawing inward and becoming quiet

These are all normal. These are all expected. These are all signs your body is doing something extraordinary.

How to Cope With Transition

Transition is intense, but it is survivable. Mothers do it every single day. And **you** will too.

Here's what helps:

1. **Low, deep breathing**
   Helps regulate your autonomic nervous system.

2. **Moaning instead of yelling**
   Low tones keep your body open; high tones create tension.
3. **Counterpressure on your back or hips**
   A partner or nurse can help stabilize you.
4. **Changing positions**
   Hands-and-knees, side-lying, leaning over the bed, birthing ball.
5. **Closing your eyes**
   Helps block visual stimuli and calm your mind.
6. **Repeating grounding phrases**
   "One contraction at a time."
   "I can do anything for 60 seconds."
   "My body knows what to do."
7. **Trusting your nurse**
   We guide your breathing, offer support, hold you steady, and help you stay grounded.

Transition With an Epidural

Even with an epidural, many women still notice:

- pressure
- shaking
- nausea
- emotional swings
- the urge to push

An epidural doesn't stop the hormonal process — it simply reduces the sharpness of the pain.

Your body still transitions because your baby is still descending.

When Transition Ends

Transition ends when:

- your cervix reaches **10 cm**
- your baby settles lower into the pelvis
- your urge to push becomes unavoidable

You may feel a sudden shift — like your body is switching gears.

Many moms say:

"Everything changed."
"I finally felt like I could do it."
"The pressure replaced the pain."

Transition may feel like the hardest part, but it is usually the shortest. Once it's over, your body is ready to push — and meet your baby.

Nurse's Note: You Are Stronger Than This Moment

Transition can make even the calmest women feel overwhelmed, frightened, or out of control.
That is normal. That is expected. That is biological.

What you may not realize is that from the outside, **you look powerful.**
You look focused.
You look like a woman doing the greatest work of her life.

You may feel like you're falling apart.
But **we see you — and you are incredible.**

Final Thoughts: Transition Is a Transformation

Transition isn't just a phase of labor — **it's a threshold.**
You enter as one version of yourself and emerge ready to bring your baby into the world.

It is the most intense, most raw, most primal part of the journey. But it is also the proof that you are close to the moment you've been waiting for.

You are not breaking.
You are not failing.
You are becoming.

The storm of transition is temporary. But the strength you discover in yourself during this phase will last a lifetime.

15

The Final Stretch: Understanding the Pushing Stage

"The moment when you want to quit, is the moment you need to keep pushing."

– Unknown

I take a lot of pride in being able to read my patients and adapt to what they need in the moment. By nature, I'm an enthusiastic, high-energy nurse — the kind who can easily turn into your personal cheerleader/motivator when the time comes.

When it's time to push, I'm not the type of nurse who simply counts for you. Honestly, I find that approach a bit mechanical. Instead, I focus on encouraging you through every push, keeping you motivated, and helping you channel your strength.

You'll probably hear me cheering you on with phrases like:

"Go, go, go — **that's it!**"
"**Right there**, that's the push!"
"**You're about to meet your baby!**"

"Get mad! You've got this!"
"I'm so proud of you!"

And I mean every word of it. Sometimes my energy spills out into the whole unit — because that moment, when you're giving everything you have to bring your baby into the world, is electric. My job is to help you feel powerful, supported, and unstoppable, because that is what you are. **Manifest it!**

The Energy Shift: Champion or Calm Anchor

But I can also be the nurse who brings calm and comfort when that's what you need. Sometimes that means:

dimming the lights
softly scented lavender
quiet voices
grounding presence

The energy shifts — it's steady, peaceful, and empowering in a different way. Whether I'm your biggest cheerleader or your quiet anchor, my goal is always the same:

To help you feel safe, supported, and completely in control as you bring your baby into the world.

In between pushes, I'll give you gentle feedback and encouragement — letting you know what's working well and guiding you if something needs adjusting. Please take this as loving, constructive coaching, not criticism. We are on the same team, working toward the same goal: **safely bringing your baby into the world.** One push at a time, we'll get there.

A Lesson From a Patient: Reading Beyond the Surface

I once had an experience helping a fellow nurse with her patient. Before pushing began, the patient seemed fired up — energized, motivated, ready to go. She was cheering herself on, almost gearing up like an athlete. My colleague immediately matched that energy, jumping in with high enthusiasm.

When I entered the room, I sensed something different beneath her intensity:
She wasn't confident — **she was terrified.**

Her excitement was a mask for uncertainty. What she truly needed wasn't hype; she needed:

calm
grounding
reassurance
steady guidance

She needed someone to slow the pace, soften the room, and help her feel safe.

That moment taught me something important:

Every woman in labor needs a different kind of nurse.

Your Role: Choosing the Energy You Need

Your next job is to figure out what kind of nurse you want supporting your birth experience.

Do you want someone:

high-energy, vocal, motivating, loud-with-love
or
calm, quiet, steady, grounding, centered

Neither option is wrong.
Only **you** know what makes you feel safe, empowered, and in control.

If You Need Something Different – Speak Up

If the nurse in the room isn't matching what you need, it's okay to speak up — or have your partner do it for you.

This does *not* need to be confrontational. Small changes shift the entire energy:

Your partner can start speaking softly → the nurse will naturally mirror that tone.
You can say:
"Could we keep things a little quieter right now?"
or
"I focus better with softer encouragement."

As nurses, we want to serve you. A simple request helps us show up in the way that honors your experience.

Remember: This Is Your Birth

Your birth.
Your moment.
Your story.

We are the guests at your party.
You get to decide how your party feels.

And any nurse worth her salt will adapt to the energy *you* need — not the other way around.

Ways to Speak Up – Respectfully and Effectively

You can express your needs without feeling uncomfortable or "difficult." Here are some gentle, powerful ways to communicate during labor:

- **"I do better with quieter encouragement during contractions."**
- **"Could we keep the lights a little lower, please?"**
- **"Can we take a minute to slow down? I need to catch my breath."**
- **"I'd like my partner to answer questions for me while I focus on pushing."**
- **"I'm feeling overwhelmed — can we talk through what's happening?"**

These small statements can completely shift the tone of the room.
You're not just participating in your birth — you're leading it.

When You Don't Feel Comfortable Speaking Up

If you're too tired, emotional, or deep in labor to advocate for yourself, this is where your support person becomes your voice.

Before labor, talk with them about:

- what calms you
- what overwhelms you
- what kind of energy you prefer
- how you cope under pressure

Give them permission to speak gently but firmly on your behalf.

> **Nurse's Tip:**
>
> Sometimes it's not what's said – it's *how* it's said.
> If your partner naturally starts speaking in a calm, soft tone, it can quietly reset the whole room. Your nurse will take that cue and shift the energy to meet your needs.

Advocating for yourself doesn't mean questioning your care — it means partnering in it. You deserve a birth experience that feels safe, respectful, and centered around you.

When Not to Push – and What to Do Instead

It's completely natural to feel a strong urge to push before it's actually time. That urge is a sign your baby is descending and your body is gearing up — but sometimes pushing too soon can cause more harm than help.

When We Ask You Not to Push

Your nurse or provider may ask you to breathe through contractions instead of pushing when:

- **You're not fully dilated yet (not at 10 cm).**
  Pushing too early can cause cervical swelling and slow things down.
- **Your baby needs more time to rotate or descend.**
  Sometimes they're still finding the right position.
- **The provider isn't in the room yet.**
  Babies come fast when they're ready, and sometimes we need 30–60 seconds to assemble the team.
- **Your baby needs a moment to recover.**
  If we see a dip in the heart rate, holding off helps baby catch their breath.

What to Do Instead of Pushing

When we tell you not to push, it's not about control — it's about keeping you and your baby safe.

Here's how to manage that intense, overwhelming urge:

1. Pant Like You're Blowing Out Candles

Short, fast breaths — in through your nose, out like you're blowing on a birthday cake.
This technique overrides the pushing reflex.

2. Focus on Breath, Not the Contraction

Channel all your energy into breathing patterns.
This gives your mind a job and helps your body stay relaxed.

3. Change Positions

If possible, move to:

- hands-and-knees
- side-lying
- leaning over the bed

These positions reduce pressure on your cervix.

4. Use Your Support Person

Have them:

- count with you
- guide your breathing
- hold your hand
- stay close and steady

That grounding presence helps keep your focus away from pushing.

Nurse's Tip

Not pushing when your body is screaming to push is *one of the hardest things you will ever do.*
I experienced this with my last son, Cooper. I went from 3 cm to 10 cm in an hour after they broke my water. He was determined to make his entrance loud and proud – **fast, furious, and full of fire,** just like the **red-headed spark** he is. No pain meds, a full bearing-down urge, and a doctor still across town. I know exactly how impossible it can feel in that moment.

But those few minutes of patience protect:

- your cervix
- your pelvic floor
- your baby's descent
- the smoothness of your delivery

Once it's truly time, your body will take over – and we'll be right there guiding you safely and confidently.

Final Thought: Timing Is Power

Labor is not just about effort — it's about timing.
Sometimes the bravest thing you can do is *wait.*

Those few minutes of controlled breathing can make all the difference in how smoothly your baby enters the world.

You're not holding back —
you're protecting the beautiful work your body is doing.

When to Push

When the time finally comes to push, you'll *know* — sometimes because your nurse or provider tells you it's time and sometimes because your body simply takes over. For many women, this moment brings a mix of relief, intensity, and a sudden surge of energy. After hours of breathing, waiting, and holding back, your body is finally ready to *work with* your contractions instead of against them.

How You Know It's Time

When your cervix is completely dilated (10 cm) and your baby has descended low into the birth canal, a few telltale signs appear.

You may notice:

- **An overwhelming urge to bear down**, like you need to have a bowel movement.
- **Deep pelvic or rectal pressure**, sometimes extending into your lower back.
- **A shift in contraction rhythm**, where your body starts directing effort downward.
- **An instinctive, primal sensation** that says: *push.*

If you have an epidural, you may feel:

- more pressure than pain
- a heavy, stretching sensation
- your nurse cueing you to push by watching the monitor

Your nurse and provider will make sure everything is aligned — your cervix is ready, baby is in position, and the room is prepared for the moment you've worked toward.

If You Have an Epidural

With an epidural, the urge to push may feel muted or unclear — and that's okay.

Your nurse will:

- watch your contractions on the monitor or palpate your belly
- guide you through when to start pushing
- help position your legs, hips, and pelvis for the most effective pushing
- encourage you to push *with the pressure* even if you can't feel much

Some women feel very strong pressure. Some feel mild pressure. Some feel almost none. Every experience is normal.

Nurse's Tip:
Focus on quality, not quantity.
Three strong, effective pushes per contraction do far more than several quick, shallow ones.

Visualize pushing your baby *down and out*, even if you can't feel the exact pathway. Your body knows what to do.

When it's truly time to push, you'll find strength you didn't know you had. Every breath brings you closer to the moment your baby enters the world.

How Long Will I Have to Push?

This is one of the most common questions women ask — and the honest answer is: it varies.

Some moms deliver in a few pushes.
Some push for hours.
Both are normal.

Average Pushing Times

First-time moms (primigravidas):
30 minutes to 2 hours
Sometimes longer with an epidural.

Moms who've delivered before (multigravidas):
Often much faster — sometimes only a few contractions.

The biggest factor isn't the clock — it's the **progress**.
As long as baby is tolerating labor well and you're moving forward, we keep going.

Formal Guideline (ACOG)

ACOG's *First and Second Stage Labor Management* (2025) guideline defines **prolonged** pushing as:

- > **3 hours** of pushing for first-time moms
- > **2 hours** for moms who've given birth before ("ACOG Clinical Practice Guideline No. 8: First and Second Stage Labor Management: Correction," 2025)

But ACOG emphasizes *individualized care*. That means we consider:

- your energy level
- fetal status
- epidural use
- your baby's position

- pelvic anatomy
- overall progress

There is no "one rule" — there is *your* labor, and *your* pace.

What Affects Pushing Time

1. Epidural Use

May reduce sensation, making it harder to feel *where* to push.
Good coaching, positioning, and patience make a huge difference.

2. Baby's Position

A baby who is:

- sunny-side up
- tilted (asynclitic)
- high in the pelvis

…may take longer to maneuver down.

3. Maternal Fatigue

You've done a marathon's worth of work before pushing even begins. Hydration, rest breaks, position changes, and encouragement help conserve energy.

4. Pelvic Anatomy

Every pelvis is shaped differently — some allow fast descent, others require more time.

5. Contraction Strength

Consistent, strong contractions (natural or Pitocin-supported) help baby move through the birth canal efficiently.

When It Takes a Little Longer and What We Do to Help

Your care team has many safe, effective tools to help progress keep moving:

Position Changes

We may help you shift into positions that open your pelvis:

- Side-lying
- Hands-and-knees
- Exaggerated runner's lunge
- Squatting bar
- Peanut ball between your knees

Small changes can create big improvements.

Laboring Down

If you have an epidural and the baby isn't quite low enough, we might pause pushing and let your uterus continue doing the work naturally. Please be advised ACOG's recommendation is to start pushing once you reach 10 cm (2025).
Nonetheless, laboring down does potentially save energy and often leads to smoother pushing later.

Adjusting the Epidural

If the epidural is too strong, anesthesia can lighten it so you can better feel pressure and direction.

Hydration & Rest

A few sips of juice, a quick rest, or a brief "reset" can help your body regain strength and coordination.

Assisted Delivery (Vacuum or Forceps)

If:

- you've been pushing for a long time
- you're exhausted
- your baby needs to be born sooner due to heart rate changes

Your provider may recommend a vacuum or forceps to help guide your baby out safely.

This is not a failure — this is precision teamwork designed to protect both of you.

> **Nurse's Tip:** Don't watch the clock. Let us do that.
> You focus on the *next contraction*, not the next hour.
> Slow progress is still progress.

Your Pushing Journey Is Unique

Whether your pushing stage is:

- 20 minutes
- 2 hours
- somewhere in between

…it does **not** define your worth, your strength, or your success.

What matters is:

- you followed your body
- you trusted your team
- you stayed present
- you brought your baby safely into the world

And that is extraordinary.

When Pushing Doesn't Work as Planned

Sometimes, even with all the effort, encouragement, and perfect timing, pushing doesn't go exactly as expected. This can happen for many reasons — and **none** of them mean you've done anything wrong. Birth is fluid, dynamic, and deeply individual. Every baby and every body have their own timeline.

When progress slows, your nurse and provider will first look at *why* and then partner with you to adjust. Our goal is always the same: **a safe delivery and a healthy mom and baby.**

> **Nurse's Tip**
>
> If progress feels slow, please don't panic – this is exactly where patience, teamwork, and thoughtful adjustments make all the difference.
>
> We'll coach you, reposition you, support you, hydrate you, and make sure you understand every option on the table.
> You are **not** doing anything wrong.
> You are **not** failing.
> Your body and your baby are still working together.

Final Reassurance

Birth rarely follows a perfect script — and that is normal.
Detours don't take away from the beauty of your experience; they are simply part of your story.

No matter what adjustments we make along the way, the outcome remains the same:

A safe, supported, empowered delivery — and the moment you finally meet your baby.

16

THE ACT OF PUSHING: Working With Your Body to Bring Your Baby into the World

"The fruit derived from labor is the sweetest of all pleasures."

– Marquis de Vauvenargues

The act of pushing is one of the most powerful, instinctive, and transformative parts of childbirth. It is the moment your labor shifts from opening your cervix to guiding your baby down and out into the world. Even though it may feel overwhelming in the moment, pushing is something your body already knows how to do — and with the right support, you'll find your rhythm, your strength, and your confidence.

This chapter will walk you through everything you need to know about how pushing works, what it feels like, what we're looking for as nurses, and how we help you through the final steps of meeting your baby.

What Pushing Really Is (In Simple Terms)

Pushing is your uterus and your abdominal muscles working together:

- Your uterus tightens from the top down, pushing your baby lower.
- Your abdominal muscles help guide baby through the birth canal.
- Your pelvic floor opens and stretches to allow your baby to pass.
- Your baby helps, too — curling and rotating through the pelvis.

You and your baby are partners in this moment — each doing your part.

Pushing usually begins once your cervix reaches **10 centimeters** and your baby's head is low enough in your pelvis.

Positions / Styles for Pushing

There are different styles of pushing and what works best often depends on:

- your body
- your baby
- your provider
- your nurse
- your pain management

Some providers use **directed pushing**, where you're coached to:

- take a deep breath
- hold it
- push for a count of ten
- repeat three times per contraction

Others encourage **spontaneous pushing** (open-glottis pushing), where:

- you follow your body's natural urge

- you exhale or make sound
- you avoid breath-holding
- you push when your body cues you

There is **no single right way** — only the way that's effective and safe for you and your baby.

Trust your instincts.
Trust your nurse.
Your body truly knows what to do.

My Preferred Coaching Method

I personally prefer this method **first** to gauge your effort and correct any ineffectiveness.

The bed is usually at a **160 degree angle (low semi-fowlers)** — this gives the baby room to tuck under your pelvic bone.

Here is the technique exactly as I teach it:

🐴 My Horse Analogy (the one ALL my patients know!)

1. **Take a deep breath in — and HOLD it.**
2. **Chin to chest.**
3. **Relax your legs out like a frog.**
4. **Grab behind your legs in the knee-fold area.**
5. **Pull back HARD — like you're trying to stop a horse.**
    - Your legs are the reins.
    - If you don't pull back, the horse won't stop.
    - If the horse doesn't stop, you'll get hit by a car.
6. **Curl your whole body around your baby.**
7. **Bear down like you haven't had a bowel movement in 5 years.**

8. **Hold it until I say: "Release, release!"**
9. **Let all the air out.**
10. **Big deep breath — hold — push again.**

I like to get **three strong pushes per contraction**.

✓ Your **feet** should NOT push against me.
✓ Your **legs** should glide toward your head without resistance.
✓ You are **curling forward**, not pushing backward. Do **not** arch your back to pick your butt up!

And yes, my coworkers laugh every time I use the horse analogy — because I use it with every single patient. Why?
Because **it works**. It creates imagery strong enough that patients instantly understand the intensity required.

You are doing ALL the work.
There is a reason they call it *labor*.
It's hard — but you are capable.

Your nurse and support person will hold the weight of your legs (especially with an epidural). Your job is direction and power — we handle the rest.

Quick Recap (Without the Story)

- Deep breath in — **hold it**
- **Chin to chest**
- **Relax legs out**
- **Grab behind your knees**
- **Pull back hard**
- **Curl around your baby**
- **Bear down**

Repeat with each contraction.

No-Nonsense Coaching: Why I Correct Ineffective Pushing

I am also not the type of nurse that is going to allow you to push ineffectively. If your pushes are not effective, **I am going to tell you that.** No sugar coating here. I'm going to have you regroup and try again.

I don't do this to be harsh — I do it to **protect you and your energy**.
Pushing is HARD work.
Like really hard.

So allowing you to use all that energy in a way that isn't getting you anywhere?
That would be a disservice on my part.

And don't get frustrated — you *will* get the hang of it.
Sometimes your body knows exactly what to do and pushes for you.
Sometimes you have to be an active participant in the activity.

Below is a summary of different pushing positions and how each one helps you and your baby.

Pushing Positions: Finding What Works for *Your* Body

Semi-Reclining

Semi-reclining is one of my favorite ways to **start** because:

- It gives me a clear view of what your pushes look like
- I can easily gauge your effort
- I can see how your body and baby respond

But it's not the only way — and it's ***definitely*** **not** where you have to stay.

Side-Lying Pushing

You can push on either side, curling your body around your baby just like I guided you earlier.
The only difference:

You'll pull back **one leg instead of two.**

This is perfect for:

- moms with an epidural
- anyone needing variety
- helping rotate a baby who's tucked in an awkward position

Closed-Knee "Cannonball" Pushing

This position is more powerful than it looks:

- Tuck your knees inward (like doing a cannonball into the pool)
- Flare your ankles outward in a "V" shape

This opens your pelvis in a totally different direction.
Sometimes that small adjustment is exactly what baby needs to navigate the birth canal.

Another cannonball pushing technique I recently learned from a fellow nurse involves bringing the knees tightly to the chest and using a sheet for added leverage. With the knees drawn in, the sheet is crisscrossed around the legs, and one end is held in each hand. As you pull firmly on the sheet, it reinforces the cannonball position and helps maximize pushing effectiveness. I was impressed by how well this worked—proof that even after all these years, this "old girl" can still learn a new trick. It's one of the many reasons I wanted to write this book while I'm still actively practicing: the bedside never stops teaching you.

Nurse's Tip

As much as your support person wants to help, **having them pull your back up during pushing actually works against you.**
It takes away from the core power *you* generate.

Your support person can:

- hold a pillow behind your head
- give counterpressure
- help guide your legs
- cheer you on

But the pushing power?
That comes from **you** – and that's why women are the most extraordinary beings alive.

Tug-of-War Pushing

Yes… your nurse might be feisty (hi, that's me!).
And yes… we *may* break out tug-of-war pushing when you need a strong, focused technique.

Here's how it works:

1. We tie knots at each end of a sheet.
2. You hold one end; your nurse holds the other.
3. Feet in stirrups or secure on the bed.
4. When the contraction starts —
   You pull that sheet toward you with everything you've got
   Curl your body around your baby

It creates **a full-body push** and can be amazingly effective. This can also be done by tying it around the squat bar instead of your nurse being an active participant. I just personally think the other way is more fun.

The Truth

This technique is **hard work** — for both of us.
(But only *your* energy matters here.)

If tug-of-war isn't giving great results, we won't waste your strength. We'll switch positions so you can shine.

> **Nurse's Tip:**
>
> Have fun with it – treat it like a challenge.
> Try to "beat" your nurse.
>
> But whatever you do...
> **Do NOT let go of the sheet mid-pull.**
>
> Trust me – I love my job, but I do *not* want to go flying across the room.

Squatting

Most hospitals have a **squat bar** that attaches to the bed. Squatting uses **gravity** to your advantage and opens your pelvis beautifully.

During each contraction:

- You grip the bar
- Lean forward
- Bear down like you have to have a bowel movement
- Let your body work with you

If you have an epidural, mobility will determine whether squatting is safe. Sometimes we modify it with:

- supported squats
- semi-squat positions
- elevated throne positions
- partner- or nurse-supported holds

Safety always comes first — but if it's an option, **squatting can be incredibly effective**.

> **Tip:** Place a **peanut ball or pillow** between your knees to keep your hips open and help baby rotate into position.

Kneeling & Leaning Forward

Kneeling while leaning over:

- the back of the bed
- a birth ball
- pillows or the raised head of the bed

...can help relieve back pressure, increase pelvic space, and give you a sense of control.
This position is also wonderful for helping your baby rotate into a better alignment.

Hands and Knees

Hands-and-knees:

- takes pressure off your back
- eases back labor

- opens the pelvis
- helps babies rotate when they're sunny-side-up (occiput posterior)

> **Tip:** Rocking gently between contractions or shifting your hips can help your baby descend more effectively.

Upright Sitting or Supported Standing

Some moms prefer pushing while sitting upright or being partially supported in a standing position — especially if:

- mobility is limited
- they want gravity
- baby's position benefits from a vertical angle

> **Tip:** Even subtle changes – pelvic tilt, leg placement, hip lift – can make a big difference. But remember, safety first. If you have an epidural, make sure you are capable.

Finding What Works for *You*

Your nurse will help you explore:

- peanut ball positions
- squat bar
- birthing stool
- side-lying

- semi-reclined
- hands-and-knees

Even with an epidural, **you can still change positions safely** — movement is key.

Birth is dynamic, not static.
Together, we'll find the rhythm and position that helps your baby make their way into your arms.

> **Nurse's Tip: Ask for a Mirror**
>
> If you'd like to better understand what your body is doing during pushing, ask for a mirror. Being able to see your baby's progress can be incredibly motivating and helps many parents coordinate their pushes more effectively by visualizing the impact of each one.

Words to the Wise: Let It Happen

When it comes time to push, I want you to **give it everything you've got** — no holding back, no tightening up, no worrying about what your body might do.

Do not be afraid to poop.
I promise you, every nurse has seen it, every nurse expects it, and every nurse understands it. In fact, I always tell my patients:

"If you poop, I'm proud of you — it means you're using the right muscles."

That's how you know you're pushing effectively.
That's how you know your baby is coming down.
That's how you know you're doing it *exactly right.*

If you hold back because you're embarrassed or worried about what might happen on the bed, your pushes won't be as strong or as effective — and that can actually **prolong the process**.

So when the time comes:

Don't hold back.
Push with power.
Use every bit of instinct your body gives you.
Trust your nurse — we've got you.

What **happens** in the delivery room, **stays** in the delivery room! **You** focus on bringing your baby into the world.
We'll take care of the rest.

The Peek-a-Boo Pushing Game: Why Your Baby Moves Back and Forth

During pushing, your baby will play what I like to call the "peek-a-boo game." As you bear down with each contraction, your baby's head descends deeper into your pelvis and begins to appear — that's the exciting part! But when the contraction ends and you stop pushing, the baby often slides back a little. It can be frustrating, especially when you're working so hard and feel like you're losing progress, but I promise — this back-and-forth movement is completely normal.

Each push helps your baby rotate, mold, and stretch the tissues that need to open to make way for birth. The baby's head is designed to shift and flex, and your body is designed to gently expand — it's truly a team effort. Think of it as your baby slowly learning how to navigate through the birth canal, getting a little closer with every round.

The goal is to help your baby get underneath the pubic bone — that bony ridge in the front of your pelvis — because once the baby's head slips past it, things move quickly. That's when the baby tends to stay visible between pushes and you'll hear your nurse or provider say, **"We're almost there!"** That is when I get really excited for you and your partner!

This process can take minutes or hours, depending on your baby's position, your pelvic anatomy, your strength, and how effectively you're pushing. Slow progress isn't failure — it's your body doing the work safely and gradually. The tissue around your perineum (the area between your vagina and rectum) is stretching, softening, and making room for your baby. Rushing that process increases the chance of tearing, so even though it feels like a cruel game of back-and-forth, it's actually your body protecting you.

Nurse's Tip:

- When you feel frustrated by the "peek-a-boo," remind yourself: every push counts. Even when the baby slips back, progress is happening beneath the surface.
- Listen to your nurse's guidance on when and how to push - sometimes breathing through a contraction instead of pushing can help tissues stretch and prevent tearing.
- If you have an epidural, your nurse or provider may use position changes or a peanut ball to help the baby find the best path under the bone.

That moment when your baby finally stays visible — when they're crowning — is the turning point. Every second of that peek-a-boo dance was worth it, leading to the first time you'll see your baby's face.

Pushing Through Exhaustion

By the time you reach the pushing stage, you've likely endured:

- hours (or days) of contractions
- interrupted sleep
- adrenaline surges and drops
- physical and emotional fatigue

You're tired. Your muscles ache. You feel like you have nothing left.

But here is what I've seen again and again:

You always find a way.
Your strength in this moment is different — deeper, instinctive, primal.

When exhaustion overwhelms you, it becomes my job to help you dig deep:

- to refocus
- to breathe
- to rest between contractions
- to believe in yourself again

If I see you starting to hit that wall, I'll help you move your body, reset your breathing, or change up our plan so you don't waste an ounce of the strength you've worked so hard to hold onto. And sometimes, a quick sip of juice is just the little burst of energy you need to keep going.

What Helps When You're Running on Empty

1. Focus on one push at a time

Not 20.
Not an hour.
Just **this** one.

2. Use your breath

Deep cleansing breaths between contractions refill your tank.

3. Change positions

Sometimes switching from semi-reclined to side-lying unlocks progress.

4. Visualize

Picture your baby moving closer with every effort.

Visualization **fuels strength you didn't know you had.**

5. Lean on your team

Let us carry the mental load.
Let us encourage, guide, and anchor you.

> **Nurse's Tip:**
> It's okay to say, "I can't do this."
> I've heard it hundreds of times –
> and every single time, **that mom did it anyway.**
>
> **I** believe in you.
> **You were made to do this!**

If you've been pushing without progress, your provider may recommend:

- a short rest
- laboring down
- a position change
- vacuum or forceps assistance

These are **not failures** — they are tools to help your baby arrive safely.

And please remember:

Sip water, juice or ice chips whenever allowed.
Dehydration makes exhaustion much worse.

You may be exhausted, but you are not done.
There is a strength that awakens in this moment — a strength born of love, instinct, and determination.
You're closer than you think. You've got this.

Assisted Deliveries: When Your Baby Needs a Little Help

Sometimes, even after all your effort and determination, your baby might need just a little extra help making their entrance into the world. This doesn't mean you've failed or that anything is wrong — it simply means your baby has worked as hard as you have, and now it's time for the care team to step in and assist.

Assisted vaginal deliveries are common, safe, and often the bridge between long pushing efforts and a successful vaginal birth. Your provider will only use these methods when it's necessary — for example, if your baby's heart rate shows signs of stress or if you've been pushing for a long time without steady progress.

When an Episiotomy May Be Needed

An **episiotomy** is a small surgical cut made in the perineum (the skin between your vagina and rectum) to make more room for your baby during birth.

Years ago, episiotomies were routine.
Today, they are **rare** and only done when absolutely necessary.

Most women tear naturally — and **that is almost always easier to heal from** than a planned cut.

Here are the main reasons an episiotomy may be needed:

1. Baby Needs to Be Born Quickly

If your baby shows signs of distress at the very end of pushing — such as a dropping heart rate — your provider may need to speed up the delivery.
A **small, controlled** episiotomy can help the baby be born faster.

2. Shoulder Dystocia (Shoulders Stuck)

If the baby's head is born but the shoulders become stuck behind the pubic bone, this is an emergency.

An episiotomy creates more room so the provider can help release the shoulders safely.

3. Use of Forceps or Vacuum

(More on these tools coming next)

Sometimes an episiotomy may be done to:

- create more space
- reduce risk of uncontrolled tearing
- help guide baby out safely

It's not always required, but sometimes it's the safest option.

4. Certain Rare Anatomical Situations

If the tissues are extremely tight, swollen, or not stretching well — or if baby's position makes deep tearing likely — your provider may recommend a small episiotomy to protect the deeper pelvic floor muscles.

What an Episiotomy Does *NOT* Mean

It does **not** mean:

you pushed wrong
you're weak
your body failed
your birth is "less than"
future births will need it

Sometimes it's simply the safest, fastest path for you and your baby.

Do All Providers Do Them?

No — most modern OBs and midwives avoid episiotomies unless there is a clear medical need.

Standard care focuses on:

controlled, slow stretching
warm compresses
perineal support
guided, slow pushing

An episiotomy is only used when these measures aren't enough for a safe birth.

How It Feels (Honest & Reassuring)

If you have:

an epidural:
You may not feel the cut at all — just some pressure or tugging.

no epidural:
Local numbing medication is used first to prevent pain.

Most women are so focused on the pressure of pushing that they don't notice the moment it happens.

Nurse's Note

Even with an epidural, if you feel *any* sharpness or discomfort when we're touching your perineum, **please tell us**.

Your sensation matters.

We can always apply additional numbing medication — your comfort and emotional safety are a priority.

You deserve to feel:

safe
relaxed
cared for

...during *every* part of your birth.

Healing From an Episiotomy

Healing is very similar to a natural tear and usually involves:

- swelling
- soreness while sitting
- stinging when urinating
- tenderness with movement

Most women heal well with:

ice pads
sitz baths
witch hazel pads
pain medication
good hygiene

Your stitches dissolve on their own.

Nurse's Reassurance

Episiotomies are **not** routine anymore. They are a *tool* — used rarely, used carefully, and only when your safety or your baby's safety requires it.

If you need one, it's because your provider is doing everything possible to protect you both in that moment.

You are not failing. Your body is not failing. You are giving birth safely — and that is the most important thing.

Vacuum-Assisted Delivery

A vacuum extractor uses a soft or rigid suction cup that's gently placed on your baby's head. When you push during a contraction, the provider applies gentle traction to help guide your baby under the pubic bone and out.

What to Expect

- **You are still the one doing the pushing.**
  The vacuum simply guides your baby's movement.
- **You may feel pressure, but not pain** (especially if you have an epidural).
- **After delivery, the cup is removed immediately, and your nurse will check for:**
  - a temporary circular mark
  - mild bruising

- slight swelling
  These typically fade within a few days.

Vacuum deliveries are common, safe, and often just the little nudge your baby needs.

Forceps-Assisted Delivery

Forceps look like large, curved spoons that cradle your baby's head to gently guide them out as you push. They're particularly helpful if:

- baby needs to rotate slightly
- baby needs help clearing the pelvic curve
- the delivery needs to happen more quickly

What to Expect

- You'll push with your contractions while your provider assists.
- Forceps are used *carefully* and usually only for a few pushes.
- You may have some extra swelling or tenderness afterward — we'll help with:
  - ice packs
  - pain relief
  - positioning support

Forceps require training, skill, and timing — and they're used only when the benefit clearly outweighs the risk.

When Assistance Is Needed

These methods may be used when:

- You've been pushing a long time without steady progress
- Baby's heart rate shows signs of stress

- You're exhausted and need support
- You have a medical condition where prolonged pushing could be risky (like certain heart conditions or severe preeclampsia)

Nurse's Tip

An assisted delivery doesn't take away from your strength or the success of your birth.
It's part of the teamwork between:

you + your baby + your nurse + your provider.

Your provider will always explain what's happening before proceeding. You always have the right to ask questions or say what you need.

Sometimes strength looks like accepting help — and in birth, that teamwork can make all the difference.

Pushing Mantras: Words of Strength for You and Your Partner

When you're deep in the pushing stage — where determination meets exhaustion — words matter. The right phrase can calm your mind, ground your body, and help you push with purpose.

Mantras for You

- "My body was made for this."
- "With every push, I'm closer to my baby."
- "I am safe. I am strong. I am doing this."
- "Breathe in calm, push out strength."

- "I am not fighting my body — I am working with it."
- "Every wave brings my baby closer."
- "I am powerful beyond measure."
- "I can do anything for one more push."
- "This pain has a purpose — it's progress."
- "I trust my body and my baby."

♡ Encouragement for Partners to Say

- "You're doing amazing — I'm right here."
- "I see your strength in every push."
- "You're not alone — we're a team."
- "You're bringing our baby into the world. You're incredible."
- "One step closer, one breath at a time."
- "You're stronger than you think — look how far you've come."
- "I'm so proud of you."
- "You are the calm in this moment."

Nurse's Tip

Pick a few phrases now – before labor – and have them ready. Write them on:

- index cards
- your phone
- a sticky note in your hospital bag

Hearing the same calming phrase during contractions builds rhythm and focus.

Mantras aren't magic words – they're reminders of your own power. During labor, they become your **anchor**, your **rhythm**, and your **strength**.

Fetal Monitoring During Pushing

Once you begin pushing, our focus turns to both you and your baby. While you're working hard, your baby is doing their own kind of work — descending through the birth canal, turning, and adjusting to the changes in pressure and oxygen that come with each contraction. Fetal monitoring helps us see how your baby is tolerating that process in real time.

What We're Watching

During the pushing phase, your baby's heart rate may go up and down. Small changes are normal — they tell us your baby is responding to contractions just like we expect.

We're looking for:

- A strong, steady baseline heart rate (usually between 110–160 beats per minute)
- Variability or small fluctuations, that show your baby is well-oxygenated
- How the heart rate changes during and after contractions

When your baby's head is squeezed during a push, you may see short dips (decelerations) on the monitor — that's often just pressure on the head or cord. What matters most is that the heart rate returns to normal quickly after each push.

How We Monitor

External Monitoring:
Most of the time, we use a soft belt around your belly that holds the fetal heart rate and contraction sensors. We can reposition these as you move and change pushing positions.

Internal Monitoring:
If the external monitor can't pick up a clear signal (especially during active pushing or if there's a lot of movement), we may use a fetal scalp electrode. It's a tiny spiral wire placed on the baby's scalp to give us a more accurate reading. It sounds scary, but it's very small and doesn't hurt the baby.

> **Nurse's Tip:**
> If you hear the monitor's rhythm change while you're pushing, don't panic – it often mirrors what we expect your baby's heart to do.
>
> Ask your nurse to explain what you're hearing. Understanding the tones and patterns can actually make you feel more involved and less anxious.
>
> Sometimes, we'll ask you to change positions (to your side, hands and knees, or with a peanut ball) to help improve oxygen flow to your baby and relieve pressure on the cord.

Remember:
The monitor isn't just a machine — it's your baby's voice during labor. Our job is to listen carefully, interpret what they're telling us, and help both of you make it safely through those final pushes.

Evaluating Your Pushing Effort

Don't be surprised if your provider or nurse uses their fingers during a contraction to help assess how effective your pushing is. This is completely normal and a very common part of guiding you through the final stage of labor.

By placing two fingers inside the vaginal canal while you push, we can feel:

- how strongly you're bearing down
- the direction of your effort
- whether the pressure is going where it needs to go
- how your baby is responding to your push
- whether a position change would help

This isn't done to cause discomfort — it's done to help you push smarter, not harder.

We use this technique only when needed and it often makes a huge difference. Sometimes a small adjustment in how you direct your energy can immediately make your push more powerful and effective.

You're not doing anything wrong if we check — it's simply one of the tools we use to help you and your baby work together beautifully in those final moments before birth.

Trust the Push

Right before your baby is born — when the pressure peaks and the "ring of fire" is close — here's something important to know:

Believe it or not, when the time comes, **pushing often feels better than fighting the contraction**.

Your instinct may be to pull away from the intensity, but when you bear down and lean into the push, many people find real relief. It helps redirect the sensation, gives your body a sense of purpose, and works *with* the contraction instead of against it.

I say this from experience — both personal and professional. Whether it's mental, physical, or a bit of both, pushing can feel empowering rather than scary.

So when your body tells you it's time, don't be afraid to push. Trust me on this one — **you will feel better.**

Crowning and the Ring of Fire

When your baby's head finally moves past that peek-a-boo stage and stays visible between pushes, we call that **crowning** — it's the moment everyone in the room has been waiting for. This is when you'll feel your baby stretching the skin and muscles at the opening of your vagina as they prepare to be born.

Many women describe a warm, burning, or stinging sensation during this phase — that's the **"ring of fire."** It happens because your tissues are stretching to their limit to make space for your baby's head. It may sound scary, but it's brief — usually lasting only a few contractions — and it's actually a good sign that you're seconds away from meeting your baby.

Your nurse and provider will help you breathe through this stage instead of pushing forcefully. Short, gentle breaths ("pant-pant-blow") or controlled exhalations help slow the delivery just enough to allow the perineum to stretch gradually, reducing the chance of tearing.

We may also use warm compresses, gentle counterpressure, or perineal support to ease the burning and help your body stretch safely. If you have an epidural, you may feel pressure instead of burning, but your team will still guide you to push carefully as your baby crowns.

Nurse's Tip:

Listen closely to your nurse and provider during this stage – how you push (or pause) makes a big difference in preventing tears.

> If you feel burning, try not to fight it. Short, quick breaths help your body stay relaxed and let the baby move through naturally.
>
> Remember: that "fire" is your body making space for your baby. It's the final threshold – and when it passes, so will your baby.

Compassion Note:
During the *ring of fire* — that intense burning as your baby's head crowns — I am going to encourage you to **push through the pain**. And I don't say that lightly. I know exactly how scary, overwhelming, and mind-blowing that moment can feel.

I experienced a fourth-degree tear delivering my first baby boy, all 10 pounds, 2 ounces of him. When I reached this point with my second son, I was terrified to push again. TERRIFIED, that would happen again. So, when I tell you I understand, I truly mean it.

In that moment, I will gently ask you to go somewhere else in your mind — to shift your focus away from the burn. Because the only way *out* of that pain is *through* it. One strong, focused push brings incredible relief... and brings your baby into your arms.

This is the moment everything changes. You've worked so hard to get here — and I'll be right there with you, helping you meet your baby.

The Last Push

The last push is unlike any other moment in labor. It's the point where exhaustion and adrenaline meet, where every ounce of strength you have rises to the surface, and where your body gathers itself for the final act of bringing your baby into the world.

By this moment, you've already done the hardest work — opening, stretching, breathing, surrendering, pushing. Your baby is right there, so close that your provider can often see hair or the outline of your baby's head. You may feel burning, stretching, pressure, or simply a deep instinct telling you that this is it.

Your nurse leans in closer. Your provider's voice softens. Your support person grips your hand.
The energy in the room shifts.

This is the push where everything changes.

You take a breath — or sometimes, you don't even think about it. You bear down with everything you have left, not from your muscles but from your heart. This is the push driven by love, instinct, and a strength you didn't know you still had.

The room goes quiet for a split second as your baby's head emerges, followed by their shoulders and tiny body. And just like that — the work transforms into wonder.

Relief washes over you. Tears flow. Laughter breaks through. Your baby cries.
And your entire world expands.

That last push is not just a physical effort — **it's a moment of becoming.**
It is the line between before and after.
It is where you meet your baby and meet a new version of yourself.

You did it.
You brought life into the world.
And nothing will ever compare to the power of that final, beautiful push.

Congratulations MaMa, you incredibly did it!

Nurse's Confession

I cry just reading those words, because how lucky am I to stand beside women in this moment of their lives? I have watched countless births and yet the power of that final push never stops moving me. Every time, I feel the same swell of emotion — awe, pride, gratitude, and the quiet privilege of being invited into a moment most people will never witness.

I get a front-row seat to the instant a woman discovers a strength she didn't know she had. I see her transform pain into power, fear into focus, exhaustion into triumph. I see her become a mother in real time.

And every single time, it hits me in the chest. Every single time, I blink away tears. Every single time, I think to myself: **How fortunate am I that this is my job?**

Being a labor nurse isn't just a profession — it's an honor. And I never take for granted the privilege of standing beside a woman as she brings her baby into the world. For that, I am truly grateful.

17

C-Sections: Planned, Unplanned, and Always Powerful

"Surgery doesn't make you less of a mother — it makes you a warrior."

A C-section, whether planned ahead of time or decided unexpectedly during labor, is still a birth — a powerful, emotional, life-changing moment. It is not a failure, not a shortcut, and not a sign that your body "didn't work."
C-sections bring babies safely into the world every single day and the mothers who undergo them demonstrate some of the fiercest strength I've ever witnessed.

In this chapter, we'll explore both planned and unplanned C-sections — what to expect, what's normal, and how your care team supports you every step of the way.

Why C-Sections Happen

There are many reasons a C-section may be recommended and **none of them mean you did anything wrong**. Common reasons include:

- previous history of C-section
- baby's heart rate concerns
- stalled labor despite all efforts
- baby's position (breech, transverse, or other malpresentation)
- placenta previa (placenta covering the cervix)
- placenta abruption
- maternal health concerns
- infection
- multiple babies
- previous uterine surgery
- shoulder dystocia risk
- preeclampsia or severe hypertension
- elective

Birth takes many forms — and each path is valid.

If You're Having a Planned C-Section: The Night-Before Checklist

If your birth plan includes a scheduled cesarean delivery, the preparation you do the night before plays a big role in how smoothly your day will go. Your care team will give you specific instructions—**and it's very important to follow them closely** for your safety and your baby's. These instructions are designed to reduce the risk of infection, anesthesia complications, and surgical delays.

You will likely be asked to stop eating and drinking at a certain time the night before. Even a small sip of water outside of your allowed window can delay surgery, so follow those directions exactly. You may also be given guidance about showering with a special soap or whether any hair removal is needed—**do not shave the area unless your provider specifically**

tells you to, as shaving too close to surgery can increase the risk of skin irritation and infection.

On the morning of your surgery, **leave all jewelry at home**, including rings, necklaces, earrings, and body piercings. Jewelry can interfere with surgical equipment and your safety in the operating room. Bring a hair tie or clip that **does not contain metal** so your hair can be secured safely for surgery.

Pack only what you truly need: your ID, insurance card, comfortable clothing for after delivery, basic toiletries, phone charger, and items for your baby. Try not to overpack—your focus should be on rest and preparation, not managing extra belongings.

Most importantly, **ask questions if anything feels unclear**. No question is too small, and your team wants you to feel informed and calm as you prepare to meet your baby. A well-prepared night leads to a smoother, safer delivery day.

Common Pre-Op and Post-Op Medications for a C-Section

Most hospitals follow a very similar medication protocol for C-sections — both planned and unplanned. These medications are not random; each one is chosen intentionally to keep you safe, comfortable, and protected during surgery and after birth.

Here's what you could expect to be given by your providers and nurse:

Pepcid (famotidine) IV

Purpose: Reduces stomach acid
Why: Protects your esophagus and reduces the risk of aspiration during anesthesia.

Sodium Bicitra by mouth

Purpose: Neutralizes stomach acid immediately
Why: Taken right before going to the OR; protects your airway in case anesthesia triggers nausea. **Warning**: Not delicious, said to be tart, bitter, and a little salty. Don't think about it, shot it!

Zofran (ondansetron) IV

Purpose: Controls nausea
Why: Helps with nausea caused by anesthesia, hormones, or intraoperative sensations.

Reglan (metoclopramide) IV

Purpose: Reduces nausea and helps empty the stomach
Why: Decreases the risk of nausea, vomiting, and aspiration during anesthesia by helping move stomach contents forward and reducing gastric volume before surgery.

Ancef (cefazolin) - Antibiotic for Surgical Infection Prophylaxis - IV

Purpose: Prevents surgical site infection
Why: Given before incision to reduce the risk of uterine, wound, and overall post–cesarean infection.

Gentamicin + Clindamycin - Antibiotic Coverage for Penicillin Allergy - IV

Purpose: Prevents surgical site and uterine infection when Ancef cannot be used
Why: This combination provides **broad-spectrum protection** against both aerobic and anaerobic bacteria for patients who are allergic to penicillin or cephalosporins.

Ofirmev (IV Tylenol)

Purpose: Improves pain control after birth
Why: Pre-loads your system to reduce post-op pain and limits need for stronger meds later.

Toradol (ketorolac) IV

Purpose: Anti-inflammatory pain relief
Why: Helps with incision pain, cramping, and overall swelling during recovery.

Pitocin (oxytocin) IV

Purpose: Helps your uterus contract after birth
Why: Prevents postpartum hemorrhage by encouraging effective uterine clamping.

Nurse's Reassurance

These medications are routine and carefully chosen to support your safety, comfort, and recovery. Nothing is given without purpose:

- some protect your airway
- some protect your stomach
- some prevent nausea
- some reduce pain
- some help control bleeding

You won't need to memorize them — your team will also explain exactly what is being given to you. At the end of the day, your caregivers simply want to ensure the smoothest, safest C-section experience possible.

Planned C-Sections: Calm and Organized

A scheduled C-section is often peaceful and structured. You know the date, you arrive prepared, and the entire process moves with intention.

What to Expect

1. Pre-op prep

You'll check in, sign consents, change into a gown, meet anesthesia and your OR team, and receive your medications. Your belly will be prepped and lower pelvic region shaved. Your partner will get their infamous "doctor outfit."

2. Epidural or spinal anesthesia

You'll be awake unless there's an emergency requiring general anesthesia.
A spinal is one shot of medication — no catheter like with an epidural.

3. A calm operating room

- Soft music may be playing as the room stays quiet, focused, and well-organized
- Your nurse gently places the foley catheter
- A grounding (Bovie) pad is applied to your leg to keep you safe while surgical equipment uses electricity
- Your baby's heartbeat is checked one last time before delivery
- Sequential compression devices (SCDs) are placed on your legs to help prevent blood clots
- Warm blankets are layered over you for comfort
- You are safely positioned and secured on the operating table

For many families, a planned C-section feels surprisingly calm and serene.

4. Finishing touches for surgery

We drape, prep, and conduct a formal "time-out" to ensure safety. Once everything is set, we bring your partner in and begin the journey to meet your baby.

5. A smooth, steady delivery

You'll feel pressure, pulling, and tugging — but not pain.
The environment is controlled, unrushed, and supportive.

6. Baby lifted into the world

Some hospitals use clear drapes or allow you to see your baby immediately.

7. Baby is shown to you

Some hospitals place your baby on your chest right away. Others may first bring your baby to the warmer after delayed cord clamping so the NICU team can do a quick assessment. Once your baby is checked and stable, they are brought right back to you for skin-to-skin and bonding.

These first moments may look a little different depending on hospital policies and your baby's needs — but the goal is always the same: **safety first, then connection.**

8. The surgical team repairs the incision

This takes longer than the birth itself — usually about 30 minutes.
Total OR time: 45 minutes to an hour and a half.

It is still **your birth moment** — powerful and unforgettable.

Nurse's Tip

Ask your physician ahead of time what closing technique they use for your incision:

- dissolvable sutures
- staples
- layered repair

Knowing this ahead of time helps you understand how your incision will look, feel, and heal – giving you confidence heading into recovery.

Unplanned C-Sections: When the Plan Needs to Change

An unplanned C-section happens when your labor did go quite as planned — and then your provider determines that a surgical birth is the safest route for you or your baby.

This does not mean anything went wrong.
It simply means your care team is responding to the needs of the moment.

Common reasons for an unplanned C-section:

- baby's heart rate dips repeatedly
- your cervix stops dilating
- baby stops descending
- baby's position makes vaginal birth unsafe
- you develop severe bleeding

- infection or fever
- cord concerns
- maternal exhaustion
- baby isn't tolerating pushing

Unplanned does not mean chaotic.
It means responsive.

Nurse Reassurance

Even if you go for an emergency C-section, we don't just send you off and disappear. Your nurse stays with you — in the OR, through the spinal, during the delivery, and into recovery.

We are right there at your side the entire time, talking you through every step, keeping you calm, watching over you, and making sure you never feel alone.

You are still our patient.
You are still our responsibility.
And **we don't leave you — not for a moment.**

Nurse's Compassion Note for her Partner and Family Members

I have been in situations where a mom needed to go to the OR quickly — sometimes very quickly — and I've seen partners and family members standing there, watching us move with urgency as we prepare for both her **safety and the baby's safety**. I know how terrifying it feels when we wheel her away and you're suddenly left alone, unsure if your partner and your baby are going to be okay. That moment of separation is one of the hardest things a parent can experience.

Please know this:
While you're waiting, we are doing **everything in our power** to keep *both* of them safe. Every nurse, doctor, tech, and anesthesiologist in that room is focused, skilled, and working together with one goal — to bring her and your baby safely back to you.

If your baby needs extra help after birth, know that the nursery and NICU teams are just as dedicated, skilled, and intentional. They will do **everything possible** to support your baby while we care for your partner.

If you ever find yourself in this situation, please remember:
The people who work in Labor & Delivery, the OR, and the NICU are truly special individuals — compassionate, highly trained, and unwavering under pressure. If there is **anything that can be done**, it **will** be done.

We operate with skill, teamwork, and a higher sense of purpose guiding every move.
Please believe that.

Unplanned C-Section: What to Expect

If your birth plan changes and an unplanned C-section becomes necessary, the overall process is **very similar to a planned C-section—just at a more expedited pace**. While things may feel like they are moving quickly, it's important to know that **your care team is following the same safety steps every time**, with precision and purpose.

- You will still be brought to the operating room and safely positioned
- Monitors, IV access, and medications are given just as they would be for a scheduled surgery
- A foley catheter, grounding (Bovie) pad, and compression devices (SCDs) are placed as quickly and safely as possible
- Your baby's heartbeat is checked up until delivery

- Warm blankets are used whenever possible to keep you comfortable
- Your partner is brought in as soon as it is safe to do so. **Be aware:** if you are being put under general anesthesia, it may be hospital policy that support people can not be in the OR. Your care team will advise on your particular situation.

The difference is not the level of care—it's only the speed.

Even though the pace may feel fast and intense, every member of the team knows their role and each step is done with **your safety and your baby's safety as the top priority**. You are never alone in that room. You are surrounded by trained professionals whose sole focus is getting you and your baby through this moment safely and confidently.

Comfort Tip: Ask for Music in the OR

If you're heading into the operating room — whether for a cesarean birth or a procedure — don't hesitate to ask if you can play music. It can make a *huge* difference.

Music helps soften the environment by drowning out some of the noises, alarms, conversations, and beeping that can feel overwhelming. It gives you something familiar and calming to focus on, and it brings a sense of control and comfort into a space that can otherwise feel clinical or intimidating.

Whether it's calming instrumental, your favorite artist, or something uplifting, let your team know — we're always happy to help create a more peaceful experience for you.

What You May Feel – And What's Normal

- tugging
- pulling

- rocking motions
- pressure under the ribs
- a sense of "my breath caught for a second"

All normal. None of it means anything is wrong.
If anything feels overwhelming, anesthesia is right at your head to help.

Nurse's Note
Sitting up for your spinal is often the moment when it all becomes real. I see it all the time — the emotions catch up, the tears start to fall, and the weight of the moment lands right on your shoulders.

And it's okay.
It's normal to cry when you're scared, excited, overwhelmed, or simply feeling everything at once.

But when you look at me with those worried eyes, this is what I will tell you:

Don't steal your own joy.
You only get so many of these life-changing moments. Let yourself experience it — not through fear, but through trust.

Trust your team.
Trust the process.
Trust that even though you don't do this every day — we do.

We've got you.
We know how to keep you safe, comfortable, and supported.
You are not alone for a single second.

Let yourself breathe.
Let yourself feel the miracle happening.
You are stronger than you know — and **we are right here with you.**

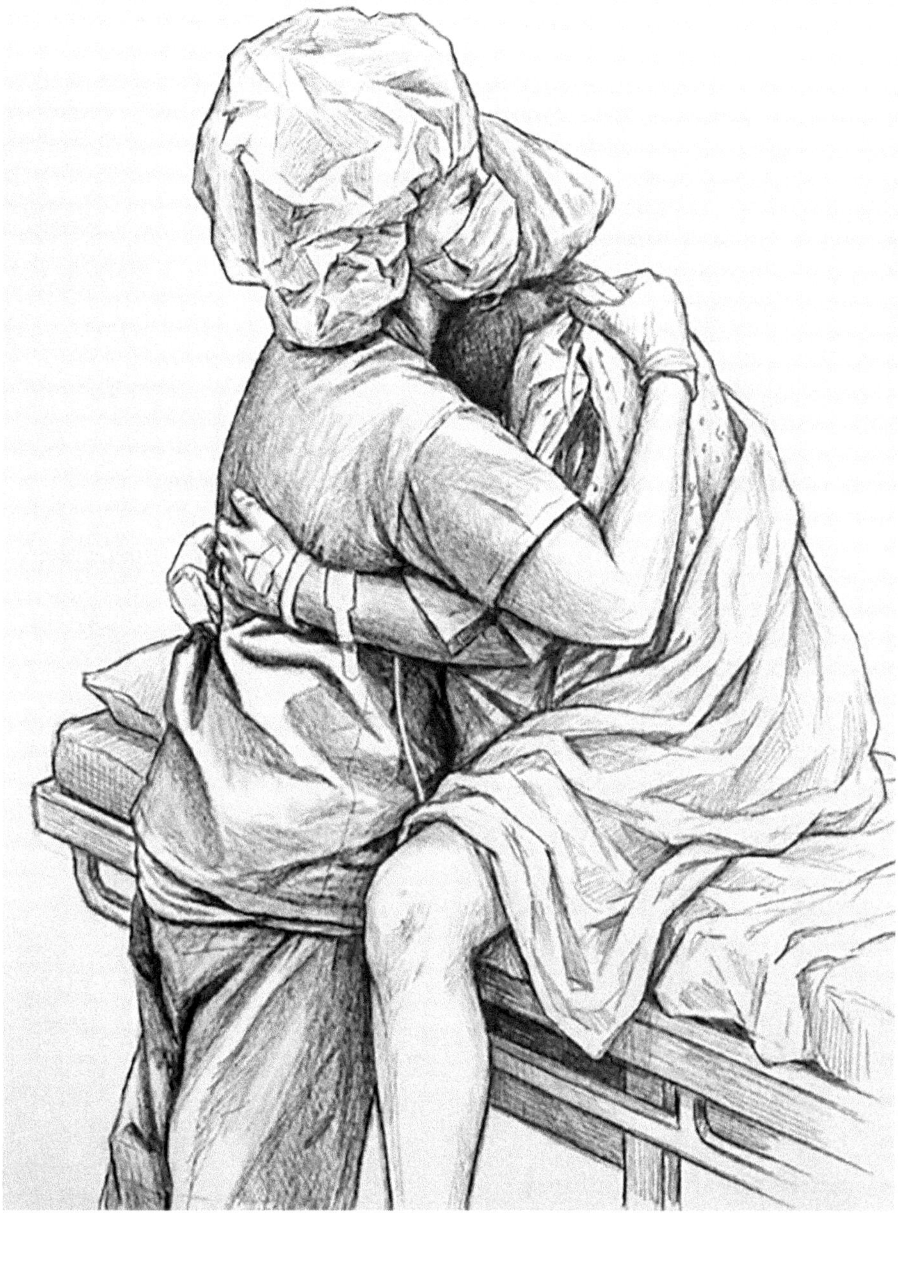

Partner's Role During a C-Section

Partners are essential:

- holding your hand
- brushing your hair
- talking to you
- announcing the gender (if you want)
- being the first to see baby
- cutting the cord **(ask your surgeon to leave cord to be cut at the warmer)**
- doing skin-to-skin if you're unable

They are your anchor in the OR.

C-Section Recovery: Honest and Encouraging

Recovery is different from a vaginal birth, but absolutely manageable:

- **Hospital stay:** 2–4 days
- **Pain level:** moderate but treatable
- **Movement:** slow but doable
- **Incision:** dissolving stitches or staples
- **Bleeding:** similar to a vaginal birth
- **Milk production:** unaffected — your body still biologically birthed

Walking as soon as it's safe helps prevent clots and speeds healing. Your nurse will help you with:

- **safe movements**
- **incision care**
- **pain control**
- **breastfeeding positions**
- **getting in and out of bed**

You are never left to navigate recovery alone.

Nurse's Note

Do not try to get out of bed or walk after your C-section until your nurse says it's safe — and until we are right there with you. Your legs may feel heavier or weaker than you expect after anesthesia and your balance won't be the same immediately after surgery.

We help steady you, support your incision, and guide you safely every step of the way.

You've just been through major abdominal surgery.
Let us protect you while your strength returns.
We've got you.

C-Sections Are Not Failures – They Are Births

This needs to be said clearly:

You didn't "fail."
You didn't "give up."
Your body didn't "quit."
You didn't get "robbed" of anything.

A C-section is an act of protection, bravery, and love.

Planned or unplanned.
Calm or urgent.

It is still the moment you met your baby.

Nurse's Tip:
You may feel shaky, cold, or emotional – that's normal and often related to anesthesia or adrenaline wearing off.

> Ask your nurse to narrate what's happening if you'd like – sometimes knowing what comes next can ease anxiety.
>
> If your baby needs to go to the nursery or NICU, we'll make sure someone stays with you and keeps you updated every step of the way.

How Nurses Support You When Things Change - Delivery Room to OR

Labor doesn't always follow the plan — and that can feel overwhelming in the moment. This is exactly where your nurse becomes your steady ground.

When things don't go as expected — whether pushing takes longer, interventions are suggested, or birth plans shift — your nurse's role becomes even more important.

We're not just there to carry out orders; we're there to **translate, reassure, and protect your experience.**

1. We Keep You Informed

When your care team discusses options, we make sure you understand what's happening, why it's happening, and what choices you have.

"Here's what's going on and what this means for you."

We explain things in plain language, answer questions honestly, and slow the process enough for you to breathe and think clearly.

2. We Watch You – and Your Baby – Closely

As you work and push, we're constantly assessing your vital signs, bleeding, and your baby's heart rate.

You may not realize how many times we quietly adjust your position or oxygen to help your baby — it's second nature to us.

3. We Protect Your Space

Labor can get busy quickly. We help keep the room calm and supportive — dimming lights, reducing noise, and advocating for quiet when you need it.

"Let's give her a moment."
One of the most powerful things a nurse can say.

4. We're Your Emotional Anchor

If you cry, panic, or feel like you can't do it anymore, we remind you that you already *are* doing it.

"You're safe. You're not alone. You're doing everything right."

5. We Celebrate Every Step

Whether your baby arrives after hours of pushing, a vacuum assist, or a C-section, we celebrate the moment you meet your child — because we've witnessed the strength it took to get there.

Nurse's Tip:
Birth doesn't have to go perfectly to be beautiful.

Let your nurse be your advocate, your translator, and your calm in the storm.

> **When plans shift, nurses are the constant – holding space for your safety, your voice, and your power.**

Your Birth Story Still Belongs to You

No matter how your labor unfolds — whether it's quick, complicated, calm, or chaotic — your story is yours. It doesn't have to look like anyone else's to be meaningful, powerful, or worthy of pride.

Sometimes birth goes exactly as planned; sometimes it takes detours you never saw coming. You might find yourself laboring longer than expected, needing interventions, or even facing a cesarean after hours of effort. But none of that changes the truth: **you did it.**

You showed up. You endured. You brought life into this world.

Reframing What "Success" Looks Like

Success in birth isn't about perfection — it's about perseverance.
It's the moment you pushed when you were exhausted.
It's the breath you took instead of giving up.
It's the courage it took to trust your team when plans changed.

Your nurse sees those victories. We witness the quiet moments — the trembling hands, the tears, the whispered *"I can't"* that somehow turns into one more push, or the *"I never wanted a C-section"* that becomes a brave choice made for your baby's safety.

That is strength.
That is motherhood already taking shape.

Why Your Story Matters

One day, when you tell your child about the day they were born, it won't be about the interventions or timelines. It will be about how fiercely you loved them from the very first moment. And no matter what your birth looked like, that love — that fight — will always be the center of your story.

Nurse's Tip:

- Write your story when you're ready – it helps you see how strong you truly were.
- Don't compare your story to anyone else's – no two births are the same.
- However your baby arrived, your body and your heart did something extraordinary.

Your birth story isn't defined by *how* it happened – it's defined by *you*.
And you, mama, are stronger, braver, and more beautiful than you realize.

Nurse's Confession: C-Section Birth

I get emotional just thinking about the miracle of a C-section birth because people don't talk enough about how powerful it truly is. I have stood at the head of the bed holding a mother's hand as the drape rises, watching her trust a room full of strangers with the most precious moment of her life. And every single time, I feel honored to witness her courage.

There is a stillness in the OR that is different from the delivery room. The lights are brighter, the temperatures are colder, and yet the moment your baby enters the world feels just as warm and breathtaking.

I watch you lie there, arms outstretched, heart pounding, unable to move but refusing to let fear win — and all I see is bravery.

I see the strength it takes to surrender control.
I see the faith it takes to let a team care for you.
I see the love pouring out of you long before we hear the first cry.

And when that cry finally echoes across the OR, when your baby is lifted into the light and shown to you for the very first time — I feel that lump in my throat every single time. I see your tears. I see your smile. I see the moment you become a mother in a room you never imagined giving birth in.

Some people say C-sections aren't "real births," and I wish they could stand where I stand. I wish they could see what I see — a woman lying on an operating table, every ounce of vulnerability on display, meeting it with more strength, grace, and love than most people will show in their entire lives.

I get emotional because I am lucky.
Lucky to witness this kind of power.
Lucky to stand beside you as you bring life into the world.
Lucky to be trusted in one of the most sacred, transformative moments of your life.

A C-section birth is not a Plan B.
It is not less.
It is not easier.
It is not weaker.

It is motherhood — raw, fierce, and extraordinary.

And I will never stop being grateful that I get to witness it and **have you to thank for that.**

18

The Placenta, Cord, and Delivering the Placenta

"The cord connected you. The placenta sustained you. Both deserve applause."

The Unsung Heroes of Pregnancy & Birth

The placenta and umbilical cord are two of the most incredible structures your body will ever create. Aside from your baby, of course. They work together every second of your pregnancy to nourish, protect, and support your baby. Even after the birth, they play an important role in completing the labor process.

Let's break down what the placenta is, what it does, what to expect when it's delivered, and common things you may hear about — including nuchal cords and true knots.

What Is the Placenta?

The placenta is a temporary organ your body builds specifically for pregnancy. It attaches to the wall of your uterus and connects to your baby through the umbilical cord.

It is your baby's lifeline.

What the Placenta Does

1. Oxygen Delivery

Your baby isn't breathing air in the womb. The placenta delivers oxygen from your bloodstream to them continuously.

2. Nutrition

It transfers all the nutrients your baby needs to grow — protein, fats, glucose, vitamins, and minerals.

3. Waste Removal

The placenta carries away your baby's carbon dioxide and metabolic waste so your body can process it.

4. Hormone Production

It produces essential hormones that:

- Support your pregnancy
- Prepare your breasts for lactation
- Regulate blood flow
- Assist your baby's growth

5. Immune Protection

It passes antibodies from you to your baby, giving them early immunity.

The placenta is truly a miracle organ.

What Happens After Your Baby Is Born?

You still have one more stage of labor — **delivering the placenta.**

This is called the *third stage of labor*, and it usually happens within:
5–20 minutes.
Sometimes a little more, rarely less.

What Delivering the Placenta Feels Like

Good news: **it's nothing like delivering your baby.**

Women often describe it as:

- A warm gush
- Mild cramping
- Pressure
- A sliding sensation

No stretching.
No burning.
No crowning.

You're often so focused on your baby that you barely notice it.

Delivering the Placenta During a Vaginal Birth

After the baby is born, your body naturally begins the process of separating and expelling the placenta.

1. Contractions Resume

Your uterus tightens to shear the placenta away from its attachment site.

2. Pitocin

Many hospitals give Pitocin after birth to help prevent hemorrhage and make the uterus contract more efficiently.

3. Gentle Cord Traction

Your provider may apply gentle guidance to help deliver the placenta after it has detached.

4. Fundal Massage

Yes, it's uncomfortable — but this helps your uterus firm up and reduces bleeding.

After delivery, your provider will examine the placenta closely to make sure it's intact and healthy.

Delivering the Placenta During a Cesarean Birth

Delivering the placenta in a C-section is **faster**, **easier**, and **completely painless** from your perspective.

Here's what actually happens behind the drape:

1. The uterus continues to contract

Just like in a vaginal birth, the uterus naturally tightens to separate the placenta from the uterine wall.

2. Your surgeon removes the placenta by hand

This is called a **manual extraction**.

- The provider reaches into the uterus
- Locates the placenta
- Gently lifts and peels it away

You only feel pressure — never pain.

3. The uterus is checked

Your surgeon inspects:

- The uterine lining
- The placental bed

- Any areas of bleeding

This ensures no tissue is left behind.

4. The uterus contracts

Pitocin is given through your IV to help your uterus tighten and prevent hemorrhage.

5. The uterus is stitched closed

Once everything is clear and firm:

- The uterine incision is sutured
- The uterus is returned to position
- Abdominal layers are closed

You don't deliver the placenta in a C-section — **your surgeon does.** It is one of the quickest steps of the procedure.

Taking Your Placenta Home

Many moms choose to take their placenta home for:

- Burial
- Planting under a tree
- Cultural or spiritual rituals
- Photography
- Keepsakes

If this is something you want, **tell your nurse early** so we can package, label, and store it properly. Hospitals have strict guidelines and early notice helps us respect your wishes without delaying anything.

Placenta Encapsulation

Some parents choose to encapsulate their placenta — drying and grinding it into pills to take postpartum.

What you should know:

- Some women report emotional or energy benefits postpartum
- Research is mixed and still very limited
- It must be handled safely by a trained, certified specialist
- Your hospital may require a release form for transport

If you plan to encapsulate:

- Bring a cooler
- Notify your nurse
- Have someone pick it up promptly
- Follow the specialist's instructions for safe handling

This is a personal choice — and it's completely yours to make.

When Placental Complications Occur

Sometimes rare complications can happen, such as:

- A placenta that doesn't separate easily (retained placenta)
- A placenta that attaches too deeply into the uterine wall (accreta spectrum disorders)

These situations sound scary but your team is fully trained to identify and manage them safely and quickly. You are never left without support.

Nurse's Note

I often explain the placenta like a scab.

When you pick a scab and don't apply pressure, it bleeds.
The same thing happens inside your uterus after the placenta is delivered.

The placenta leaves behind a **large, scab-like wound**, and your uterus must contract to put pressure on that area to stop bleeding. That's why:

- postpartum contractions
- fundal checks
- uterine massage
- and postpartum Pitocin

are all so important.
They help your uterus clamp down, protect you, and prevent hemorrhage — the most serious postpartum risk.

The Umbilical Cord: Your Baby's Lifeline

The umbilical cord connects your baby to the placenta and carries:

- Oxygen
- Nutrients
- Blood
- Immune cells

It is cushioned by **Wharton's jelly**, a thick, protective substance that prevents the cord from being compressed.

This design is why most babies stay perfectly safe — even if the cord loops or twists.

Nuchal Cords (Cord Around the Neck): Common & Usually Harmless

A nuchal cord simply means the umbilical cord is looped around your baby's neck or another part of their body.

It might look like:

- One loop around the neck
- Multiple loops
- Loops around the arm, torso, or leg
- A draped cord across the shoulder or chest

Here's the important truth:

Nuchal cords are extremely common — about 1 in 4 births — and usually do NOT harm the baby (Cleveland Clinic, 2025).

Why?

Because:

- Babies aren't breathing through their necks
- They are oxygenated through the cord
- The cord is thick, slippery, and protected
- Wharton's jelly prevents compression
- Cords are designed to handle movement, flips, and twists

Most nuchal cords never affect labor at all.

What Happens if Baby Has a Nuchal Cord at Birth?

Your provider will simply:

Slip it over the baby's head

If it's loose, it's removed like a scarf.

Deliver the body through the loop

If it's snug but not tight.

Perform the "somersault maneuver"

If the cord is tight, baby may be guided out close to your body so the cord stays relaxed.

Rarely: clamp and cut early

Only if absolutely necessary and your provider explains everything in real time.

We do this all the time — calmly, safely, and without emergency.

True Knots & False Knots

True knots (1% of pregnancies) (Gaikwad et al., 2023):

A real knot formed when baby swims through a loop in early pregnancy.

Most true knots are loose and harmless.

We only become concerned if the knot tightens or compresses during labor, and the fetal heart rate will show us that quickly.

False Knots

False knots are *not* real knots.
They're simply thicker or looped areas of the umbilical cord where extra Wharton's jelly collects. They look dramatic on ultrasound but they're **completely harmless**.

Your Baby Is Designed for This

Babies are experts at navigating the womb. Throughout pregnancy, they move through:

- Nuchal cords
- Loops around limbs
- Cord variations
- True knots
- Long cords
- Short cords

And they do all of this safely because they're protected by:

- **Wharton's jelly** (a thick, cushioning gel inside the cord)
- **Amniotic fluid**
- **Continuous placental oxygenation**

Most cord variations **never cause a single problem**.

Nurse's Note: Nuchal Cords Are Normal

If your baby has the cord around their neck or body, it is almost always **safe and manageable.**
A nuchal cord does not mean your baby is choking — babies don't breathe air in the womb. Their oxygen comes through the cord itself.

Providers gently and routinely handle nuchal cords during birth.
This is a normal, common variation of pregnancy — not an emergency.

Honoring the Body That Created This Life System

Your body built an entire life-support system from scratch:

- Your **placenta** nourished your baby.
- Your **umbilical cord** carried oxygen and nutrients back and forth.
- Your **uterus** protected the entire process.

And when labor ended, your placenta completed its mission — a final, powerful act before your postpartum journey begins.

Whether you choose to keep it, encapsulate it, honor it, or let us take care of it,
your placenta is a testament to everything your body accomplished.

19

The First Moments After Birth

"Let choice whisper in your ear and murmur in your heart. Be ready. Here comes life."

– Maya Angelou

The instant your baby is born, the room shifts — all the intensity of labor melts into relief, awe, and emotion. Whether your baby lets out a loud cry right away or takes a quiet moment before breathing, your nurse and provider will be right there making sure everything is okay.

Whenever possible, we place your baby directly on your chest — this is called **skin-to-skin contact**. It helps your baby stay warm, regulates their heart rate and breathing, and strengthens the bond between you. Those first few minutes are powerful: your baby knows your voice, your scent, and your heartbeat. It's the beginning of everything you've worked for.

If you've chosen **delayed cord clamping**, your team will wait to cut the cord for 30–60 seconds (sometimes longer), allowing extra blood to flow from the placenta to your baby. This gives your newborn an added boost of oxygen and iron. If your baby needs a little extra help after birth, the cord may be clamped earlier so we can move quickly — but either way, we'll keep you informed every step of the way.

While you're meeting your baby, your provider will deliver the placenta and your nurse will gently massage your belly (the uterus) to help it contract and minimize bleeding. This might not be comfortable, but it's an important safety step. You might also notice a small amount of shaking or shivering — that's completely normal and will pass quickly.

Nurse's Tip:

- Try to soak in those first moments. Everything else can wait – the weighing, the visitors, even the photos.
- If skin-to-skin isn't immediately possible (for example, after a C-section or if the baby needs extra attention), don't worry. As soon as it's safe, your nurse will make sure that connection happens.
- Ask your nurse to dim the lights and lower the noise – a calm environment helps both you and your baby adjust gently to life outside the womb.

These first few minutes are sacred.
The world narrows to just you and your baby — two hearts that worked together for months, finally beating side by side.

Delayed Cord Clamping: What It Means and Why We Do It

If baby allows it, delayed cord clamping means we wait a short period of time—usually 30 seconds to 2 minutes—before clamping and cutting your baby's umbilical cord. This small delay allows extra blood from the placenta to flow into your baby, giving them a boost of oxygen-rich, iron-rich blood that supports their transition into life outside the womb. Research shows that delayed cord clamping can improve iron stores for months, help stabilize newborn breathing and circulation, and reduce the risk of anemia. For preterm babies, it can even lower the risk of complications in the NICU. During this time, your baby is either on your chest or held close to you and the delay does not interfere with bonding in any way. It's a simple, powerful step that supports your baby's health from their very first moments.

What Babies Look Like When They Come Out

One of the biggest surprises for new parents is realizing that babies don't always come out looking like the clean, pink newborns you see in photos. Birth is messy, magical, and very real — and your baby's first moments will reflect that. Everything you see is normal, expected, and nothing to worry about.

Here's what you may notice:

Vernix: The Newborn "Lotion"

Some babies are covered in vernix, a thick, creamy, white coating that protected their skin in the womb.

- Early babies often have a lot
- Full-term babies may have a little
- Post-dates babies may have almost none

It's completely normal and actually great for their skin — many hospitals rub it in instead of wiping it off right away.

A Little Blood (Totally Normal)

Birth is a big transition, so don't be shocked if you see:

- streaks of blood
- a little on their skin

- some on the blankets

None of this means your baby is hurt — it's simply from the birth canal or C-section incision area. Babies themselves rarely have any injuries or bleeding of their own.

Skin Color: It Changes Rapidly

Many babies come out looking:

- blue-ish
- purple
- red
- blotchy
- a little swollen
- sometimes even bruised, especially if they descended quickly or were in an odd position

This is all part of adjusting to life outside the womb.

Pink color comes once they start crying and breathing on their own.

Head Shape: Cone Heads Are Normal

If your baby takes a long journey through the birth canal, their head may be:

- cone-shaped
- elongated
- a bit misshapen

That's thanks to the skull bones molding to fit through the pelvis — and they go back to normal within hours or days.

C-section babies often have beautifully round heads because they didn't have to squeeze through the birth canal.

Lanugo: The Soft "Fuzz" Some Babies Are Born With

Lanugo is the **fine, downy hair** that sometimes covers a newborn's back, shoulders, ears, or cheeks. It can be surprising if you've never seen it before, but it's completely normal.

Lanugo develops in the womb to help protect your baby's skin and regulate their temperature. Most of it sheds before birth, but some babies — especially those born a little earlier — still have it when they arrive.

It's soft, harmless, and **fades on its own** over the first few days or weeks of life. Nothing needs to be done about it.

Think of lanugo as one more sign of the incredible way your baby has grown and developed inside of you. ♡

How Babies Behave Right After Birth

Some babies cry loudly right away — others don't and both are normal.

Babies may:

- cry briefly
- whimper
- gasp
- cough
- stay quiet but alert
- take a few seconds to establish a rhythm

What you won't see: perfectly calm, smiling Gerber babies.
That's commercial life — not real life.

What Nurses Do Right Away

Your nurse and the delivery team watch your baby closely in the first seconds and minutes after birth. Here's exactly what we do:

1. Dry and Stimulate
Rubbing them with warm blankets helps:

- warm them up
- clear their airway
- encourage a strong first cry
- stimulate breathing

Drying is one of the most important steps we do right away.

Sometimes I gently rub their little feet to get them real vigorous.

2. Suction if Needed
If your baby has extra fluid or mucus, we may:

- suction their mouth
- suction their nose
- gently clear any obstructions

This helps them breathe more easily.

3. Assess Their Breathing and Tone
We look for:

- a strong cry
- good movement
- color improving
- chest rising and falling normally

If baby needs extra help, we respond immediately and expertly.

4. Place Baby Skin-to-Skin

If medically appropriate, we place your baby directly on your chest. This:

- warms them
- stabilizes their breathing
- regulates their heart rate
- calms them
- helps bonding begin instantly

If baby needs a few moments of assistance first, we bring them to you as soon as it's safe.

What Does APGAR Stand For?

A newborn gets assessed in five areas — each scored from 0 to 2.
This gives a total score between 0 and 10.

Here are the five categories:

A – Appearance (skin color)
0 → Blue or pale
1 → Pink body, blue hands/feet (very common!)
2 → Completely pink

P – Pulse (heart rate)
0 → No heartbeat
1 → Below 100
2 → Strong heartbeat over 100

G – Grimace (reflex irritability)
How they respond to stimulation.
0 → No response
1 → Grimace
2 → Crying/moving/grimacing

A – Activity (muscle tone)
0 → Limp
1 → Some flexing of arms/legs
2 → Active, good movement

R – Respirations (breathing)
0 → Not breathing
1 → Slow or irregular breathing
2 → Good cry and regular breaths

What the Scores Really Mean

7–10:
This is normal. Most healthy babies fall in this range at 1 and 5 minutes. Even a 7 is perfectly fine — especially at the 1-minute mark when many babies are still adjusting.

4–6:
Your baby may need a little extra help:

- Stimulation
- Suctioning
- Positioning
- Supplemental oxygen

These babies usually respond quickly.

0–3:
This means your baby needs immediate resuscitative support from the NICU or delivery team.
Even babies with very low initial scores often improve dramatically with intervention.

APGARs are about *right now*, not long-term outcomes.

Why Babies Don't Always Score a 10

Most babies born vaginally will *not* score a perfect 10 at one minute — and that's okay.

Common reasons include:

- Blue hands and feet (acrocyanosis) — very normal
- Being a bit stunned from delivery
- Taking their time to get that big first cry out
- Needing a little suction or stimulation

A 9 is often the highest possible score because many babies keep blue feet in the first couple of minutes.

What You Will See as a Parent

You might notice the nurse rubbing your baby's back, suctioning their mouth, or drying them vigorously.
This isn't because anything is wrong — it's how we help them transition.

Sometimes:

- Baby comes out crying loudly → high score
- Baby comes out quietly but breathing well → normal
- Baby is sleepy from medications or long labor → needs stimulation
- Baby born via C-section → may take a moment to clear fluid

Everything you're seeing is part of a very normal process.

Nurse's Reassurance

APGAR scores are simply a snapshot of your baby's first moments — not a prediction of their future.

They don't define health, intelligence, development, or who your baby will become.

I've seen babies start with low APGARs and thrive beautifully.
I've seen babies start with high APGARs and also do wonderfully.

What matters most is how your baby *responds* and we are trained to support that transition every second of the way.

Nurse's Thoughts

Everything you see in those first few seconds — the vernix, the swelling, the color changes, the cries, the quiet moments — is part of your baby's perfect transition from womb to world.

Every baby arrives in their own way, in their own time, and in their own style.
Your nurse will explain everything as it happens, reassure you, and make sure your baby is transitioning beautifully.

This is birth — real, raw, beautiful.
And your baby is absolutely perfect.

If Your Baby Needs a Little Extra Help

Most babies transition beautifully with just drying, stimulation, and a good cry. But sometimes — especially after a long labor, a fast delivery, or a C-section — your baby may need a little more assistance. And that does *not* mean anything is "wrong." It simply means your baby needs a moment to adjust to life outside the womb.

Here's what happens, step by step:

1. Baby Might Go to the Warmer for a Quick Assessment

If your baby isn't crying strongly or needs more help clearing their airway, we may bring them to the warmer just a few feet away.

This is done so we can:

- see them clearly
- access equipment
- keep them warm
- work efficiently as a team

You can still see your baby the entire time. They are never "taken away" — just moved to the safest place to assist them quickly.

2. Extra Stimulation and Suctioning

We may:

- rub their back more firmly
- gently rub the bottoms of their feet
- suction deeper in the mouth or nose
- clear extra fluid they swallowed on the way out

This often does the trick within seconds.

3. Blow-by Oxygen

Sometimes babies need a little extra oxygen right after birth. We don't put anything on their face — we simply hold oxygen close so they can breathe it in.

It is safe, gentle, and very common.

4. CPAP or Positive Pressure Breathing

If your baby needs help opening their lungs or taking deeper breaths, we may use a tiny mask to give a few gentle puffs of air.

This helps:

- open the air sacs
- clear fluid
- establish a strong breathing pattern

Many babies perk up immediately.

5. NICU Team Involvement

If we think your baby could benefit from an expert set of eyes, we may call the NICU team.

This does *not* mean your baby is in danger — it means we want specialists to support your baby right from the very beginning.

The NICU team can:

- evaluate breathing
- assess tone and color
- provide advanced support if needed

They are calm, skilled, and move with confidence and reassurance.

6. You Will Be Updated Every Step of the Way

Your nurse *and* your provider will tell you:

- what we see
- what we're doing
- what it means
- what's coming next

You are never left in the dark.
Your support person can stand right between you and baby so you can hear everything and stay connected.

7. Skin-to-Skin Happens as Soon as It's Safe

Even if baby needs some extra help, our goal is always to stabilize them quickly and bring them right to you.

Skin-to-skin is powerful and healing — and we never delay it unless your baby truly needs those first moments to transition safely.

Nurse's Reassurance

Babies are incredibly resilient and needing a little extra help in the first minutes is far more common than you might think.

It does *not* mean your baby is unhealthy.
It does *not* mean you did anything wrong.
It does *not* mean your birth went poorly.

It simply means your baby needed a moment — and you had an entire team ready to step in.

And once they are safe, stable, and breathing beautifully, nothing will stop us from placing your baby right in your arms where they belong.

The NICU Team: Who They Are and What They Do

Hearing that the NICU team is coming into the room can sound scary, but I promise you — their presence is one of the biggest safety nets we have for newborns. They are the specialists who care for babies who need a little extra help transitioning in those first moments after birth.

Most of the time, they are called as a precaution, not because something is wrong.

Here's who they are and what each person does:

Neonatal Nurse Practitioner (NNP) or Neonatologist

These are the true baby experts — advanced practitioners or physicians trained exclusively in newborn care.

They can:

- assess breathing and heart rate
- make immediate medical decisions
- provide advanced resuscitation if needed
- oversee newborn stabilization

They are calm, skilled, and incredibly reassuring.

NICU Nurses

NICU nurses are some of the most detail-oriented, gentle, and highly trained nurses in the hospital. They specialize in:

- assisting with newborn breathing
- warming, drying, and stimulating baby
- providing CPAP or oxygen
- monitoring vital signs
- supporting the NNP or neonatologist

They work seamlessly as a team — quick, quiet, and completely focused.

Respiratory Therapist (RT)

If a baby needs help clearing fluid or taking stronger breaths, the respiratory therapist steps in.

RTs may:

- assist with CPAP
- provide blow-by oxygen
- support babies who have extra fluid in their lungs (common, especially with C-sections)

They are experts in newborn breathing and move with confidence and precision.

Why the NICU Team Might Be Called

The NICU team may be present when:

- baby is born early
- baby is very small or very large
- meconium-stained fluid is present
- baby has heart rate changes during labor
- baby needs more stimulation than expected
- vacuum or forceps-assisted delivery
- the provider simply wants extra hands "just in case"

Many babies perk up quickly and never leave your room — the NICU team simply observes, supports, and steps back.

What They Actually Do in the Room

If needed, they will:

- dry and stimulate the baby
- assess breathing and tone
- clear the airway
- give oxygen or a few gentle breaths
- monitor color and heart rate

- ensure safe transition to life outside the womb

They move efficiently but gently, narrating what they're doing and speaking softly to the baby throughout.

Most parents are surprised by how fast everything happens — often within the first minute or two of life.

Your Baby Is Never "Taken Away" Without Explanation

If your baby needs to go to the NICU for closer monitoring, you will be told:

- why
- what we're concerned about
- what the plan is
- how long it might take
- when you can see them

Your nurse stays with you and your partner can accompany the baby when stabilized.

But here's the truth:

Most babies who need the NICU team at birth stay right in the room and go straight to their parents as soon as they're stable.

🌼 Nurse's Reassurance

The NICU team is not a sign that something is wrong.
They are a sign of protection, preparation, and readiness.

When they walk into the room, it isn't panic — it's expertise. It's calm. It's layers of safety.

And the moment your baby is breathing well, warm, and stable, we place them right into your arms.

Nurse's Insight

A heartfelt shout-out to our NICU teams — truly some of the most respected clinicians in the hospital. Labor nurses trust them completely. When they walk in, the room settles. Their skill, precision, and compassion make all the difference for babies who need just a little more help.

We couldn't do this work without them.

20

NICU Admission – What It Means for Baby and Mom

"The NICU is a place where the tiniest fighters begin their journey toward life."

When a baby is admitted to the Neonatal Intensive Care Unit (NICU), it can feel like an overwhelming whirlwind of emotion for parents. For mothers, this moment may bring confusion, fear, and helplessness. For babies, it is a critical step in receiving the specialized care they need to thrive.

The NICU is a world of hope, medicine, and progress — a place where fragility and resilience exist side by side.

The NICU Journey for Baby

When a baby is admitted to the NICU, it's because they need monitoring, specialized equipment, or expert care that cannot be provided in a standard nursery. Reasons may include:

- premature birth
- respiratory issues

- low birth weight
- low blood sugar issues
- infections or complications
- difficulty transitioning after birth

The NICU is designed to give babies their strongest possible start.

Nurse's Note:

I know this is a difficult time and seeing your baby surrounded by monitors and equipment can be overwhelming. But please be rest assured — your baby is in the best hands possible. The NICU team is here to support your little one every single minute of every single day.

The NICU is not a place where babies are left alone. It is a space of constant, expert care, whether the baby needs:

- help breathing
- temperature support
- help feeding
- continuous monitoring

Nurse Reassurance:

Even if your baby is in an incubator or under lights, they are *never* alone. They are watched closely, cared for constantly, and supported by a team that specializes in giving fragile babies exactly what they need to grow stronger.

For parents, the equipment and tubes can be startling — incubators, ventilators, IV lines, and monitors. But they represent the safest, most advanced care available. Even the tiniest humans need a tremendous amount of love and medical support to thrive and the NICU provides both.

The NICU Journey for Mom

For a mother, NICU admission can feel like an emotional earthquake. You may have envisioned holding your baby right away, nursing immediately, or going home together within a day or two. Suddenly, your reality is different:

waiting
watching
hoping
healing
and longing for the moment you can hold your baby freely.

> **Nurse's Note:**
>
> You are still your baby's source of comfort, love, and security – even if you can't hold them yet. When it's safe, we will help you do skin-to-skin, because it strengthens bonding, stabilizes temperature, improves breathing, supports blood sugar, and even boosts brain development.
>
> If breastfeeding isn't possible immediately, we will help you begin pumping so your milk is ready the very moment your baby is able to receive it. Your connection to your baby is not delayed – it simply looks different right now.
>
> Many mothers struggle with guilt, wondering if they did something wrong. Please hear this clearly:
> You did not cause this.
> Most NICU admissions happen for reasons completely outside a mother's control. Your baby is receiving the exact care they need to grow stronger, and your love, your voice, and your presence are still shaping their journey every single day.
>
> Please don't blame yourself.

Your Feelings Are Valid

Your feelings — all of them — are valid.
Fear, sadness, frustration, guilt, numbness, anger, confusion…
Every emotion has a place here.
You do not have to navigate this alone.

Your NICU nurses will guide you through every step with compassion, patience, and unwavering support.

How You Can Be Involved

Many NICUs encourage parents to participate in their baby's care from Day 1, even when babies are fragile or in an incubator. Your involvement matters and it strengthens your bond.

You may be able to:

- provide gentle touch through the incubator
- learn and follow your baby's unique cues
- participate in diaper changes when allowed
- help with temperature checks
- practice kangaroo care (skin-to-skin) when it is safe

Breastfeeding or pumping is also encouraged — even drops of colostrum are incredibly powerful for NICU babies, offering antibodies and immune protection that only you can give.

You Are Still Their Mother. They Still Know Your Love.

Even in the NICU, even behind tubes or wires, your baby knows your voice, your scent, your touch, and your presence. You are still the person they recognize, rely on, and feel comforted by.

And we — your NICU team — are here to support both of you, every step of the way.

Building a Bond in the NICU

The NICU experience is unique — parents and babies learn how to connect in ways that go beyond immediate holding or cuddling. For mothers, there may be an emotional longing to hold their baby right away, but in the NICU, bonding may look different at first. This does **not** mean the bond isn't happening — it's simply happening in new, beautiful ways.

Nurse's Note:

Although it may not feel the same as holding your baby at first, you *are* creating an incredibly important bond. Your baby can hear your voice and your presence is comforting. Speak to them, sing to them, gently touch their hands or feet. These actions are powerful for their development and emotional security.

Parents can bond through:

- voice
- touch
- scent
- presence

Speaking softly, singing, and touching their tiny fingers or toes through the incubator walls all foster connection. These moments matter more than you could ever imagine — babies recognize their parents' voices and respond to their touch, even in the NICU.

Parents should also lean on their support networks during this time. Feeling overwhelmed, uncertain, or even scared is normal. Connecting with:

- other NICU parents
- NICU nurses and doctors
- support groups
- counseling resources

...can help mothers and families navigate both the emotional and physical challenges of the NICU journey.

What NICU Admission Means for the Family

The NICU journey is often one of the hardest and longest a family will ever face. It demands patience, strength, and trust in the healthcare team. For many parents, it feels like a waiting game:

waiting for weight gain
waiting for stable breathing
waiting for test results
waiting to finally bring their baby home

Nurse's Note:

Celebrate the small victories. Every ounce gained, every tube removed, every stable day — these are BIG wins. Your baby is showing strength every single day and we will be with you every step of this journey.

The NICU is ultimately a place of **healing, hope, and progress**. Each day your baby spends there is a day closer to coming home. It is often the place where families witness just how strong their little one truly is.

The NICU team becomes part of your extended family — offering expert medical care, emotional support, and constant reassurance. They don't just care for the baby; they care for the parents, too. Their goal is to guide your family toward a safe, successful homecoming.

The Road to Home

After days, weeks, or even months in the NICU, discharge day is one of the most emotional milestones. Your baby has fought hard, grown stronger, and is finally ready to continue their journey in the comfort of home.

It may feel bittersweet to leave the safety of the NICU behind, but it is also a sign of how far your baby has come.

Nurse's Note:

When it is time to bring your baby home, we will help you prepare. You'll leave with the knowledge, training, and confidence you need — including follow-up appointments, feeding plans, developmental recommendations, and any special care your baby may require.

The NICU journey is a testament to the strength of both the baby **and** the parents. It is a chapter you will never forget, and the bond formed during this time will stay with you for a lifetime. Families who weather the NICU journey emerge more connected, more resilient, and more grateful than ever before.

21

Immediate Postpartum Recovery – Vaginal and C-Section Births

"The postpartum period is a time of healing, rest, and adjustment for both mother and baby."

The birth of your baby marks the beginning of an entirely new chapter — one filled with joy, emotion, and massive transformation. While all eyes naturally gravitate toward the newborn, your body is also going through one of the most important transitions of your life. Postpartum recovery, whether following a vaginal or C-section birth, is a time of **healing**, **recovery**, and **rediscovery.**

Understanding what happens in the hours and days after giving birth can help you feel more confident, prepared, and supported during this vulnerable period.

This chapter will walk you through the **universal recovery experiences** that happen after both vaginal and cesarean births. In the chapters that follow, we'll dive deeper into the **specific recovery details** for each birth individually.

The Medication We Give After Birth: Pitocin

Right after your baby is born, we give you a dose of **Pitocin** — either through your IV or as an injection into your thigh. This is standard care for all vaginal and cesarean births. Pitocin helps your uterus contract firmly after delivery, which is essential for preventing **postpartum hemorrhage**. A well-contracted uterus squeezes the blood vessels where the placenta detached, reducing bleeding and helping your body begin its immediate recovery.

You may notice your uterus tightening or feeling "crampy," especially if this isn't your first baby — that's the Pitocin doing exactly what it's supposed to do. These after-birth cramps can feel intense at times, but they are temporary, normal, and an important part of keeping you safe.

Why Uterine Contraction Matters After Birth

Think of the placenta like a scab.
When it detaches after delivery, it leaves behind a raw, open area inside your uterus. If pressure isn't applied to that spot, it will continue to bleed. Your uterus stopping that bleeding is **just like applying firm, steady pressure to a wound.**

That pressure comes from **uterine contractions.**
When your uterus firms up, it clamps down on the blood vessels where the placenta was attached — protecting you from postpartum hemorrhage.

When your uterus becomes soft or "boggy," it can't clamp those vessels closed. That's when bleeding becomes dangerous.

That's why your nurse will:

- Check your belly frequently
- Massage your fundus (even though it's uncomfortable)
- Give medications like **Pitocin, Cytotec, Hemabate, or Methergine** to help your uterus contract

Nurse's Tip:

- A firm uterus feels like a **hard grapefruit** just below your belly button – this is exactly what we want.
- If it feels soft or mushy, we massage it until it firms up.
- It may not feel pleasant, but it is absolutely lifesaving.

Your uterus carried your baby; now it protects **you.** It knows what to do — and we're simply helping it along.

What We're Checking When We Press on Your Belly

Every time your nurse presses on your abdomen postpartum, we're assessing your **fundus** — the top of your uterus.

We're checking for three things:

1. Is it firm?

A firm uterus = good contraction = less bleeding.

2. Is it midline?

If it's shifted to one side, your bladder might be full and blocking it from contracting properly.

3. Is it shrinking?

Each day, your uterus moves lower in your abdomen as it returns to its pre-pregnancy size.

Nurse's Tip:

- Emptying your bladder makes fundal checks easier and safer.
- Fundal checks are uncomfortable, especially right after birth – breathing through the discomfort helps.
- Ask us to guide your hand so you can feel it too. It's incredible to feel the home that held your baby for months.

When we press on your belly, it's not random — it's one of the most important assessments to ensure you're healing safely.

Bleeding (Lochia)

Postpartum bleeding — called **lochia** — is normal after both vaginal and cesarean births.

You may see:

- Heavier bleeding in the first few days
- Small clots
- Gradual tapering over the next several weeks
- Color changes (red → pink/brown → yellow/white)

When to Be Concerned:

- Soaking through **more than one pad per hour**

- Passing clots larger than a golf ball
- Bleeding that suddenly increases
- Fever or foul-smelling discharge

Nurse's Note:

We'll be monitoring your bleeding closely — but *your* awareness matters too. If something feels off, looks unusual, or seems like "too much," please tell us immediately. Early recognition saves lives.

Postpartum Bleeding (Lochia): What's Normal and What's Not

After birth, every woman experiences vaginal bleeding called **lochia** — your body's natural way of cleansing and healing the uterus after the placenta detaches. Because that placental site is like a large internal wound, bleeding is expected and normal. What helps is knowing *what's normal*, *what's not*, and *when to call for help.*

Let's walk through it together.

The Normal Stages of Lochia

1. Lochia Rubra (Days 1–3) (Cleveland Clinic, 2025)

Deep red, heavy, and similar to a very heavy period.
You may notice:

- Bright red bleeding
- Small clots (no larger than a quarter)
- Increased flow when standing after resting
- A gush when breastfeeding (oxytocin makes the uterus contract)

All of this is normal — gravity and hormones are hard at work.

2. Lochia Serosa (Days 4–12) (Cleveland Clinic, 2025)

The flow begins to lighten and change color:

- Pink, brown, or lighter red
- Smaller clots or none at all
- Steadier, more manageable flow

This is your uterus shrinking and healing beautifully.

3. Lochia Alba (Days 12 up to 6 weeks) (Cleveland Clinic, 2025)

Your discharge shifts into:

- Creamy white
- Pale yellow
- Minimal spotting

This phase can last **up to six weeks** and signals that your uterus is almost completely healed.

When to Call Your Nurse or Provider

Postpartum bleeding should *steadily improve.*
Reach out immediately if you experience:

- Soaking **more than one pad per hour**
- A sudden gush of bright red bleeding after it had already lightened
- Clots larger than a golf ball
- Bleeding with a foul odor (possible infection)
- Fever or chills
- Feeling dizzy, faint, or weak
- Bleeding that just "doesn't feel right"

Your instincts matter — trust them.

Nurse's Tip

- Change pads frequently (no tampons or menstrual cups until cleared).
- Rest as much as possible – heavy activity can trigger bleeding to increase again.
- Breastfeeding causes your uterus to contract, so don't be alarmed if bleeding increases while feeding.
- Keep track of your bleeding pattern. Your nurse will want to know what's normal for *you*.

Postpartum bleeding is a natural, healthy part of recovery. It should taper, lighten, and shift in color – not worsen. If anything concerns you, please reach out. Your safety is our priority.

Afterbirth Cramps: Why You Still Feel Contractions

Just when you're ready to celebrate the end of contractions… your uterus has one more job to do.

Afterbirth pains — or postpartum contractions — are your uterus shrinking back to its pre-pregnancy size. These cramps:

- Happen in the first few days after birth
- Are stronger with each subsequent baby
- Intensify during breastfeeding or pumping
- Feel similar to menstrual cramps or early labor
- Are completely normal and necessary

Why?

Because your uterus is clamping down on the placental site, putting pressure on the area to stop bleeding — just like pressing on a wound.

This is healing.
This is recovery.
This is your uterus doing exactly what it was designed to do.

Why They Happen

After you deliver, your uterus — which expanded to hold your baby and placenta — begins shrinking back to its pre-pregnancy size. Every time it contracts, it squeezes down on those open blood vessels inside, preventing bleeding and promoting healing.

So those cramps? They're your uterus doing its job.

Think of it as your body's natural way of saying, **"Okay… time to heal now."**

Fun Fact: The more babies you have, the stronger these afterbirth cramps tend to feel. With each pregnancy, the uterus has to work a little harder to regain its tone — and you'll definitely notice the difference. Ask for pain management!

When You'll Notice Them Most

During breastfeeding or pumping

Oxytocin — the same hormone that helps with your milk let-down — also triggers uterine contractions.
So if you feel a sudden wave of cramping right as your milk begins to flow, that's totally normal.

When standing up or moving around

Gravity shifts blood inside your uterus, which can trigger more cramping.

In the first few days postpartum

They are strongest in the first 48–72 hours, then gradually settle as your uterus heals.

How to Find Relief

Pain medication

Take ibuprofen, acetaminophen, or narcotic as ordered — they're safe, effective, and commonly used postpartum.

Heat therapy

A warm compress or heating pad across your lower abdomen helps soothe tight muscles.

Deep breathing

The same slow, controlled breathing you used during labor can help ease this discomfort too.

Empty your bladder regularly

A full bladder can push on the uterus and make cramps feel much worse.

> **Nurse's Tip:** If your cramping suddenly becomes severe, is paired with **heavy bleeding**, or doesn't improve after several days, let your nurse or provider know.
> Discomfort is normal.
> **Sharp, severe, or worsening pain is not.**

Every twinge and tightening means your body is healing. The contractions that helped bring your baby into your arms are now helping your uterus recover and protect you.

How the Uterus Shrinks After Birth (Involution)

Your uterus is an extraordinary organ. It grew from the size of a pear to the size of a watermelon over the course of your pregnancy — and now it begins the process of shrinking back down. This process is called **involution**, and it's one of the most important parts of postpartum healing.

What's Happening Inside

As your uterus contracts, it squeezes down on the open blood vessels where the placenta was attached. Those contractions — the same ones that cause afterbirth cramps — gradually make the uterus smaller, firmer, and lower in your abdomen each day.

Immediately after birth, your uterus weighs about **2 pounds** and can be felt at or just below your belly button. By the end of the first week, it's half that size, and within about **six weeks**, it returns to its pre-pregnancy weight of just a few ounces (Chauhan & Tadi, 2022).

What You'll Notice Day by Day

Right after delivery

The fundus (top of the uterus) sits at or slightly below your belly button and feels firm, like a grapefruit.

12 hours postpartum

It may rise slightly above the umbilicus — totally normal and expected.

Each day after

It moves about one fingerbreadth lower as it continues to shrink.

By 10–14 days

The uterus has usually slipped back behind the pubic bone and can no longer be felt through your abdomen.

(Berens, 2025)

How You Can Help

Breastfeed or pump

Oxytocin helps your uterus contract efficiently, speeding healing.

Empty your bladder regularly

A full bladder can push the uterus upward and interfere with contraction and may lead to unnecessary postpartum bleeding. Go pee!

Rest and hydrate

Fatigue and dehydration can slow the natural healing process.

Call your provider if:

- Your bleeding suddenly increases
- You develop a fever
- Your uterus feels soft, boggy, or unusually tender

Ask your provider about a belly band

These can make you feel more supported — many women describe it as feeling "put back together."

> **Nurse's Tip:** It's normal for your uterus to feel a little sore or crampy as it works its way back down. Think of it as your body **"tidying up"** after doing the biggest job it will ever do.
>
> Your uterus brought life into the world – and now it's gently guiding you back to yourself.

Why We Check Your Vital Signs After Birth

After giving birth, your body goes through major changes — fast. For the first few hours, your nurse will check your vital signs frequently: **blood pressure, heart rate, temperature, and respirations**. It might feel repetitive, but each number tells us something important about how your recovery is going.

We're not just being thorough — **we're being protective**. Frequent vital sign checks help us catch subtle warning signs early, long before they become serious.

Here's What We're Watching For

Blood Pressure (BP)

We monitor for both high and low readings.

- **High BP** may be a sign of postpartum preeclampsia.
- **Low BP** can signal excess bleeding or fluid loss.

If your BP is abnormal, we may recheck frequently or draw labs to keep you safe.

Heart Rate (Pulse)

A rising heart rate can indicate:

- pain
- anxiety
- infection
- bleeding

We look for patterns — not just one number.

Temperature

A fever after birth may indicate infection:

- uterine infection (endometritis)
- urinary tract infection
- breast infection (mastitis)

Even a mild temperature can matter, especially after a long labor or prolonged rupture of membranes.

Respirations (Breathing)

We monitor your breathing closely — especially if you had:

- magnesium sulfate
- an epidural
- certain pain medications

Shallow or slowed breathing can indicate a medication side effect that needs quick attention.

What the Schedule Looks Like

In most hospitals, your vital signs follow a structured pattern designed to catch any early warning signs while letting you rest and bond with your baby. A typical schedule looks like this:

- **Every 15 minutes for the first 2 hours**
- **Every hour for the next 2 hours**
- **Every 2 hours for two checks**
- **Then every 4 hours for the next 24 hours**

This pattern can vary depending on:

- your hospital's policies
- whether you had a vaginal birth or a C-section
- how your body is recovering
- any medications or interventions you received

Think of it as a gradual widening of the safety net — close monitoring at first, then less frequent as you stabilize and heal.

> **Nurse's Tip:** If you start to feel off – dizzy, sweaty, shaky, lightheaded, unusually anxious, or just "not right" – speak up immediately. You know your body better than anyone and your instincts are powerful.
>
> Don't hesitate to ask what we're looking for or what your numbers mean. Nurses love to teach and understanding your own care helps you feel confident and in control.

These checks aren't interruptions — they're our quiet, steady way of keeping you safe while your body recovers from one of the most intense experiences it will ever go through.

Emotional Recovery: The First Days After Birth

The days following birth come with a swirl of emotions — joy, relief, exhaustion, overwhelm, tenderness, tears, pride. Your hormones shift dramatically after delivery and that can create emotional highs and lows.

This is incredibly common.

The Baby Blues

Up to 80% of mothers experience:

- mood swings
- tearfulness that comes out of nowhere
- irritability
- feeling overstimulated or overwhelmed
- moments of sadness mixed with joy

These usually peak around days 3–5 postpartum and improve within two weeks as hormone levels stabilize and your body finds its rhythm (American Pregnancy Association, 2025).

When It's More Than the Blues

For some, emotions become heavier. Postpartum depression (PPD) can appear anytime in the first year and may include:

- persistent sadness or hopelessness
- feeling disconnected from your baby
- overwhelming anxiety
- loss of interest in things you normally enjoy
- guilt or thoughts like "I'm not a good mother"
- difficulty sleeping even when baby sleeps
- feelings of panic, dread, or fear

Nurse's Note:

These feelings are not your fault — not even a little bit.
PPD is a medical condition, not a reflection of your strength or your ability to parent.

Talking about your feelings is an act of courage, not weakness. Tell your nurse, doctor, or midwife if you're experiencing:

- excessive crying
- intrusive thoughts
- persistent sadness
- difficulty bonding with your baby

We're here to protect *you*, not just your baby.

You deserve joy, support, and healing — and there is help for every mother who needs it.

22

Vaginal Birth Recovery

"The postpartum recovery after a vaginal birth is a time of healing, rest, and finding strength in the journey ahead."

The recovery process after a vaginal birth is both physical and emotional. While the birth of your baby is a momentous occasion, it's important to remember that your body needs time to heal from the effort of bringing new life into the world. Understanding what to expect during your recovery will help you navigate the days and weeks ahead with confidence.

The Perineum

One of the most immediate areas of recovery after a vaginal birth is the perineum—the area between the vagina and anus. Whether you had a tear or an episiotomy, this area can be sore and swollen for several days. It's normal to feel discomfort, but there are ways to manage and soothe the area as it heals.

Perineal Care and Comfort Measures

After birth, it's normal to feel sore, swollen, or tender in your perineal area — the space between your vagina and rectum. This area stretches (and sometimes tears) during delivery, and if you've had stitches or an episiotomy, it needs gentle care while healing.

Just like the rest of your body, your perineum deserves attention, patience, and comfort measures to help you recover smoothly.

How We Help You Heal

Your nurses will guide you through perineal care, which includes:

Ice packs: Used for the first 24 hours to reduce swelling and numb discomfort.

Peri bottle: A small squeeze bottle filled with warm water that you'll use every time you go to the bathroom instead of wiping. Gently rinse from front to back to keep the area clean and reduce stinging.

Warm sitz baths: After the first 24 hours, soaking your bottom in warm water (with or without Epsom salt or a healing solution) promotes circulation and soothes soreness.

Witch hazel pads (Tucks) and Dermaplast spray: Calm burning and numbs area which helps with inflammation.

Perineal pillows or donut cushions: Reduce pressure when sitting.

Nurse's Tip:

Change your pad frequently – at least every few hours.
Avoid perfumed sprays or wipes – they can irritate healing tissue.
Pat gently dry after using the peri bottle – don't rub.
Keep stitches clean and dry; they'll dissolve on their own.

What's Normal:

Mild to moderate soreness and swelling for the first few days

A bruised or heavy sensation, especially when sitting

Light bleeding or pink discharge

Tenderness around any stitches or repaired areas

Discomfort usually improves significantly within the first week, but full healing can take several weeks.

What's Not Normal:

Perineal Hematoma: What It Is and What You Need to Know

A perineal hematoma is a collection of blood under the skin of the perineum — the area between the vagina and rectum. It happens when a blood vessel breaks during birth and bleeds into the surrounding tissue instead of outward. Hematomas are **not common**, but when they occur, they can be **very painful** and need quick recognition so we can treat them.

Think of it like a deep bruise that forms suddenly… but grows quickly and creates intense pressure.

Why They Happen

A perineal hematoma can occur after:

- a fast or forceful birth
- baby coming out in an unusual position
- a vacuum or forceps-assisted delivery
- a larger baby
- prolonged pushing

- trauma to delicate tissue
- a laceration that bled internally instead of externally

Most of the time, it is **not caused by anything you did or didn't do.** It's simply anatomy, pressure, and the mechanics of birth.

What It Feels Like

Patients often describe:

- **severe, deep, throbbing pain** in the perineum
- pain that feels **much worse** than expected for their degree of tearing
- intense pressure that doesn't ease, even with medication
- difficulty sitting, standing, or walking
- a feeling of **fullness or heaviness** in the perineum

A major red flag is pain that **suddenly worsens instead of improving** after birth.

What It Looks Like Clinically

As nurses, we may see:

- one-sided swelling of the perineum
- purple, blue, or dark red discoloration
- a tense, firm, or tight area under the skin
- a distinct "ball-like" bulge
- the swelling increasing in size quickly

A hematoma may stay small and stable… or it may expand rapidly, which requires immediate intervention.

How We Treat It

Treatment depends on size, rate of growth, and symptoms.

Small Hematomas

These may be managed conservatively with:

- ice packs
- pressure
- pain medication
- bed rest
- close monitoring
- perineal support

Most small hematomas **reabsorb on their own** over time.

Large or Expanding Hematomas

These require more aggressive treatment:

- draining the hematoma
- suturing the bleeding vessel
- applying pressure dressings
- IV pain management
- sometimes surgery (rare but possible)

Quick treatment brings relief and prevents complications.

Nurse's Reassurance

Perineal hematomas can feel shocking because the pain is so sharp, deep, and sudden — but your team is trained to recognize and treat them **immediately**.

Your nurse will:

- listen carefully to your concerns

- assess your pain seriously
- examine the area thoroughly
- monitor for changes
- call your provider promptly if anything seems unusual
- stay with you through the process

You are never expected to determine what's normal and what isn't. **That's our job — and we take postpartum perineal pain very seriously.**

With treatment, rest, and supportive care, most women recover quickly and fully. Be sure to ask for pain management to alleviate discomfort. Hematomas can be quite painful.

Nurse's Note

Use your peri bottle every time you use the bathroom after a vaginal birth — warm water eases discomfort and keeps the area clean. Apply witch hazel pads and Dermaplast for cooling relief and don't worry about your stitches — they will dissolve on their own. Follow all care instructions from your nurse or provider and speak up if your pain feels "different," deep, or out of proportion to what you expect.

Pain Relief Medications

Postpartum recovery may come with some pain, especially in the early days. Fortunately, there are medications available to help manage discomfort, including over-the-counter pain relievers and any prescribed medications from your care team.

Ibuprofen (Motrin): This medication helps reduce inflammation and alleviates soreness. It is often prescribed to manage general postpartum pain, especially in the perineum and lower back.

> **Nurse's Note**: Motrin is effective for managing moderate pain and inflammation. You may be instructed to take it regularly for the first few days to help with swelling and soreness. Be sure to take it with food to avoid an upset stomach.

Tylenol (Acetaminophen): Tylenol can help with general pain relief, especially if you're experiencing headaches or mild discomfort. It's typically used in conjunction with Motrin but make sure to follow your doctor's instructions regarding dosing.

> **Nurse's Note**: Tylenol is often used alongside Motrin to control pain. Always check with your healthcare provider to ensure you're taking the right medications at the right times. It's safe to take them together, but it's important to follow your healthcare provider's specific recommendations.

Pitocin highlight: If you were given Pitocin during delivery to help stimulate uterine contractions and deliver the placenta, you may feel some continued uterine cramping or afterpains, especially while breastfeeding. This is a normal part of the recovery process.

First Time Out of Bed

One of the first challenges after a vaginal birth is getting out of bed and moving around. It's important to take things slowly and be gentle with your body as it heals. When you first stand up, do not be surprised if your body feels out of whack, you feel like you've been hit by a car, or your internal organs just feel out of place. That baby took up a big part of you and things are readjusting.

> **Nurse's Note**: If you had an epidural during your delivery, it may take a little while for the numbness to wear off. You'll be monitored carefully as the anesthesia wears off and we'll help you stand up when you're ready. The first time you get out of bed, we'll make sure you have support and can move safely. Do not walk around with the baby unless you are positive your legs work and your nurse has cleared you to do so.

Moving Around for the First Time: After delivery, you'll be encouraged to get out of bed as soon as it's safe and as often as possible. This helps prevent blood clots and promotes circulation. However, your first time out of bed should be slow and steady—don't rush the process.

> **Nurse's Note**: When you're ready to get out of bed, I'll be here to help you. Start by sitting on the edge of the bed for a few minutes before standing. You may feel a little lightheaded at first, but don't worry, I'll be right here to support you. Take your time and move at your own pace.

Continued Care and Support

As you recover from vaginal birth, your care doesn't end once you're out of bed. Ongoing support is key to your physical and emotional well-being during this period.

Nurse's Note: If you experience any additional discomfort, bleeding, or feel unwell, please let us know. It's important that we monitor your progress and adjust your care as needed. We want to ensure you have the best possible recovery.

23

C-Section Birth Recovery

"Stitched on the outside. Unstoppable on the inside."

A C-section (cesarean section) is a surgical procedure that requires a longer recovery time compared to a vaginal birth, as the body needs time to heal from the incision made in the abdomen and uterus. While the baby is delivered safely, the mother's healing process is more complex and deserves patience, care, and understanding.

After the C-Section

After surgery, you'll move into the recovery area where your nurse will monitor:

- your vital signs
- your pain level
- your incision
- your bleeding
- your response to anesthesia

You will still have:

- your IV
- your foley catheter
- compression devices on your legs (to prevent blood clots)

As soon as you're stable, we help you begin skin-to-skin and feeding — **even if you can't fully sit up yet**.

About the Monitors

You may still be attached to:

- an EKG
- a blood pressure cuff
- a pulse oximeter
- IV fluids
- sometimes oxygen

I know it can feel frustrating — wires everywhere when all you want is to hold your baby, feed your baby, and sink into that moment. It's normal to feel like the monitoring equipment is "in your way."

But those monitors aren't there to inconvenience you — they're there to keep you safe as:

- anesthesia wears off
- your blood pressure stabilizes
- your uterus begins contracting
- your circulation changes
- your incision begins healing

As soon as it's appropriate, we begin removing them so you can move more freely.

And don't worry — your nurse will help you position pillows, elevate the bed, and adjust everything so you can comfortably **snuggle, feed, and bond** with your baby while still connected to the necessary equipment.

Expect Soreness and Fatigue

A C-section is major abdominal surgery. It is absolutely normal to feel:

- soreness
- weakness
- burning sensation on your incision
- pressure
- fatigue
- difficulty sitting up
- discomfort when coughing or laughing

Your nurse will guide you through:

- safe ways to move
- breathing exercises
- pain management
- early walking to prevent clots and promote healing

> **Nurse's Tip**
>
> It's completely normal to shake after a C-section or an epidural. This shaking can be intense – sometimes so strong that the blood pressure cuff can't pick up a reading.
>
> Here's a bedside trick:
>
> **Stick your tongue out slightly and gently bite down.**
>
> It activates a nerve reflex that often reduces the shaking just enough for the cuff to get a good reading.
>
> The shaking itself is **not dangerous** – it's simply your body reacting to anesthesia, hormones, adrenaline, and the sudden shift in temperature and circulation.
>
> This is not evidence based, just a Kimism. I heard it, used it, and it works.

Abdominal Incision Care

Your incision will feel tender, sore, or even numb in certain spots — all normal.

To protect your incision:

- keep the area clean and dry
- wash gently with mild soap and water (don't scrub)
- pat dry
- avoid tight waistbands
- avoid lifting anything heavier than your baby
- look daily for signs of infection

Call your provider if you notice:

- increasing redness
- warmth
- swelling
- separation of the incision
- drainage that is thick, yellow, foul-smelling, or pus-like
- fever or chills

Nurse's Note

You'll be given detailed instructions on caring for your incision. If something doesn't look or feel right, trust your instincts and reach out. Early attention prevents complications.

A Cesarean Birth Is Not a Lesser Birth

Your birth is still powerful.
Your story is still valid.
Your motherhood is still real.

How your baby enters the world does **not** define your strength.

C-section recovery is simply a different journey — one that requires patience, support, and grace.

Nurse's Note

Rest as much as possible.
Avoid heavy lifting.
Ask for help.
Be gentle with yourself — this is major surgery layered on top of becoming a mother.

Your body just brought life into the world. It deserves time, care, and compassion as it heals.

Pain Management After a C-Section

After a C-section, the spinal anesthesia used during surgery continues to provide pain relief for a period of time during recovery. As that medication begins to wear off, it's important to have a pain-management plan already in place. One of the most helpful things you can do for your recovery is to stay ahead of the pain rather than waiting for it to escalate. When pain becomes severe, it is much harder to control. Your comfort plays a vital role in your ability to breathe deeply, bond with your baby, breastfeed, walk, and heal.

Here's what to expect:

What Medications You'll Likely Receive
Most hospitals use a combination of medications that work together:

Ofirmev (IV Tylenol)

- Helps decrease baseline pain

- Reduces the need for stronger narcotics
- Works beautifully when given on a schedule

Toradol (Ketorolac) IV

- A powerful anti-inflammatory medication
- Helps with incision pain, cramping, and overall discomfort
- Think of it as "super ibuprofen," but stronger and IV

Narcotics (as needed) IV

- Provided only if necessary
- Helps ease deeper or breakthrough pain
- Used safely and in small doses to keep you comfortable

You are not expected to "tough it out." Your comfort is part of your recovery plan.

If You Had General Anesthesia

If your C-section required general anesthesia, your team will already have:

- pain medication ordered, usually in the form of a Patient-Controlled Analgesia (PCA) pump
- a plan ready for the recovery room
- a timeline for dosing
- monitoring in place to keep you safe and comfortable

The goal is for you to not wake up in severe pain — managing that is part of our job.

Why Staying Ahead of Pain Matters

There's a reason pain control is so important after surgery:

Fundal checks are very uncomfortable without medication.
We massage your uterus to help it clamp down and prevent postpartum bleeding and depending where you are at in your recovery, will determine how frequently we do this. This can be incredibly painful without adequate pain control — especially after a C-section.

Moving early helps prevent complications.
Good pain control helps you:

- breathe deeply
- sit up
- stand (when permitted)
- walk (when permitted)
- reduce the risk of blood clots
- feel steady on your feet

Pain affects bonding and feeding.
If you're in too much pain to move, hold your baby, or position yourself comfortably, everything becomes more difficult. Pain management supports both you and your baby.

Nurse's Reassurance

You just went through major abdominal surgery — while becoming a mother. You deserve good pain control. You deserve comfort. And you deserve a plan that supports your healing.

Tell your nurse when your pain starts to creep up. Don't wait. Your body heals better when it isn't fighting pain.

And we are here to help you every step of the way.

Mobility and Movement:

While it's important to rest, it's also crucial to start moving around as soon as possible to prevent complications like blood clots. You'll be encouraged to get out of bed and take short walks with help in the hours after surgery.

Nurse's Note 📝:

Moving as much as you can after your C-section will help prevent complications and speed up your recovery. We'll help you with your first steps and encourage you to walk around the room and eventually down the hallway. Take it slow, but don't be afraid to get moving.

Why You Might Feel Nauseated After a C-Section

It's very common to feel **nauseated** during or after a C-section, and it doesn't mean anything is wrong. The combination of anesthesia, changes in blood pressure, a suddenly empty uterus, and all the movement happening around your abdominal organs can trigger a wave of nausea. Some people feel it immediately; others feel it in recovery.

To help you stay comfortable, we use safe, effective medications like:

- **Zofran (Ondansetron)** — works quickly and gently to settle the stomach
- **Phenergan (Promethazine)** — stronger and longer-lasting for more intense nausea

Both medications are routinely used and very reliable. If you start to feel sick at any point, just tell us — we can treat it fast so you can focus on meeting your baby and settling into recovery.

Why You Might Feel Itchy After a C-Section

Itching after a C-section is **very common** and it doesn't mean you're having an allergic reaction. Most of the time, the itchiness comes from the **opioid medication** that's placed in your spinal or epidural to provide long-lasting pain relief after surgery. These medications can activate the itch receptors in your skin, especially on your face, chest, arms, and scalp.

It can be mild or surprisingly intense — but it's temporary and very treatable.

Medications We Use to Help

We have several safe and effective options to calm the itching quickly:

Nubain (Nalbuphine)

This is one of the most effective treatments for spinal-induced itching.

- Works fast
- Relieves itching **without** taking away your pain control
- Often the first medication we give

Benadryl (Diphenhydramine)

Great for itchiness that has a more histamine-like feel or for patients who want something extra calming.

- Helps take the edge off
- May make you sleepy, which many moms don't mind during recovery

Other Options We May Use

Depending on the cause and intensity of the itching, your provider may also use:

- **Zyrtec or Claritin** — non-drowsy antihistamines for milder itching
- **Low-dose Narcan** — used rarely, but can reverse the itching effects of spinal opioids **without** taking away your pain relief (a very tiny dose)

The Bottom Line

Itching after a C-section is normal, common, and completely manageable. Just let your team know — we can treat it quickly so you're comfortable, calm, and able to focus on your baby and your recovery.

A Gentle Heads-Up About Shoulder Pain After a C-Section

One of my favorite anesthesiologists used to gently prepare patients for a strange but very common sensation after a C-section: **shoulder pain**. It happens because, during surgery, a small amount of air can get trapped under the diaphragm. As your body adjusts, that air irritates a nerve that sends pain up into your shoulder — even though nothing is wrong there.

He always reassured patients ahead of time so they wouldn't panic or fear something serious like a heart attack. This shoulder pain is uncomfortable, but it's temporary, harmless, and very normal during recovery.

Knowing it can happen often brings a huge sense of relief. You're not in danger — it's just your body settling after surgery.

> **Nurse's Tip: Eating After a C-Section**
>
> After a C-section, anesthesia can temporarily slow down your digestion. This is completely normal and expected. You may be hungry but the key is to **start slow and listen to your body**. There is no rush – your body has just done something big. 🩷

> Eating too much or too quickly can lead to nausea or vomiting, which is especially uncomfortable with a fresh incision. Taking a gradual approach helps keep you comfortable and supports healing.

Simple Progression Chart

Ice chips / sips of water

Clear liquids (broth, apple juice, tea, popsicles)

Light foods (crackers, toast, soup, applesauce)

Regular diet as tolerated

ALWAYS FOLLOW YOUR PROVIDER'S ORDERS REGARDLESS

Nurse Reassurance:

If your appetite is low at first, that's okay. Your hunger will return as your body recovers. Small bites, slow pacing, and gentle choices go a long way in keeping you comfortable. When in doubt, ask your nurse — we're here to help you every step of the way.

Getting Feeling Back in Your Legs After a C-Section

After a C-section, it's completely normal for your legs to feel heavy, numb, or impossible to move. The spinal or epidural anesthesia wears off **gradually**, and your body needs time to regain full control. For many patients, this is the part that feels the most vulnerable — lying in bed while others reposition you, clean you, or help with the baby.

Most people begin getting feeling and movement back **about two hours after arriving in the recovery room**. You may notice tingling, warmth, or little bursts of sensation before full movement returns — all completely normal signs that the anesthesia is wearing off.

But here's the truth: **you are not useless.**
You just had major abdominal surgery and brought a human being into the world. Your only job in these first hours is to rest, recover, and let the medication clear from your system.

As sensation returns, your nurses will guide you step by step — helping you sit up, stand, and walk when it's safe, usually within the first 6–12 hours.

You are **not** a burden.
You are **not** helpless.
You are healing and you're already doing the most important job — loving and caring for your newborn in every way that matters.

Emotional Recovery:

Like a vaginal birth, a C-section birth can bring about a variety of emotions. You may feel disappointed if you had planned for a vaginal birth or be overwhelmed by the length of your recovery. It's normal to feel a mix of emotions after surgery.

Nurse's Note:

It's okay to feel frustrated or sad after a C-section. Your recovery may take longer, but that doesn't lessen the love you feel for your baby. Lean on your support system and talk to your nurse or doctor about any emotional struggles you might face.

24

Your First Moments Together

"I didn't just hold you. I finally held the piece of me I'd been missing."

The moment your baby is placed on your chest is the moment everything changes. After all the anticipation, all the work, all the waiting, this is where your story together truly begins. These first moments aren't about doing anything "right" — they're about simply being with your baby.

Breathing them in.
Feeling their warmth.
Hearing their tiny sounds.

Letting your heart adjust to the fact that this little person you've carried is finally in your arms.

Bonding isn't a performance or a timeline. It's a quiet unfolding and it looks different for every family. All that matters is that you are here, together, beginning your journey one gentle moment at a time.

First Skin-to-Skin Moments & Feeding Cues

Those first moments of **skin-to-skin contact** are powerful — and they matter more than many parents realize. Placing your baby directly on your bare chest right after birth (and often in the hours and days that follow) helps your baby feel safe, regulated, and ready to feed.

Why skin-to-skin is so important:

- Helps regulate your baby's temperature, heart rate, and breathing
- Promotes calmness and reduces crying
- Encourages natural feeding behaviors and improves latch
- Supports bonding and emotional connection
- Stimulates milk production and colostrum release

When babies are skin-to-skin, they are more likely to show **early feeding cues** — like rooting, bringing hands to mouth, and opening their mouth — before they ever cry.

Leading into feeding cues:

Skin-to-skin helps you *see* and *respond* to hunger cues sooner. A calm, regulated baby feeds more easily than a crying one. Crying is a **late hunger cue**, so feeding during those early signs often leads to a smoother, more relaxed feeding experience for both you and your baby.

Remember:

There is no "wrong" way to do skin-to-skin. Even short moments count. Whether it's immediately after birth, after a diaper change, or before a feeding, holding your baby close helps set the stage for successful feeding and a confident start together.

Nurse Reassurance: Feeding Cues (Crying Is a Late Sign)

Babies communicate hunger long before they cry. Crying is actually a **late hunger cue**, and once a baby is crying, feeding can be harder because they may need calming first. Learning early feeding cues can help feeds go more smoothly and feel less stressful for both you and your baby.

Early hunger cues (best time to feed):

- Smacking or licking lips
- Sticking out the tongue
- Bringing hands to mouth
- Turning head side to side (rooting)
- Opening the mouth or making soft sucking motions

Mid hunger cues:

- Stretching or increased movement
- Mild fussing
- Facial tension

Late hunger cue:

- Crying

Reassurance:

If your baby starts crying, it doesn't mean you've missed your chance or done anything wrong. Simply pause, cuddle, swaddle, or offer skin-to-skin to help calm them — then try feeding again. Feeding at early cues often leads to a calmer baby, easier latch, and a more relaxed feeding experience overall.

Your First Time Breastfeeding

That first time you bring your baby to your chest isn't just about feeding — it's about connection. Whether it happens right after birth or a little later, it's one of the most natural and emotional moments of your journey.

Your baby is born with an incredible instinct to find and latch onto the breast. During skin-to-skin contact, many newborns will bob their heads, open their mouths, and make rooting movements as they search for your nipple. Don't worry about doing it perfectly — your nurse or lactation consultant will be there to help guide you.

What to Expect

In those first moments, your baby may:

- lick
- nuzzle
- or suckle gently

before truly latching on. That's all part of learning.

A **good latch** feels like firm tugging — *not* pinching or biting. You might feel cramping (afterpains) as your uterus contracts — that's oxytocin at work, helping your body heal.

If your baby doesn't latch right away, take a breath. Sometimes it takes a few tries. We may help you try different positions — the football hold, cross-cradle, or side-lying — to find what's most comfortable for you and your baby.

How I Help You Start Breastfeeding

When it's time for that first feed, I'm going to guide you through it step-by-step — calmly, gently, and without rushing you. Breastfeeding is a skill **you and your baby learn together**, and I promise, you are not expected to know how to do it on your own.

Here's exactly how I help you start:

1. Wake up the colostrum (Manual Expression)

I'll have you massage all four quadrants of your breast — top, bottom, inner, and outer.
This helps stimulate your milk ducts and encourages the colostrum to start moving forward.

2. Shape your breast for your baby

Cup your breast like a hamburger (long ways across, not up and down). Then gently **pull backward toward your chest wall** and **roll forward**. You should see little drops of colostrum appear — this is your baby's "gold," and it's exactly what they're looking for. And when your baby gets a taste, they will know what they are working for.

3. Get *your* body comfortable first

You cannot breastfeed well if you're uncomfortable.
Your shoulders should be relaxed, your back supported, and your baby brought **to you** — not you leaning down to them.

4. Help your baby get a deep latch

When you bring your baby to the breast, keep the "hamburger hold" and aim your nipple slightly upward toward the roof of their mouth.

The goal is for **a good portion of your areola to go into their mouth**, not just the nipple.
A deep latch = comfortable feeding.
A shallow latch = pain, cracking, and sore nipples.

5. What a good latch looks like

Once your baby latches, here's what we want to see:

- Their jaw moving in a smooth, rhythmic motion
- Their cheeks flat (not puffing in and out)
- You hearing or seeing little swallows
- No pinching, sharp pain, or burning

A newborn may take a while to latch — that's normal. We're not rushing anything.

6. What you should feel

You might feel **a tugging, pulling sensation**, but you should not feel sharp pain.
If it hurts, we stop, breathe, and relatch. Pain is a sign the latch needs adjusting — not a sign that you need to "push through it."

Colostrum: Liquid Gold

At first, your body produces **colostrum**, a thick, golden-yellow fluid packed with antibodies and nutrients. It's small in volume but mighty in protection — exactly what your baby's tiny stomach needs.

Within a few days, your milk will:

- thin out
- turn white or bluish
- and increase in amount

Nurse's Tip:

- Don't stress about timing – let your baby lead the way.
- Keep your baby skin-to-skin as much as possible; warmth and closeness stimulate milk production.

- If it hurts, stop and reposition – pain usually means the latch needs adjustment.
- Ask for help – nurses and lactation consultants *love* helping new moms succeed.

Every feeding is a conversation between you and your baby — full of cues, connection, and comfort. You're both learning together.

Nurse Reassurance: "Is My Baby Getting Enough?"

It's very common to worry that your baby isn't getting enough colostrum or milk — especially in the first day or two. A helpful thing to remember is just **how tiny your baby's stomach really is**.

In the **first 24 hours of life**, your baby's belly is only about the **size of a marble**. That means **small amounts are not only normal — they're exactly right**.

Newborn belly size progression:

- **Day 1:** *Marble / small cherry* — about **5–7 mL per feeding**
- **Day 2:** *Walnut* — about **10–15 mL**
- **Day 3:** *Apricot* — about **20–30 mL**
- **By Day 7:** *Golf ball*

Colostrum is thick, concentrated, and powerful — a little truly goes a long way. Frequent feeding does **not** mean your baby isn't getting enough; it means your baby is doing exactly what newborns are designed to do.

In the first few days of life, one of the **best and simplest signs** that your baby is getting enough milk is what's showing up in their diaper. Newborn stomachs are tiny, feeds are frequent, and output gradually increases as milk transitions from colostrum to mature milk. Ask your nurse what their particular telltale diaper sign is that your baby is getting enough.

Reassurance:

If feeds seem short, amounts seem small, or your baby wants to eat often, take a breath — this is normal. Trust your baby, trust your body, and know your nurse is always there to support you, answer questions, and help you feel confident every step of the way.

Nurse's Tip:

Skin-to-skin and manual expression are powerful partners - one builds connection, the other builds confidence.

If your baby is in the NICU or can't go skin-to-skin yet, even holding a blanket or hat that smells like them while expressing can help trigger that same hormonal response.

Remember: your body knows what to do - sometimes it just needs a little warmth, touch, and reassurance to get started.

Common Breastfeeding Challenges and How Nurses Help

Breastfeeding is natural — but that doesn't mean it's always easy. Every mother-baby pair is unique, and it can take time, patience, and practice to find your rhythm together. You're learning just as much as your baby is and that's completely normal.

Here are a few common challenges new moms face — and how your nurses and lactation team can help.

Sore or Cracked Nipples

Tenderness is normal at first but pain or cracking usually means the latch needs adjusting. Your nurse or lactation consultant will help you position your baby so their mouth covers more of the areola, not just the nipple. We can also provide nipple creams, hydrogel pads, or saline soaks to soothe soreness while healing.

Tip: Air-dry your nipples after feeds and apply a little expressed breast milk — it's naturally healing.

Sleepy Baby

Some newborns are so relaxed — especially after a long labor — that they don't wake to feed often. Your nurse will help you recognize feeding cues (like hand-to-mouth movements or lip smacking) and show you gentle ways to wake your baby, such as unwrapping them, changing their diaper, or rubbing their back.

Tip: Skin-to-skin contact helps wake sleepy babies and stimulates their feeding instincts naturally.

Engorgement

When your milk first comes in, your breasts may feel full, firm, warm, and uncomfortable. This swelling is called **engorgement** and it can make latching more difficult for your baby.

Your nurses can help you:

- hand express a small amount of milk
- pump briefly (just 1–2 minutes) before feeding
- soften the areola to help baby latch
- use warm compresses **before** feeds to encourage flow
- use cool compresses **after** feeds to decrease swelling

Engorgement is temporary — and manageable — with frequent draining of the breast.

Tip: Frequent feeding is the best cure.
The more milk that's removed, the quicker the swelling improves.

Latch or Position Problems

Sometimes all it takes is a small adjustment in position to make breastfeeding more comfortable and effective. Your nurse will help you try different holds:

- cradle
- cross-cradle
- football
- side-lying
- laid-back breastfeeding

We'll look for signs of a good, deep latch:

- rhythmic sucking
- audible swallows
- relaxed hands and body
- minimal nipple pain

Tip: Bring your *baby* to the breast — not the breast to the baby.
This protects your back and helps your baby latch deeper and more effectively.

Worrying About Milk Supply

Almost every new mom worries she's not making enough — especially before her milk fully comes in. But your nurse will reassure you that **your body knows what to do**.

Signs your baby is getting enough:

- frequent feeding (8–12 times per day)
- several wet diapers
- softening of your breasts after feeds
- content periods between feeds
- steady weight gain

Supplementation isn't always necessary — but if it is, we'll walk you through safe methods that **protect your milk supply**, like paced bottle feeding or using a supplemental nursing system.

Tip: Trust your body.
Milk supply runs on a simple system: **the more your baby nurses, the more milk you make.**

Breastfeeding is a journey, not a test.
Some days will feel natural and easy and other days may take patience, learning, and teamwork. Your nurses and lactation consultants are here for both you and your baby — every step of the way.

For Moms Who Choose Not to Breastfeed

Let me start with this — loud and clear:

How you feed your baby is your choice.

Breastfeed, formula feed, or do both — what matters most is:

- your baby is fed
- your baby is loved
- *you* are supported

There are many reasons a mother may choose not to breastfeed: personal preference, medical considerations, past trauma, lifestyle needs, mental health, or simply knowing formula is the best fit for her family.

Whatever your reason — **it is valid.**

Modern formulas provide complete nutrition for healthy growth and development. Your nurse will help you learn:

- how to prepare formula safely
- how to store it
- how often to feed
- what hunger and fullness cues look like

And bottle-feeding can be *just as bonding* as breastfeeding.

Hold your baby close, talk to them, gaze into their eyes — this is connection, and it has nothing to do with how milk enters their tummy.

Nurse's Tip:

- Feed your baby without guilt or pressure.
- Hold your baby skin-to-skin during bottle feeds for added closeness.
- Choose what works best for *your* body, *your* recovery, and *your* family.

A fed baby is a thriving baby - and a confident, supported mother is the best gift you can give your child.

Breast Care and Mastitis Awareness

Even if you decide **not** to breastfeed, your body may still produce milk for a short time — that's completely normal. Caring for your breasts during this period helps keep you comfortable and prevents complications like mastitis (a breast infection).

Caring for Your Breasts

Supportive Bra

Wear a comfortable, supportive bra — not too tight.
Avoid binding your breasts; compression can make things worse and lead to clogged ducts.

Cold Compresses

If you feel engorged or uncomfortable, use:

- cold packs
- chilled cabbage leaves (Kimism)

Apply for **15–20 minutes** at a time to reduce swelling and soothe discomfort.

Avoid Stimulation

Try not to pump or express milk unless absolutely necessary — stimulation signals your body to **keep making milk**, which prolongs discomfort.

Pain Relief

Over-the-counter medications like ibuprofen (if approved by your provider) help reduce discomfort and inflammation.

If You *Are* Breastfeeding or Pumping

Keep the breasts emptied regularly.
Skipping feeds, wearing tight clothing, or going long periods between pumping sessions can trap milk and cause clogged ducts.

Signs of Mastitis

Mastitis happens when milk gets trapped and becomes infected.
It can occur whether you're:

- breastfeeding
- pumping
- weaning
- or not nursing at all

Watch for:

- **Red, warm, swollen area** on one breast
- **Pain or tenderness** that worsens instead of improves
- **Fever, chills, or flu-like symptoms**
- **Fatigue or feeling unwell**

If you notice these signs, **call your provider right away.** Most cases resolve quickly with antibiotics, continued milk removal (if lactating), and rest.

Nurse's Tip:

- Rest and hydration are just as important as medication when you're healing.
- If you're not breastfeeding and your breasts suddenly feel full, swollen, or painful, use **ice and a supportive bra** – the discomfort will pass in a few days as your body adjusts.
- Mastitis doesn't mean you did anything wrong – it simply means your body needs a little extra care.

Your breasts have worked hard — whether they fed your baby or simply prepared to. Treat them with the same kindness and patience you're giving the rest of your body.

Skin-to-Skin with Your Partner: The Power of Presence

No matter who your partner is — dad, mom, spouse, or support person — they are one of your baby's most important sources of love and comfort.

Skin-to-skin isn't just for birthing mothers — it's an evidence-based, powerful bonding tool that helps **both** baby and partner adjust emotionally and physiologically to this brand-new world.

Why It Matters

When your partner holds your baby skin-to-skin, incredible things happen:

- Baby's temperature stabilizes — your partner's body warms or cools to meet their needs
- Heart rate, breathing, and oxygen levels become more regular
- Stress hormones decrease in *both* baby and parent
- Oxytocin rises in your partner, increasing bonding and confidence

This moment is grounding and reassuring — especially when you're recovering, nursing, or simply catching your breath. It helps your partner feel involved, capable, and deeply connected from the start.

When It's Especially Helpful

- If you're in recovery after a **C-section**
- If baby needs the **nursery or NICU** temporarily
- During nighttime feeds
- While you're showering, resting, or being assessed
- Any time you need a moment to breathe, regroup, or recover

Nurse's Tip: Have your partner:

- remove their shirt
- place the baby (in just a diaper) directly on their bare chest
- cover both with a warm blanket
- and speak softly – babies recognize familiar voices and find comfort in them

Skin-to-Skin with Dad: The Biological Bond You Didn't Know Existed

While skin-to-skin contact benefits any loving partner, **fathers experience something uniquely powerful on a biological level**. Holding their newborn against bare skin doesn't just strengthen emotional connection — it triggers real, measurable changes in the father's body and brain.

The Science Behind the Bond

When a father holds his baby skin-to-skin:

Oxytocin Surges

- The same "love hormone" that rises in mothers during labor and breastfeeding floods dad's system too.
  It helps him bond, relax, and become more attuned to his baby's cues.

Temporary Drop in Testosterone

- This shift softens aggression and heightens nurturing instincts — a natural biological adjustment toward caregiving and protection.

Lower Stress (Cortisol Decreases)

- Dad becomes calmer, more grounded, and less anxious.
  Baby feels that calm instantly.

Dopamine Increases

- The "reward hormone" spikes, reinforcing joy, pride, and bonding — making dad want to hold, protect, and care for his baby again and again.

- In other words, **dad's body biologically transforms** to meet his newborn's needs.
  Nature designed fathers not just to protect — **but to nurture**.

Partner Reflection: "The First Time I Held You"

The first time I held you against my chest, everything else disappeared.
I could feel your heartbeat against mine — small, steady, perfect.

I didn't realize how much I needed that moment until it happened.
The warmth, the stillness, the way your body melted into mine…
it was as if the world had stopped to let us meet.

They told me skin-to-skin would help you breathe better and stay warm. What they didn't tell me was how it would change me — how it would make me feel connected, protective, and completely in awe of you.

In that moment, I wasn't just a bystander to your birth.
I became part of your story.

Nurse's Note

- Encourage your partner to take their time.
  These first quiet moments — **no screens, no distractions** — are powerful for both of them.
- That warmth.
  That stillness.
  That love.
  It becomes the first memory your baby carries into the world.

25

Baby Care in Recovery

"Every tiny act of care is a big act of love."

Once you and your baby are together in the recovery room — whether after a vaginal birth or a C-section — there are a few important things we do to make sure your newborn is transitioning safely into life outside the womb. These steps are routine, gentle, and designed to keep your little one warm, stable, and healthy while you get those first precious moments together.

Measurements: Getting to Know Your Baby

After your skin to skin time, we'll take your baby's:

- Weight
- Length
- Head circumference

These numbers become part of your baby's birth record (and usually the stats that everyone wants to text to family immediately!).

We try to do this **in the room** so your baby never has to leave your side unless absolutely necessary.

Be sure to take a picture of your beautiful baby next to their birth weight on the scale. Memories for a lifetime!

Vital Signs: Making Sure Baby Is Transitioning Well

We check baby's vitals frequently in the first hours. Here's what we look for — and what's considered normal for a newborn:

- **Heart Rate:** 110–160 beats per minute
- **Respiratory Rate:** 40–60 breaths per minute
- **Temperature:** 97.7–99.5°F (36.5–37.5°C)

Color & Tone: Pink lips, warm skin, good muscle tone

These checks help us make sure your baby is adapting beautifully outside the womb.

Footprints & Identification

Your newborn will receive:

- Footprints (keepsake + part of the medical chart)
- ID bands for baby, you, and your support person
- A security tag (usually on the ankle) — it alarms if someone tries to remove baby from a secure area

We double-check band numbers with you **every single time** we move baby or perform care — your baby's safety is our top priority.

Visit From the NICU or Pediatric Provider

Even if everything looks perfect, it's common for a pediatrician, neonatal nurse practitioner (NNP), or neonatologist to stop by.

They'll do:

- A quick but thorough physical exam
- Check muscle tone, reflexes, breathing, and color
- Listen to heart and lungs
- Make sure baby's transition is smooth
- Answer your questions

This visit is usually gentle, fast, and done right at your bedside.

Vitamin K & Erythromycin: What They Are and Why They Matter

Right after birth, there are two medications we routinely offer newborns to protect them as they transition into the world:

- **Vitamin K (the vitamin K shot)**
- **Erythromycin eye ointment**

Both have been used safely for decades, and each plays a very specific — and very important — role in newborn health.

These aren't "shots and ointments just because."
They are **evidence-based, preventative, and lifesaving when needed.**

Vitamin K Injection

What It Is

Vitamin K is a vitamin we all need in order to help our blood clot properly. Adults and older children get Vitamin K naturally from food and from healthy bacteria in the gut.
Newborns don't have these bacteria yet and breastmilk alone doesn't provide enough Vitamin K.

Why Newborns Need It

Babies are naturally born with very low levels of Vitamin K, which puts them at risk for a serious condition called:

VKDB – Vitamin K Deficiency Bleeding, which can cause:

- unexpected bruising
- gastrointestinal bleeding
- bleeding after circumcision
- dangerous internal bleeding
- **brain bleeding (most feared complication)**

VKDB can happen days or even weeks after birth — even in healthy breastfed babies.
Vitamin K is given to almost every newborn to prevent bleeding that you cannot predict or prevent on your own.

How It's Given

- A single injection into the baby's thigh
- Takes less than 2 seconds
- Typically causes only a brief cry
- Protects against VKDB for months

Does it hurt?

Like any shot, it stings briefly. But it's fast, safe, and incredibly important.

Can parents decline it?

You *can* — but it's strongly discouraged because VKDB is unpredictable and potentially fatal. Many hospitals require informed consent and documentation if refused.

Nurse's reassurance:

Vitamin K is one of the simplest, safest, and most effective ways to protect your newborn.

Nurse's Note

When it's time for your baby's shot, you don't have to step back. Your partner can come hold your baby's hand or we can give the shot while your baby is lying right on your chest. Being close to you helps calm them, steady their breathing, and makes the moment more comforting for everyone. You are part of your baby's care and we'll always give you the option to stay involved and keep them close.

Warning

Most hospitals will **not perform a circumcision** if your baby does **not** receive the **Vitamin K shot**.
Rationale: Vitamin K is essential for helping your baby's blood clot. Without it, newborns are at a higher risk for bleeding — including bleeding during a circumcision. The Vitamin K shot protects your baby from potentially serious complications and ensures the procedure can be done safely.

Erythromycin Eye Ointment

What It Is

Erythromycin is a gentle antibiotic ointment placed in your baby's eyes shortly after birth.

Why It's Used

Its purpose is to prevent **ophthalmia neonatorum**, a serious newborn eye infection caused by exposure to **gonorrhea or chlamydia** during birth.

Even if you tested negative during pregnancy, infections can happen later or go unnoticed. The ointment provides a protective barrier "just in case."

Without treatment, these infections can cause:

- severe eye swelling
- pus drainage
- corneal damage
- **blindness**

Erythromycin dramatically reduces these risks.

How It's Given

- A thin ribbon of ointment is placed inside each eye
- Baby may look blurry or "glazed" for a little while — totally normal
- It does **not** hurt
- It does **not** affect long-term vision
- You may wipe around the eyes after 1–2 hours — just don't wipe the ointment out right away

Does the ointment interfere with bonding?

Not really — but if you prefer, you can ask for it to be given after the first hour of skin-to-skin as long as baby is stable.

Can parents decline it?

Yes, in most states. But most hospitals require signing a refusal form because this protects against a potentially severe infection.

Nurse's reassurance:

This ointment is preventative — not a sign that anything is wrong. It simply protects your baby's eyes from infections that can be harmful if they happen.

Nurse's Note

If your baby gets erythromycin eye ointment, don't worry if they wipe their eyes or put their hands in their mouth afterward. The ointment is completely safe and won't harm them if a little gets on their skin or in their mouth. It's normal for babies to rub their eyes or seem a little "blurry-eyed" at first — it wears off quickly and everything is just fine.

Bringing It All Together

Both Vitamin K and Erythromycin are routine because they work. They protect newborns during the most vulnerable hours and days of life, and they allow parents to focus on bonding, feeding, and settling in — not worrying about complications.

Whether you choose one, both, or delay the timing, your nurse will explain everything, answer your questions, and help you make the decision that feels right for your family.

Your baby's safety is our priority, and these simple steps are part of that care.

Hepatitis B Vaccine: What It Is and Why It's Offered

The Hepatitis B vaccine is another routine newborn medication offered in the hospital — usually later in the postpartum period, after the first hours of bonding, feeding, and settling in. Unlike Vitamin K or Erythromycin, this one isn't urgent, which is why many hospitals give it toward the end of your stay or before discharge.

Here's what you need to know:

What Hepatitis B Is

Hepatitis B is a virus that affects the liver. It can be passed from person to person through:

- blood
- bodily fluids
- unsterile needles
- unexpected injuries later in childhood
- and, less commonly, from mother to baby

It can lead to chronic liver disease if contracted early in life.

Why We Give the Vaccine at Birth

Babies are vaccinated early because:

- Infants who contract Hep B have a greater chance of developing chronic infection.
- Newborns respond extremely well to the vaccine and build strong immunity.
- Not all exposures are predictable — siblings, caregivers, daycare settings, or accidental contact can all be sources.
- The birth dose acts as the first layer of protection, even if mom tests negative.
- For babies born to Hepatitis B–positive mothers, the birth dose is essential and given immediately.

But for most families, the vaccine is offered in the hours or days after delivery, not right away.

When It's Given

Timing varies by hospital, but usually:

- Before discharge from the postpartum unit
- Sometimes on the first or second postpartum day
- After parents have had time to bond, rest, and ask questions

It's not urgent, and your nurse will explain your options.

How It's Given

- A small injection in the baby's thigh
- Quick, safe, and well-tolerated
- No major side effects other than brief fussiness or mild soreness
- Most babies cry for a moment, then settle easily with skin-to-skin, feeding, or cuddling.

Do You Have to Get It?

You can:

- say yes
- delay it
- or decline and have it done at the pediatrician's office.

However, most pediatricians strongly recommend the birth dose because it provides the earliest protection during a period when babies are most vulnerable.

Your nurse will provide the information — and you make the decision that feels right for your family.

Nurse's Reassurance

The Hepatitis B vaccine isn't about assuming risk — it's about building protection early, when your baby's immune system is brand new. It's safe, it's well-studied, and it gives your baby a head start against a virus that can be serious later in life.

But the choice is always yours. We're here to educate, not pressure. You'll never be rushed and your questions will always be welcomed.

If Your Baby Is a "Sugar Baby"

If your baby is considered a "sugar baby," it simply means they are at risk for low blood sugar (hypoglycemia) after birth. Babies who fall into this category may include: infants of diabetic mothers, babies who are smaller or larger than expected, late-preterm babies, babies of mothers who have taken certain medications, or those who had a stressful delivery.

If your baby fits one of these groups, we'll check their blood sugar in the first hours of life. It's a quick heel stick that gives us an immediate reading. Newborns rely on stable blood sugar to stay warm, calm, alert, and able to feed well — so these checks help us make sure your little one is transitioning smoothly.

If a sugar level is low, we'll respond right away with feeding, glucose gel, or additional support. It's not a sign that anything is "wrong" with your baby — just an extra layer of safety to keep them healthy while their body learns how to regulate its own sugars.

Nurse's Note

If your baby is a "sugar baby," keeping them warm is extra important. When newborns get cold, they burn through their stored sugar to generate heat — and that can put them at higher risk for hypoglycemia. Keeping your baby skin-to-skin, wrapped in blankets, and wearing an approved hat helps them conserve energy and maintain stable blood sugars. Warmth isn't just comfort — it's part of their care.

Nurse's Reassurance

These early steps all have one purpose: **to keep your baby safe while keeping your baby with you.**

You will never feel rushed, separated without explanation, or left wondering what's happening. Everything we do — every measurement, every vital check, every tag and footprint — is to ensure your baby is healthy, stable, and right where they belong: in your arms.

Circumcision: To Choose It or Not – Understanding Your Options

Circumcision is one of the most common newborn procedures, but it's also one of the most personal decisions a family can make. There is no right or wrong choice — only the choice that feels right for your baby, your beliefs, and your family.

My goal as your nurse isn't to sway you but to give you the information and reassurance you need to feel confident in whatever you choose.

Why Some Parents Choose Circumcision

Families may decide to circumcise for:

- Cultural or religious traditions
- Family preference or wanting baby to "match" a parent
- Perceived hygiene benefits
- Reduced risks of certain infections later in life
- Provider recommendation for medical reasons (rare)

If you choose circumcision, it is typically done:

- In the hospital
- Within the first 24–48 hours
- With pain control (usually a numbing injection + oral sucrose)
- In just a few minutes

Your baby may be sleepy after the procedure — that is normal.

Why Some Parents Choose Not to Circumcise

Families may decide not to circumcise because:

- They prefer to keep the penis intact
- No cultural or religious reason to do it
- They want their child to decide later
- They feel comfortable with caring for the foreskin
- They prefer to avoid any unnecessary procedures

Intact care is simple:
Do not retract the foreskin.
Just wash the outside gently with water during baths.
It naturally separates on its own over time.

If You Choose Circumcision – What to Expect

The procedure is quick. During and after, many places use:

- Numbing cream or injection
- Sucrose (sweet drops) for comfort
- Swaddling and soothing
- Careful bleeding checks afterward

Afterward, you'll see:

- A small amount of blood (like a scraped knee)
- A raw, wet appearance (normal)
- Swelling that generally improves over 24–48 hours

How to Care for It

- Use petroleum jelly with gauze each diaper change to prevent sticking
- Keep the area clean and dry
- Healing complete within 4 weeks (Warees et al., 2024)
- Call your provider if you notice continuous bleeding, unusual swelling, or pus

If You Choose Not to Circumcise – What's Normal?

The foreskin is attached at birth and protects the penis. Over time, it will naturally loosen — sometimes years later.

What to know:

- Never retract the foreskin
- Clean the outside only
- It will separate on its own as your child grows
- Redness at the tip from urine is harmless and common

Nurse's Reassurance

Circumcision is a choice, not a requirement. Babies do equally well circumcised and uncircumcised. What matters most is:

- You feel comfortable
- Your questions are answered
- Your baby is cared for gently, respectfully, and safely

Whatever you choose, your nurses will guide you every step of the way — with no judgment, no pressure, and full support.

26

Transition from Immediate Recovery to Postpartum: The Hand-Off of Care

"New phase, new nurses, same incredible care."

After your initial recovery period in Labor and Delivery, you'll transition to the postpartum unit — a quiet, healing space designed for rest, bonding, and learning your new baby. During this handoff, your labor nurse will give a thorough report to your postpartum nurse, sharing everything about your birth, your recovery so far, your preferences, and any special needs you or your baby may have. This ensures your care continues seamlessly, without you ever needing to repeat a single detail. Your postpartum nurses will take over from there, guiding you through pain control, feeding support, newborn care, and helping you settle into your new role as a parent. It's a smooth, compassionate relay — one team passing you gently to the next, all with your comfort and safety at the center. But before that, we help you with:

Your First Time Out of Bed

Once your delivery is complete and your nurse has confirmed that your bleeding and vital signs are stable, it'll soon be time for one of the biggest milestones after birth — **getting out of bed for the first time.**

Whether you've had a vaginal birth or a C-section, this is the moment your physical recovery truly begins. Your nurse will be right beside you, helping you move slowly, safely, and with confidence. If you had an epidural or were on magnesium sulfate, we'll first make sure you have full strength and sensation in your legs before standing.

We'll start by gently raising the head of your bed, helping you sit upright, and allowing your legs to dangle over the edge. This gives your blood pressure time to adjust and helps prevent dizziness. You might feel weak, shaky, or lightheaded — and that is *completely normal* after hours of labor, blood loss, anesthesia, and lying flat.

Step-by-Step Support

When you first get out of bed — especially after an epidural or C-section — I'm going to guide you through the process one step at a time. First, I'll have you stand up and look **straight up**, not down. Lifting your gaze helps stabilize your blood pressure and decreases dizziness.

Please tell me *immediately* if you feel:

dizzy
lightheaded
like you're "going underwater"
or if you start seeing stars

If you're feeling steady, I'll ask you to **march in place** so we can make sure both legs are supporting your weight equally. If that goes well, then we'll take our first slow, supported walk to the bathroom together.

If You Feel Unsteady – You're Still Safe

If your legs feel wobbly or unsure, don't worry — that's exactly why we have equipment to help you. One of my favorite tools is **Sara Stedy**, a supportive standing transfer device that keeps you upright, balanced, and safe. She lets us get you to the bathroom without risking a fall, especially when your body is still adjusting.

The First Rush of Bleeding

When you stand for the first time, you may feel or see a sudden **gush of blood**. This is completely normal — it's simply gravity pulling down everything that pooled while you were lying in bed.

It can look like more than it actually is, so don't be alarmed.
You're not hemorrhaging — your body is just shifting, releasing, and doing exactly what it's supposed to do.

And remember:
You are never doing this alone.
I will be there, hand on your back, steadying your arm, and guiding you safely through every moment.

Your First Bathroom Trip

Your first trip to the bathroom after giving birth can feel a little intimidating, but I'll be right there to help you through it. What you see in the toilet may surprise you — **blood and small clots are completely normal** in the first hours after delivery. Your body is clearing out everything it needs to and the amount can look like a heavy period.

It's common to feel a little off when you first sit or stand — your muscles may feel heavy, sore or not quite connected yet. If you had a Foley catheter, your bladder can take some time to "wake up," and starting to urinate may feel difficult at first. This is expected.

You may also notice some burning the first few times you urinate after a catheter is removed. That sensation is normal and usually improves quickly.

We do like to see you urinate within about six hours after your last time. An overly full bladder can increase bleeding and make it harder for your uterus to contract the way it should, which is why your care team keeps a close eye on it.

I'll help you get cleaned up and comfortable. We'll place your pads, spray **Dermoplast** for soothing relief, and line your pad with **Tucks** to reduce swelling. I'll show you how to use a **peri bottle** — a small squirt bottle filled with warm water — to gently rinse instead of wiping. This keeps things clean and minimizes burning, especially if you have stitches, swelling, or tenderness around your perineum.

If you had an episiotomy or tear, I'll check the area after your first bathroom trip to make sure bleeding and swelling are under control. We'll move slowly, take deep breaths, and make this first visit as comfortable and reassuring as possible. **You are never doing this alone.**

Nurse's Tip

- Move slowly and ask for help – even if you feel okay. Standing too quickly can make you dizzy or faint.
- Use your peri bottle every time you go to the bathroom for the first few days. It keeps you clean and helps prevent stinging.
- Mild burning the first time you urinate is normal and improves each day.
- If you pass clots larger than a golf ball or soak a pad in under an hour, call your nurse right away.

Necessary Intervention

If English is not your first language, make sure **translation services** are available during your **first time out of bed and your first trip to the bathroom** after birth. These moments can feel overwhelming and if you feel something or need something, you must be able to communicate it clearly to your nurse. Having an interpreter present — in person, by phone, or through a translation device — ensures your safety, comfort, and confidence as you take those first important steps in recovery.

This first walk and bathroom trip may seem small but it's a major milestone. It's proof that your body is already healing, adjusting, and finding its rhythm again — one careful, supported step at a time.

Transitioning to Postpartum Care

After that, we'll either get you settled into a wheelchair or transport you in the bed if you've had a C-section. We'll move slowly and carefully, making sure you're steady and comfortable — sitting up too fast can make you dizzy or strain your incision and your safety is everything in these first tender moments.

If your baby was admitted to the NICU, we'll make a stop there first so you can see your little one, touch them, and know exactly where they are and how they're doing before we take you to postpartum. **You will never be left wondering** — you will see your baby, meet their NICU team, and take a moment together before we continue on.

Once you're ready, I'll bring you to the amazing postpartum nurses who will continue your care and walk with you through the next stage of recovery.
And while my time as your labor nurse may be ending, the bond we formed — through every contraction, every decision, every moment of trust — will stay with me forever.

How Long You'll Stay in the Hospital

In general, most families stay with us for:

2 nights after a vaginal birth
3 nights after a C-section

—as long as there are no complications. This gives us time to monitor your recovery, help with feeding, manage pain, check your baby's progress, and make sure you are both safe and stable before going home.

Every recovery is different but these time frames are typical — and we'll guide you every step of the way until you're ready to take your little one home.

27

Common Infections in Labor & Delivery: What They Are & How We Treat Them

"Most infections are small problems.
Ignoring them is the big one."

Infections in pregnancy or during labor are more common than people realize — and most are very treatable. We screen for certain infections throughout pregnancy because they can affect you or your baby during labor, and we want to be ahead of them, not behind.

This chapter explains the most common infections we see in Labor & Delivery, how we monitor them, and how we keep you and your baby safe.

1. Group Beta Strep (GBS)

What it is:

A naturally occurring bacteria that lives in the vagina or rectum of a good percentage of healthy women. It is **not** an STD, **not** caused by poor hygiene, and **not** dangerous to you.

Why it matters in labor:

Baby can be exposed during birth and a small percentage of babies can develop serious infections if GBS is not treated.

How we test:

A quick vaginal/rectal swab around 36–37 weeks

How we treat:

IV penicillin (or an alternative if allergic) during labor
Given every 4 hours until delivery

What it feels like:

Just an IV medication — you won't feel "sick" or any different.

Reassurance:

With proper antibiotics, the risk to your baby drops *dramatically.* GBS-positive labors are routine — we handle them every single day.

Nurse's Tip: IV Penicillin Sensation

IV penicillin can sometimes cause a temporary burning or stinging sensation at the IV site. If you feel any discomfort, let your nurse know right away—we can often slow the infusion or take steps to make it more comfortable for you.

2. Chorioamnionitis ("Chorio")

What it is:

An infection of the amniotic fluid, membranes, and sometimes the placenta.

How it starts:

Prolonged rupture of membranes
Bacteria entering the uterus
Long labor with many vaginal exams
And sometimes… it just happens — **not your fault**

Signs & symptoms:

Fever
Fast heart rate (mom and/or baby)
Uterine tenderness
Foul-smelling fluid (sometimes)

How we treat:

Broad-spectrum IV antibiotics
IV fluids
Tylenol for fever
Delivery if infection is progressing

What it feels like:

You may feel tired, chilled, achy, or feverish.

Reassurance:

Once antibiotics begin and baby is delivered, symptoms usually improve quickly.
Baby may need a NICU evaluation depending on the situation.

3. Urinary Tract Infection (UTI) & Pyelonephritis

Why it matters in pregnancy:

UTIs are more common when pregnant because hormones relax the urinary tract. If untreated, they can progress to kidney infection (pyelonephritis).

Symptoms:

- Burning/urgency with urination
- Fever
- Flank pain
- Chills
- Contractions (UTIs can irritate the uterus)

Treatment:

Oral antibiotics
IV antibiotics if severe
Hydration

Reassurance:

UTIs are simple to treat and often detected early. We screen and respond quickly so you and baby stay safe.

4. Gonorrhea & Chlamydia

Why we test:

These infections are common and often have no symptoms but can pass to the baby during delivery.

How we test:

A vaginal swab or urine test early in pregnancy

Symptoms (if any):

- Discharge
- Pelvic discomfort
- Burning with urination

Treatment:

- **Gonorrhea:** one-time injection of ceftriaxone
- **Chlamydia:** oral antibiotics (azithromycin)

Effect on baby:

Untreated, these can cause **eye or respiratory infections** — which is why erythromycin eye ointment is routinely given at birth.

Reassurance:

With treatment, these infections are resolved and rarely cause complications.

5. BV (Bacterial Vaginosis) & Yeast Infections

These are **common, uncomfortable, but typically harmless** in pregnancy.

BV Symptoms:

- Strong odor
- Thin, grayish discharge
- Mild irritation

Yeast Infection Symptoms:

- Itching
- Thick, white discharge
- Burning

Treatment:

- **BV:** oral or vaginal antibiotics
- **Yeast:** antifungal medication

Reassurance:

These rarely affect labor but can make pregnancy miserable — we treat quickly so you can be comfortable.

6. Herpes Simplex Virus (HSV)

What matters in labor:

Active lesions can transmit HSV to the baby during vaginal birth.

What we do:

- **No active lesions** → vaginal birth is safe
- **Active lesions** → scheduled or urgent C-section to protect baby

Prevention:

Many providers prescribe **daily antiviral medication at 36 weeks** to suppress outbreaks.

Reassurance:

You are not alone. HSV is common, manageable, and safely monitored. With antiviral therapy and close attention during labor, risks are extremely low.

7. HIV & Hepatitis B/C

Why we test:

To keep both mom and baby safe.
Not for judgment — ever.

HIV

With medication throughout pregnancy and precautions after birth, transmission can be reduced to **less than 1%**. Babies may receive medication after birth as part of prevention.

Hepatitis B

If mom is positive, babies receive:

- **Hepatitis B vaccine**
- **HBIG injection (Hepatitis B Immune Globulin)** for extra protection

These two together dramatically reduce the chance of transmission.

Hepatitis C

There is **no vaccine yet**, but babies born to Hep C–positive moms are monitored carefully and tested at specific intervals after birth. Interventions are standardized and evidence-based.

Reassurance:

You will **never** be judged.
You will be cared for with dignity, privacy, and compassion.
Testing positive for any condition does **not** define you — and it does not define your ability to be an incredible parent.

8. Fever During Labor

Sometimes a fever happens for reasons that have nothing to do with infection — and certainly nothing you did wrong.

Common reasons:

- Epidural-related temperature rise
- Viral infections
- Dehydration
- Prolonged labor
- Early chorioamnionitis
- Medications given (Cytotec)

We respond quickly by:
treating the underlying cause
hydrating you
checking baby's heart rate
monitoring closely for any changes

Even a mild fever can cause baby's heart rate to rise — so we stay ahead of it.

Nurse's Note: You Did Nothing Wrong

Nurse's Note
Infections happen. Hormone changes happen. Fevers happen.
None of these make you "dirty," irresponsible, or unsafe.

As your nurse, my only goal is to keep you and your baby healthy — without judgment, without shame, and without assumptions.

If an infection or fever is present, we treat it quickly, calmly, and compassionately.
Your only job is to tell us how you're feeling.
We've got you. Always.

28

Hypertensive Disorders including Pre-Eclampsia and her Ugly Sisters: What You Need to Know

"There will be roadblocks but we will overcome them."

– DJ Khaled

As you can see, I have dedicated a whole chapter to hypertension and preeclampsia with her sisters because, unfortunately, she shows up far too often in Labor and Delivery. She's unpredictable, complicated, and sometimes silent until she's already caused chaos. Over the years, I've seen her in many forms — from the mom who comes in with just a headache to the one whose blood pressure is dangerously high before she even realizes something is wrong.

This chapter is for every woman whose pregnancy took an unexpected turn — into magnesium drips, frequent blood pressure checks, and continuous monitoring. It's for the mothers who felt the grief of losing the "normal" pregnancy experience they envisioned, and for the nurses who stand at the bedside each day, balancing vigilance with compassion.

My goal is to explain these conditions in a way that **empowers rather than frightens**. Because understanding what is happening — and why — can help you reclaim a sense of control in the middle of uncertainty.

High blood pressure during pregnancy is more common than many people realize and it's something we take seriously — not to scare you, but because early recognition and timely care can make a meaningful difference for both you and your baby. These conditions fall under what we call **Hypertensive Disorders of Pregnancy**, which include:

- Chronic Hypertension
- Gestational Hypertension
- Preeclampsia
- Preeclampsia with Severe Features
- Superimposed Preeclampsia
- Eclampsia
- HELLP syndrome

Each one looks a little different but they all share one important theme:

They are conditions we manage together, with close monitoring, clear communication, and a focus on keeping both you and your baby safe.

Chronic Hypertension in Pregnancy: What It Is & What It Looks Like

Chronic hypertension means high blood pressure that **existed before pregnancy** or is diagnosed **before 20 weeks of gestation**. For some women, this is a known condition they managed prior to becoming pregnant; for others, it's discovered early in pregnancy during routine prenatal visits.

What it looks like:

- Blood pressure readings consistently **140/90 or higher**
- Often present **before pregnancy** or noted early on
- Many women feel completely **normal** and have **no symptoms**
- May require **more frequent monitoring**, labs, and ultrasounds
- Some women continue or start **blood pressure medications** that are safe in pregnancy

Reassurance:

Having chronic hypertension does **not** mean something will automatically go wrong. Many women with chronic hypertension go on to have healthy pregnancies and healthy babies. The goal is awareness, close monitoring, and early intervention when needed. Knowledge gives us a plan — and a plan brings confidence, safety, and peace of mind.

Gestational Hypertension

What It Means, Why It Matters, and How We Care for You

Gestational hypertension is high blood pressure that develops after 20 weeks of pregnancy in a patient who previously had normal blood pressure. It can feel scary to hear the words "high blood pressure," but the important thing to know is this:

We catch it early. We monitor it closely. And most patients do very well with the right care.

This condition does not automatically mean you're in danger — it simply means your body is asking for closer watching.

What Gestational Hypertension *Is* (and Isn't)

Gestational hypertension is defined as:

- Blood pressure ≥140/90, taken twice, at least 4 hours apart,
- After 20 weeks of pregnancy,
- Without signs of protein in the urine or organ involvement.

It is *not* the same as chronic hypertension (blood pressure that starts before pregnancy), and it is *not yet* preeclampsia — but it can progress, which is why we stay on top of it.

Common Symptoms

Many people have no symptoms, which is why routine prenatal visits are crucial.

When symptoms do show up, they can include:

- Persistent headaches
- Vision changes (blurry, spots, flashing lights)
- Sudden swelling in the hands, face, or feet
- Right upper abdominal pain
- Rapid weight gain due to fluid retention

If you ever feel "off," swollen, or can't shake a headache — call. You know your body better than anyone.

How We Diagnose and Watch It

Once blood pressures rise, your care team will monitor you more closely. This may include:

- More frequent blood pressure checks
- Urine testing
- Bloodwork to check liver and kidney function
- Growth ultrasounds to check on baby

- Non-stress tests (NSTs) to watch baby's heart rate
- Fetal movement monitoring at home

We're not just watching numbers — we're watching you and your baby as a whole.

How It Can Affect Your Pregnancy

Most patients with gestational hypertension go on to have healthy births, but the risks increase if the condition progresses. Untreated high blood pressure can affect:

- Placental blood flow, which may impact baby's growth
- Fluid levels, sometimes causing low amniotic fluid
- Your well-being, if the condition becomes preeclampsia

This is why we treat and monitor early — prevention is powerful.

How We Manage It

Your plan depends on your blood pressure, symptoms, and how far along you are.

Management may include:

- Rest and reduced stress
- Staying hydrated
- Medications for severe or persistent high blood pressure
- Close fetal monitoring
- Possible early delivery after 37 weeks (recommended by ACOG)

If your blood pressures are severely elevated or symptoms develop, we may recommend:

- Magnesium sulfate to prevent seizures
- Induction of labor if the condition becomes dangerous to you or baby

Our goal is always:
Healthy mom. Healthy baby. Safe delivery.

What It Means for Delivery

Most patients with gestational hypertension will:

- Deliver at 37 weeks or later
- Have a vaginal birth (if it's safe)
- Be monitored closely during labor
- Have blood pressures checked frequently
- Have medications adjusted as needed

This isn't a "failure" of your body — it is a condition we manage together.

Nurse's Note

Your job is not to perfect your blood pressure. Your job is to listen to your symptoms and let us care for you.
High blood pressure in pregnancy can feel unpredictable, but I promise you: we are watching you closely, listening to your body, and doing everything we can to keep you and your baby safe.

You're not facing this alone — you have an entire team behind you, every step of the way.

What Preeclampsia Is

Preeclampsia is a condition that can develop during pregnancy, usually after 20 weeks. It's when your blood pressure gets too high and your organs — especially your kidneys and liver — start showing signs of stress.

You might notice symptoms like:

- swelling in your face or hands
- headaches that don't go away with Tylenol
- vision changes (spots, blurriness, flashing lights)
- pain under your ribs (your liver getting very unhappy)

Other times, you may feel completely normal — which is why those routine blood pressure checks at prenatal visits are so important.

No one can say for certain what causes preeclampsia, but we believe it starts in the placenta. For reasons we still don't fully understand, the blood vessels that form the placenta sometimes don't develop or function the way they should, leading to poor blood flow and a lot of stress on your body.

Preeclampsia With Severe Features

What It Means & Why We Act Quickly

Preeclampsia with severe features is a more serious form of preeclampsia where your body begins to show signs that the condition is affecting your organs — most commonly your liver. It doesn't mean something terrible is happening right this minute, but it *does* mean your pregnancy needs closer monitoring and, often, delivery sooner rather than later.

Severe features can include:

- Very high blood pressure (160/110 or higher)
- Severe headache that doesn't go away
- Blurry vision or seeing spots
- Pain under the right ribs
- Low platelets
- Abnormal liver or kidney labs
- Fluid in the lungs
- Signs that baby isn't tolerating the pregnancy well

When these signs appear, the safest plan is usually delivery, because preeclampsia only resolves once the placenta is out. In the meantime, we may give medications such as magnesium sulfate (to prevent seizures) and antihypertensives to control blood pressure.

The most important thing to know:
You are not in this alone. We act quickly not because we're alarmed, but because we know early intervention keeps you and your baby safe.

Superimposed Preeclampsia

When Chronic Hypertension Develops New Symptoms in Pregnancy

Superimposed preeclampsia happens when a patient who already has chronic hypertension (high blood pressure before pregnancy or before 20 weeks) develops new signs of preeclampsia later in pregnancy. It can be confusing, because these patients already start with elevated blood pressures — but the key difference is the *new* symptoms or lab changes that appear.

This is a condition we take seriously, not because it always becomes an emergency, but because we know how quickly it can change. You'll never go through it alone — we monitor both you and your baby closely and act swiftly if anything starts to shift.

What Superimposed Preeclampsia Means

To diagnose it, a patient with chronic hypertension must develop one or more of the following:

- New protein in the urine (protein–creatinine ratio ≥ 0.3)
- New or worsening high blood pressures
- Abnormal labs (liver or kidney function)

- New symptoms suggestive of preeclampsia
- Sudden changes in fetal growth or fluid levels

In simple terms: It's chronic hypertension + preeclampsia symptoms layered on top.

Signs and Symptoms We Watch For

Many of the symptoms mirror classic preeclampsia:

- Persistent or severe headache
- Blurry vision, flashing lights, or spots
- Upper right abdominal pain
- Nausea/vomiting that isn't normal for you
- Sudden swelling of face, hands, or feet
- Rapid fluid gain
- Shortness of breath
- Decreased fetal movement

You might feel completely fine — or you might feel like something is "off." If something feels wrong, tell us. You never need to justify your instincts.

How We Monitor You and Your Baby

Because this condition can progress quickly, we typically increase monitoring:

- More frequent prenatal visits
- Blood pressure checks at home or in clinic
- Urine testing for protein
- Bloodwork (platelets, liver enzymes, kidney function)
- Growth ultrasounds (to check baby's size and blood flow)
- Non-stress tests (NSTs)
- Biophysical profiles (BPPs)

The goal is to catch changes early before symptoms become dangerous.

How We Manage It

Your care plan depends on gestational age, symptom severity, and lab results.

Management may include:

- Blood pressure medications
- Rest and hydration
- Close lab monitoring
- Fetal monitoring in late pregnancy
- Magnesium sulfate if severe features develop
- Delivery if your health or baby's health is at risk

For many patients, we aim for delivery at 37 weeks, but earlier delivery may be safest if severe symptoms appear.

This is not a failure — this is your body letting us know it needs help and your medical team stepping in to keep you both safe.

What It Means for Labor & Delivery

During labor, we monitor you closely:

- Frequent BP checks
- IV access
- Continuous fetal monitoring
- Possible magnesium infusion
- Possible antihypertensive medications
- Careful watching for postpartum progression

You may hear the team using words like "severe features," "stabilize," or "trend the labs." That doesn't mean something terrible is happening — it means we're being thorough.

And I promise you: You will never be left alone to guess what's happening. We explain every step.

Nurse's Note

Superimposed preeclampsia can feel overwhelming because you're dealing with a condition *on top of* something you were already managing. I want you to know this:

We take this seriously because we care about you — not because we're trying to scare you.

We watch you closely because we want:

- Your baby safe
- You safe
- Your birth story to end with both of you healthy

Your team is not reacting to danger — we're preventing it. And you are never navigating this alone.

Eclampsia: When Preeclampsia Crosses the Line

Eclampsia is a rare but serious complication that occurs when preeclampsia progresses to seizures. It can happen before delivery, during labor, or even postpartum.

You might hear your team say:

- "Putting her on Mag"
- "Give a Mag bolus"

This is magnesium sulfate — our frontline defense for preventing and treating seizures.

What Happens If a Seizure Occurs

Your care team moves **fast** and with purpose:

- You'll be turned onto your side to protect your airway.
- Oxygen will be applied.
- We'll keep you safe from injury.
- Magnesium will be started or increased immediately.
- Your vital signs, reflexes, and urine output will be monitored continuously.

Delivery is often recommended once you're stabilized, because the **only true "cure"** for preeclampsia and eclampsia is delivering the baby and placenta.

HELLP Syndrome: Another Ugly Stepsister of Preeclampsia

HELLP syndrome is a severe and potentially life-threatening complication related to preeclampsia. The name comes from the three major things happening inside the body:

H — Hemolysis: the breakdown of red blood cells
EL — Elevated Liver Enzymes: showing the liver is under stress or injury (a *very* angry liver)
LP — Low Platelets: your blood has a reduced ability to clot

HELLP can develop **suddenly** — sometimes even before high blood pressure or protein in the urine appear. That's what makes it so dangerous. It hides in plain sight.

Symptoms May Include:

- severe right upper abdominal or epigastric pain (just below your ribs)
- nausea or vomiting

- headache
- vision changes (spots, flashing lights, blurriness)
- **unexplained nosebleeds** or
- **broken blood vessels in the eyes**

Those last two aren't always in textbooks — but they're absolutely real. They can signal low platelets, something I've personally seen more than once.

A Story From the Bedside

I'll never forget a patient who came in for a scheduled, routine C-section. On the outside, she looked absolutely perfect:

- normal blood pressure
- no swelling
- no headaches or vision issues
- normal fetal movement

But she mentioned a nagging pain under her ribs. Something in my gut told me it wasn't normal. I asked my doctor to run labs "just to be safe."

She was in full-blown HELLP.

If we hadn't checked, if we had brushed it off as "pregnancy discomfort," things could have gone very differently.
This is why nurses listen to more than symptoms — we listen to you.

HELLP often **mimics normal pregnancy symptoms**, which is why lab work and close monitoring matter so much in women with preeclampsia.

What We Do When HELLP Is Suspected

Your care team will move quickly and calmly:

- Draw bloodwork to check your liver enzymes, platelets, and hemolysis markers

- Start **magnesium sulfate** to prevent seizures
- Manage blood pressure with IV medications
- Discuss timing of delivery — because the only true cure is delivering the baby and placenta
- Give blood products (platelets, plasma) if counts are dangerously low
- Monitor reflexes, urine output, breathing, and vital signs **nonstop**

HELLP requires expertise, teamwork, and vigilant nursing — and you will be surrounded by all of that.

HELLP Can Progress Quickly – But Outcomes Are Often Excellent

With close monitoring, early recognition, and the right treatment, we are usually able to stabilize both mom and baby quickly. The key is *listening to your body* and acting early — and that's exactly what your care team is trained to do.

Magnesium Sulfate: What It Is and Why We Use It

Magnesium sulfate — "mag" — is one of our most powerful tools in Labor & Delivery. It has **two major purposes**, depending on your situation:

1. To Prevent Seizures in Mothers with Preeclampsia

When blood pressure reaches severe ranges (160/110 or higher), the brain becomes at risk for electrical misfiring — meaning seizures.

Magnesium sulfate dramatically lowers this risk and is considered the gold-standard medication worldwide.

It protects:

- the brain
- the nervous system
- and reduces the chance of eclampsia

2. To Protect the Baby's Brain in Very Preterm Labor

If labor is happening much earlier than expected, magnesium sulfate is often used for **neuroprotection**.

It helps lower the risk of:

- cerebral palsy
- neurological injury
- damage from early, rapid delivery

In these cases, mag is given for the baby, not the mother.

How Magnesium Sulfate Is Given

Magnesium sulfate begins with a **loading dose**, given through your IV over about **20–30 minutes**.
After that, you'll receive a **continuous drip**, which runs for several hours to 24+ hours depending on:

- whether you're on it for **preeclampsia**
- whether you're on it for **seizure prevention postpartum**
- or whether it's being used for **preterm neuroprotection for your baby**

During this time, you'll have:

- frequent vital sign checks
- close monitoring of your reflexes and breathing
- regular assessments of your urine output
- labs drawn as needed to monitor magnesium levels and organ function

It's a medication that requires *attentive care* — and that's exactly what your nurses will provide.

Nurse's Tips: Being on Magnesium Sulfate

Here's what you can expect – and what helps.

Eating & Drinking

Depending on your hospital and how your body responds:

- You **may or may not** be allowed to eat.
- If eating is allowed, choose **light, bland foods** – magnesium can make you nauseous and slows down digestion.

Hydration helps with headaches and flushing, but your team will guide you based on your status.

Stay Cool

Magnesium often causes:

- flushing
- sweating
- a warm, heavy feeling

Ask for a cool washcloth, a fan, or lower room temperature if needed.

Blood Clot Prevention

Because magnesium keeps you in bed, you'll usually wear **SCDs** (sequential compression devices). These gently squeeze your legs to prevent blood clots – a crucial part of safety during bedrest.

Bathroom Assistance

Depending on your condition:

- Some providers place a foley catheter to monitor urine output. If not, we will measure using a bedpan or bedside commode. **Do not get out of bed without your nurse.**

Magnesium affects coordination, balance, and reflexes. Always call your nurse before getting up.

Communication

Mag can make you feel:

- groggy
- foggy
- slow
- disconnected

Tell your nurse right away if you feel:

- dizzy
- short of breath
- extremely drowsy
- unable to stay awake
- weak
- or if your vision changes

Your nurse is monitoring closely, but your feedback is essential.

Rest When You Can

Magnesium is exhausting. Your body is working incredibly hard – both to stay safe and to support your baby. Rest is medicine.

Low Down on How Mag Makes You Feel

Real Deal Mag Vibe:

- This is a **bedrest** situation — it's not safe to get up.
- Most patients describe it as feeling warm all over, like a full-body hot flash.
- You may feel flushed, groggy, or foggy-headed.
- A patient once told me it felt like a **heavy weighted blanket** was lying over her body.
- You might feel like everything is happening in slow motion — that's normal.

Nurse's Tip: Create a Calm Space

Being on magnesium can make you feel:

- flushed
- overwhelmed
- overstimulated
- heavy
- mentally foggy

A calm environment makes a world of difference.

Your nurse will help create a soothing space by:

- dimming the lights
- minimizing noise
- limiting unnecessary interruptions
- encouraging visitors to keep voices soft

You can also bring:

- a cozy blanket

- headphones
- a calming playlist
- lavender or another gentle scent

A peaceful room helps:

- lower blood pressure
- reduce headaches
- ease anxiety
- support your body's response to the medication

Remember: Magnesium isn't designed to make you *feel good.* It's designed to keep your brain protected and your body safe — and that makes it one of the most important medications we give.

If you ever feel:

- too hot
- too sleepy
- short of breath
- confused
- or "not right,"

tell your nurse immediately. We're watching you closely — but your voice matters most.

How It Affects the Baby After Birth

If you receive magnesium sulfate during labor, your baby may show a few temporary effects right after birth. This is completely expected and not a sign that anything is wrong. Magnesium crosses the placenta so baby gets a small dose too — just enough to make them a little more relaxed than usual.

You may notice your newborn is:

- **Sleepier at birth**
- **A little less "perky" or floppy in tone at first**
- **Slower to transition or feed in the first couple of hours**

This is *temporary.*
As the medication wears off, your baby wakes up, perks up, feeds better, and settles into their normal rhythm. Most babies bounce back beautifully within a few hours.

Because magnesium sedation can make babies a little slower to transition, the **NICU team or pediatric provider may be present at delivery** — not because we expect a problem, but because we want every layer of safety in place for you and your baby.

Nurse's Reassurance

Magnesium sulfate can *sound* intimidating, especially when you're already tired, scared, or overwhelmed — but it's one of the most protective medications we have in all of obstetrics.

It saves lives.
It prevents seizures.
It keeps your brain safe.
It protects premature babies' developing brains.

Yes, you may feel awful for a little while — hot, heavy, foggy, or wiped out — but your nurse will be there with you the entire time:

- monitoring your breathing
- checking your reflexes
- helping you stay cool

- supporting you emotionally
- and watching baby's transition closely

Magnesium is given with intention, precision, and constant care. You are never left alone with the medication or with the fear of it.

We don't just treat you — we stay with you.

You may feel terrible.
But you are safe.
Your baby is safe.
And you are surrounded by a team whose entire purpose is to protect both of you through this chapter.

Blood Pressure Management: Keeping Mom Safe

When blood pressure climbs too high during pregnancy, it can strain your heart, kidneys, and liver — and reduce blood flow to your baby. Our goal is always the same: **lower your pressure safely and steadily** without dropping it too fast. We want both you and your baby well-perfused, well-oxygenated, and stable.

Treatment depends on how high your readings are and what symptoms you're experiencing.

IV (Intravenous) Medications – For Immediate Control

If your blood pressure reaches dangerously high levels (often **≥160/110**) or if you're showing warning signs — headache, visual changes, pain under your ribs — your team will act quickly with IV medications.

Common IV medications include:

Labetalol

- Works fast to lower blood pressure
- Relaxes blood vessels
- May cause a brief warm sensation or lightheadedness

Hydralazine

- Relaxes arterial walls
- Lowers pressures steadily

Nifedipine (oral)

- Relaxes smooth muscle in the vessel walls
- Can help rapidly bring pressures back into a safe zone

Your nurse will check your blood pressure every few minutes during treatment. The goal is **not** to make your pressure "perfect" — it's to bring it out of the dangerous zone and into a safer, more stable range.

PO (By-Mouth) Medications – For Maintenance Control

Once you're stable — or if your blood pressure is only mildly elevated — your provider may start or switch you to oral medications.

Common oral medications include:

Labetalol (oral)

- Safe in pregnancy
- Safe in breastfeeding
- Usually taken multiple times a day

Nifedipine (extended release)

- Keeps blood pressure consistently controlled
- Taken once or twice daily

Oral medications help maintain safe pressures over the long term, sometimes even **after delivery** until your body finishes recalibrating.

> **Nurse's Tip**
>
> - Take your blood pressure medication **exactly as prescribed**, even if you feel fine.
> - Stand up slowly – these meds can cause sudden lightheadedness.
> - If you're asked to check your pressures at home, keep a simple log.
> - While you're receiving IV meds, let your nurse know right away if you feel dizzy, faint, or notice a racing heart – those are signs your pressure may have dropped too quickly.

In Summary

- **IV medications** = act fast when pressures are dangerously high
- **Oral medications** = maintain stability over time
- **Both** = protect your brain, heart, kidneys — and keep your baby safe

> **Nurse's Tip: Connection Overload**
>
> When you're being treated for high blood pressure or any of the preeclampsia-related conditions, it can feel like you're connected to *everything*.

Between the:

- blood pressure cuff cycling every 10–15 minutes
- pulse oximeter glowing on your finger
- IV tubing
- magnesium drip
- fetal monitors
- SCDs on your legs

...it can feel overwhelming, tangled, or even claustrophobic.

That's **completely normal.**
And it's okay to say so.

Each connection has a purpose – to keep track of your breathing, your heart, your pressure, your reflexes, and your baby's safety while your body stabilizes.

Pro Tips:

- Ask your nurse to reorganize or reposition cords so they're less intrusive.
- If the BP cuff hurts or leaves marks, we can often switch arms.
- The pulse ox can be moved to a different finger – or even a toe.
- Slow breaths help ease the overstimulation of beeping monitors.
- Focus on your baby. You're doing this for both of you.

You are *not* just a patient hooked up to wires – you are a person being carefully protected. Every line and connection has a purpose, and none of them define you.

What Magnesium Does to Labor

One thing I want you to know is that **magnesium sulfate can slow down or even stall labor.** This medication relaxes muscles — and your uterus is one big muscle. While magnesium's main purpose is to protect your brain and prevent seizures, it can also push back against your body's attempts to contract efficiently.

If you're being induced or augmented, you may notice that progress is slower than expected or that we need to increase your Pitocin more often. That's because magnesium and oxytocin work in opposite directions:

- **Magnesium** = relaxes the uterus
- **Oxytocin/Pitocin** = stimulates contractions

It can feel frustrating, especially when you're so ready to meet your baby, but please know that we're watching your progress closely and adjusting everything safely.

Magnesium doesn't stop labor completely — it just makes your uterus a little "lazy" while it's busy protecting your body.
You'll still get there. Slow and steady wins the race.

The Tug of War: Magnesium vs. Pitocin

When you're on magnesium sulfate for preeclampsia or HELLP syndrome, your team often also needs to induce or augment labor with Pitocin or other induction agents.

Here's the tricky part:

- **Magnesium** is trying to *calm* and relax your muscles
- **Pitocin** is trying to *activate* your uterus and build contractions

Your uterus ends up caught in a gentle tug-of-war.
Magnesium says, "Shhh, relax,"
while Pitocin says, "Okay uterus, let's work!"

Because of this:

- Labor may progress more slowly
- We may need to adjust your Pitocin multiple times
- We move more cautiously to balance **safety + progress**

If things aren't moving quickly, please don't get discouraged — the slow pace is intentional. We're protecting your body while still working toward a safe, healthy birth for both you and your baby.

Magnesium and Postpartum Bleeding

Something else to know: magnesium sulfate can make your uterus a little "lazy" **after birth too.**

Since magnesium relaxes muscles, it can interfere with your uterus's ability to clamp down firmly once the baby and placenta are delivered. This increases the risk of:

Postpartum Hemorrhage (PPH)

— heavy bleeding after birth.

That's why your nurse will check your uterus frequently after delivery — pressing firmly on your belly to make sure it feels like a firm grapefruit. It's not comfortable but it's one of the most important steps for preventing excessive bleeding.

And for moms with HELLP syndrome:

The risk is even higher because platelets — the cells that help your blood clot — can be very low. When platelets are low, even normal postpartum bleeding can become heavy quickly.

What We Do (Nursing + Provider Interventions)

We take postpartum bleeding seriously — and we take *you* seriously. Aside from the two IVs that you should already have, here's what you may see us do:

Extra uterotonics

To help your uterus contract if Pitocin alone isn't enough.
This may include medications like:

- Methergine (depending on blood pressure)
- Hemabate
- Misoprostol
- Tranexamic Acid (TXA), depending on bleeding and risk factors

Frequent assessments

- Checking your fundus (uterus) for firmness
- Monitoring pad saturation
- Watching for clots
- Checking your vital signs

Additional interventions if needed

If bleeding becomes heavier:

- **Bakri balloon** (a small balloon placed inside the uterus to apply pressure)
- **Jada device** (newer device that uses gentle suction to help the uterus contract)

- **D&C** (to remove retained tissue)

Blood products

In rare cases:

- Platelets
- Plasma
- Packed red blood cells

...may be needed to restore your blood volume and clotting function.

> **Nurse's Tip:** Don't be alarmed by how often your nurse checks your belly or bleeding – it's part of keeping you safe. Magnesium can make your uterus slow to respond so we're extra watchful.
>
> If you feel **dizzy**, **weak**, or notice **increased bleeding or clots**, tell your nurse immediately.
>
> Know that even if things get intense, you're surrounded by a team that's highly trained and ready to act fast.

Compassion Note: I know this probably isn't the pregnancy journey you pictured for yourself. When you imagined bringing your baby into the world, magnesium sulfate was probably never part of the plan — and I understand that. It can be disappointing, even scary, to have your birth story take a turn you didn't expect.

Please know this: even though the circumstances may be different, my goal — and the goal of every nurse caring for you — is still the same. **We want you to have the best possible experience while keeping you and your baby safe.**

You can still have a meaningful, empowering birth even when things don't go exactly as planned. You're strong, capable, and doing an incredible job — and we'll walk beside you through every step of it.

For Partners and Visitors: Supporting a Loved One on Magnesium

If your loved one is on magnesium sulfate, you might notice the room is quiet, dimly lit, and almost spa-like — that's on purpose. Magnesium can make your girl feel hot, flushed, sleepy, or foggy. A calm environment helps reduce stress, stabilize blood pressure, and prevent overstimulation.

Here's how you can help:

- Keep the room peaceful. Speak softly, silence phones, and limit visitors.
- Offer gentle reassurance. A light touch, a calm voice, or just being present makes a difference.
- Don't take it personally if she's too tired to talk or seems out of it. It's the medication, not you.
- Be patient. This phase is temporary — once the magnesium is discontinued, she'll feel more like herself.
- Let the nurse know if you notice trouble breathing, confusion, or excessive sleepiness.

Your calm presence can be one of the most powerful medicines in the room.

After the Magnesium Is Turned Off

When the magnesium infusion is finally stopped — usually about 24 hours after delivery — your body begins to transition back to its normal rhythm. Most patients describe this moment as a huge relief, both physically and mentally.

At first, you may still feel a little groggy or heavy, like moving in slow motion. Magnesium takes time to leave your system, so it may be several hours before you feel fully clear-headed. Your nurse will continue checking your reflexes, urine output, and blood pressure while your body "wakes up."

You might notice:

- **Feeling lighter and clearer:** the fog begins to lift
- **More energy:** alertness returning quickly
- **Increased urination:** your body releasing extra fluid
- **Mild headache or fatigue:** common as you readjust

If you had a catheter, we usually remove it a few hours after the infusion ends. Your nurse will help you get up slowly for that first trip to the bathroom.

Nurse's Tip:

- Take your time getting up – magnesium + bed rest = weak, wobbly legs.
- **Wait at least one hour** after the infusion ends and do **not** get up without your nurse.
- Eat something light and sip fluids to restore energy.
- Ask for help with your baby if you're tired – this is recovery, not a performance.
- Don't feel discouraged if you're emotionally drained – it's normal after days of stress and monitoring.

The moment magnesium is turned off often feels like freedom — the fog lifts, your strength returns, and the first real breaths of motherhood begin. You did it, and you did it safely.

29

Postpartum Hemorrhage (Pph): What It is, Why It Happens, And How We Respond

"PPH is powerful, but your team is stronger."

Postpartum hemorrhage (PPH) is one of the most serious complications we watch for during labor and birth. It occurs when a mother bleeds more than **1,000 mL after delivery** (vaginal or C-section) or when bleeding is heavy enough to cause symptoms like dizziness, weakness, or low blood pressure.

PPH can happen **immediately after birth** (primary hemorrhage) or **hours later** (secondary hemorrhage).

The most important thing to know is this:

We train for this constantly.
We recognize it early.
We never ignore heavy bleeding.
You will not face it alone.

This chapter explains what we look for, why it happens, and exactly what we do to keep you safe.

WHY PPH HAPPENS (THE FOUR T's)

We categorize causes of PPH into four major groups:

1. Tone – a good majority of the culprit.

The uterus doesn't contract well after birth. We call this **uterine atony**.

When the uterus is firm, it clamps down on open blood vessels. When it's soft, those vessels stay open and bleeding continues.

Risk factors include:

- Induction or augmentation with Pitocin (especially prolonged inductions)
- Long labor or precipitous labor
- Multiple gestation
- Big baby (macrosomia)
- High parity (many previous births)
- Magnesium sulfate use
- Infection / chorioamnionitis
- Retained placenta

Tone-related bleeding is the **most common — and the most treatable**.

2. Tissue – Placenta or clots left behind

If any portion of the placenta remains inside the uterus, bleeding continues. This happens because the uterus does not know how to behave when things are left in it.

This includes:

- Retained placental fragments
- Retained clots
- Placental abnormalities (accreta, increta, percreta)

3. Trauma – Tears or injury

Bleeding can come from:

- Vaginal tears
- Cervical tears
- Perineal lacerations
- Episiotomy extensions
- Uterine rupture (rare)
- Instrumental delivery (vacuum/forceps)

4. Thrombin – Clotting problems

Conditions where the blood doesn't clot properly:

- Pre-eclampsia / HELLP syndrome
- DIC (disseminated intravascular coagulation)
- Severe abruption
- Severe infection
- Abnormal labs

These are less common but taken extremely seriously.

WHAT PPH LOOKS LIKE

PPH isn't always dramatic. Sometimes it's slow but continuous and we catch it early because we're trained to recognize subtle changes.

Signs include:

- Heavy vaginal bleeding
- Passing large clots
- Feeling faint, dizzy, or "off"
- Rapid heart rate
- Low blood pressure
- Pale or sweaty appearance
- Uterus feeling "boggy" during a fundal exam

You may not notice early signs — **your nurse will**.

FIRST-LINE INTERVENTIONS: WHAT WE DO RIGHT AWAY

If you begin bleeding heavily, we move quickly and in a coordinated order. No chaos — just rapid teamwork.

1. Fundal Massage ("Uterine Massage")

This is not comfortable — but it's effective.
We massage the top of your uterus to help it contract. Don't be surprised if we put a sand bag on your uterus. That is to create constant stimulation for it to contract.

Think of it as *waking the uterus back up.*

2. Increase IV Fluids

We open up the IV rate to support your blood pressure and help stabilize circulation.

3. Medications to Help the Uterus Clamp Down

Pitocin (oxytocin)
Given to every mother after birth per evidence-based practice.
If bleeding continues, we increase the rate.

Methergine
Helps the uterus contract strongly.
Not used for moms with high blood pressure unless benefit outweighs risk.

Hemabate (Carboprost)
A powerful uterotonic.
Can cause diarrhea and bronchospasm.
Avoided in asthmatics.

Cytotec (Misoprostol)
Placed rectally, orally, or buccally to stop bleeding — extremely effective.

Tranexamic Acid (TXA)
Helps blood clot and reduces blood loss by preventing clot breakdown.
Most effective if given within **3 hours** of birth.

Nurse's Note: Hemabate, Cytotec, and What to Expect

If you need medications to help your uterus contract after birth, you may receive **Hemabate** or **Cytotec** — both are safe and effective but they can come with side effects you should be aware of.

Hemabate can commonly cause **diarrhea** because of how it stimulates smooth muscle in the body. If we're giving Hemabate, we'll be prepared and often have **Imodium on board** to help manage that side effect and keep you comfortable.

Cytotec, especially in **larger doses**, can sometimes cause a **fever or chills**. This doesn't necessarily mean you have an infection — it can simply be a reaction to the medication. Your team will monitor you closely, keep you informed, and make sure you understand what's medication-related versus what needs further evaluation.

These side effects are temporary, expected, and manageable — and we will always keep you informed so nothing catches you off guard.

🩸 IF BLEEDING CONTINUES: NEXT STEPS

If the bleeding doesn't slow quickly, we escalate care while keeping you calm and supported.

1. A Second IV Line

If not already recognized as a risk, we place a second IV for:

- Blood transfusions
- Additional medications
- Rapid fluid administration

This is standard.
It's preparation — not panic.

2. Bloodwork

We check:

- Hemoglobin/hematocrit
- Blood loss
- Coagulation labs
- Type & crossmatch for blood products

3. Ultrasound

We perform a quick bedside ultrasound to check for clots or retained placenta.

BLOOD TRANSFUSIONS: WHAT YOU NEED TO KNOW

Sometimes a transfusion is the safest choice.

We may give:

- **Packed red blood cells** – to restore oxygen-carrying capacity
- **Plasma or platelets** – if clotting issues are present
- **Cryoprecipitate** – if fibrinogen levels are low

Transfusions today are extremely safe, thoroughly screened, and continuously monitored.

Nurse reassurance:

A transfusion is **not** failure — it is life-saving, stabilizing, and protective.

PROCEDURES IF BLEEDING CONTINUES

If medical management isn't enough, there are more advanced options your care team may use. These interventions are part of a **highly coordinated, step-by-step response — not signs of panic**.

1. JADA® System (Vacuum-Induced Uterine Hemorrhage Control)

A soft silicone device is placed inside the uterus and connected to gentle suction. Instead of pushing outward like a balloon, JADA helps the uterus **collapse and contract**, which is what naturally stops bleeding. It often works quickly and can reduce the need for more invasive procedures.

2. Bakri Balloon (Uterine Tamponade)

A special balloon is placed inside the uterus and filled with fluid to apply pressure from the inside. It's very effective and often avoids the need for surgery.

3. Manual Removal of Placental Tissue

If placental fragments remain inside the uterus, the provider may remove them manually. If you don't already have pain management on board, ask for it — this should **not** be done without adequate comfort.

4. D&C (Dilation & Curettage)

A small surgical procedure used to clear the uterus of any remaining tissue or clots.

5. Interventional Radiology (Uterine Artery Embolization)

A radiologist blocks the blood vessels feeding the uterus, decreasing blood flow. This is used when bleeding continues despite first-line measures.

6. Emergency Surgery

Very rare, but may include:

- Laparotomy
- Hysterectomy *(only as a last resort to save your life)*

These decisions are **never taken lightly**. They are life-saving measures used only when absolutely necessary.

WHAT PPH FEELS LIKE FOR YOU – AND HOW WE CARE FOR YOUR EMOTIONS

PPH can feel frightening because it often happens quickly. But you will **never be left alone.**

Your nurse will:

- Stay right beside you
- Talk you through every step
- Maintain grounding touch (hand holding, a firm hand on your shoulder, etc.)
- Reassure you constantly
- Keep you warm and physically supported

- Explain what's happening in calm, simple terms

This is where nursing shines — presence, compassion, and protection.

NURSE'S NOTE: YOU DID NOTHING WRONG

PPH is **not your fault.**
It is **not** caused by:

- Pushing wrong
- Breathing wrong
- Not being "fit enough" or "healthy enough"
- Anything you did or didn't do

It is a medical event that can happen to *any* woman — even those with perfect pregnancies and perfect labors.

We train relentlessly so that when PPH happens, we respond instantly and effectively.
You are not a complication.
You are a mother deserving of safety, dignity, and compassion.

AFTERCARE AND RECOVERY

After a PPH, we monitor you closely for:

- Vital signs
- Urine output
- Uterine tone
- Additional bleeding
- Dizziness, fatigue, or weakness
- Signs of anemia

You may need:

- Iron supplementation
- Repeat bloodwork
- Rest
- Extra hydration
- Nutrient-dense meals

We will **not** send you home until we are absolutely certain it is safe for you.

FINAL REASSURANCE

PPH is one of the **most practiced, most rehearsed, and most research-driven** emergencies in obstetrics.

When PPH happens, you will have:

- A nurse at your bedside
- A provider giving clear, rapid orders
- Extra team members assisting
- Medications ready
- Blood available
- Equipment on standby

It is teamwork at its absolute finest — and every movement is for **you**.

You are safe.
You are supported.
And you will never go through this alone.

Nurse's Note

Please make sure to tell your healthcare providers **if you've ever had postpartum hemorrhage before.**
This information truly matters.

A previous PPH increases your risk for another one and your team can take important precautions when they know your history — such as preparing medications, including blood early, having extra staff available, or placing your IV sooner.

Sharing your history helps us keep you safe.

Nurse's Compassion Note for Partners

I have been in situations where a mom was bleeding and her partner stood at the bedside watching in absolute fear. I know how terrifying it is when we whisk her — or you — away, and suddenly you're left alone wondering if your person is going to be okay. Please know that in those moments, we are doing **everything in our power** to bring her safely back to you.

If something like this ever happens to you, remember that the people who work in Labor and Delivery are truly special, dedicated, professional, and incredibly skilled. If there is **anything** that can be done, it **will** be done.

We operate with skill, intention, and a sense of higher purpose. Please believe that.

30

Other Pregnancy Complications

"Complications are detours, not dead ends."

Gestational Diabetes Mellitus (GDM): What It Means for You and Your Baby

Gestational Diabetes Mellitus (GDM) occurs when your body can't regulate blood sugar effectively during pregnancy. It's more common than many people realize and many women who develop GDM had **no risk factors at all**. With good management, mindful eating, and close monitoring, most moms with GDM have safe pregnancies, healthy babies, and smooth deliveries.

But it's important to understand *why* we take GDM seriously — especially around the time of birth.

What GDM Does During Pregnancy

When glucose levels stay higher than normal, that extra sugar crosses the placenta. Your baby's pancreas reacts by making more insulin to manage the extra sugar.

Because insulin is a hormone that moves sugar into cells, babies exposed to high glucose levels end up producing **more insulin than they should**.

This can lead to:

- Larger babies (macrosomia)
- Extra fat storage (especially shoulders and trunk)
- Increased risk of shoulder dystocia
- Babies getting used to receiving "high sugar" fuel from the placenta

But the biggest impact happens **right after birth**.

What Happens to Your Baby at Birth

When your baby is born, the umbilical cord is cut — and your glucose supply stops instantly.

But your baby's pancreas may still be working overtime, producing **too much insulin** because that's what it was used to.

This can cause a **sudden drop in their blood sugar**, known as **neonatal hypoglycemia**.

This is why babies born to moms with GDM are lovingly nicknamed **"sugar babies."**

Signs Your Baby's Blood Sugar May Be Low

Some babies look completely normal — which is why we check their blood sugar even if they appear perfect.

Others may show signs like:

- Jitteriness or tremors
- Low body temperature

- Poor feeding
- Sleepiness or difficulty waking
- Rapid breathing
- Pale or bluish skin (in more severe cases)

These symptoms are uncommon, especially with good monitoring — but this is why we watch closely.

Why We Check Your Baby's Blood Sugar

All babies born to mothers with GDM — whether *diet-controlled* or *insulin-dependent* — will have scheduled blood sugar checks starting within the first few hours of life and continuing until proven stable.

Our goal is simple:

Prevent a sudden and dangerous sugar drop.

Every hospital has a different policy or protocol as to when they intervene regarding blood sugars. It's simple, just ask!

If your baby's sugar is low, we will:

- Encourage immediate breastfeeding or formula feeding
- Give **glucose gel** if needed
- Continue monitoring until stable
- In some cases, administer IV glucose in the NICU

Stabilizing sugars early helps babies:

- Feed better
- Stay warm
- Maintain energy
- Transition smoothly into life outside the womb

Why We Check *Your* Blood Sugar Too

Even after delivery, your body is still recalibrating. Some moms who were diet-controlled go right back to normal glucose levels once the placenta is delivered — sometimes within hours. Others still see elevated sugars for a short period while hormones shift and the body adjusts.

If you were on insulin or oral medications during pregnancy, we will often:

- Check your blood sugar during your postpartum stay
- Teach you signs of high or low blood sugar
- Review your medication plan before discharge

Most women's blood sugar levels return to normal quickly — but because GDM increases your lifetime risk of developing Type II Diabetes, postpartum monitoring and follow-up are essential.

Your Diet Still Matters During Your Stay

Even once the baby is born, the hormones that influenced your blood sugar don't disappear instantly. Eating in a way that keeps your sugar stable can help you feel better, heal faster, and support your baby's glucose levels too.

We'll encourage you to choose:

- Lean proteins
- Complex carbohydrates
- Healthy fats
- Balanced meals instead of sugary snacks
- Avoiding juice unless it's necessary for a low sugar

No need for a strict diet — just gentle awareness of what helps your body stay steady while it transitions out of pregnancy mode.

How GDM Affects Feeding After Birth

Feeding is *incredibly* important for GDM babies because **milk = sugar stability**.

We will help you:

- Breastfeed early and frequently
- Supplement safely if sugars are low
- Pump if needed to stimulate production
- Keep your baby warm (cold stress burns glucose)

Your baby is **not** sick — their pancreas simply needs time to adjust. A few extra checks and early feeds help prevent dips and keep everything stable.

Nurse's Reassurance

Gestational diabetes does **not** mean:

- you did something wrong
- your baby is unhealthy
- your birth will automatically be complicated

What it *does* mean:

We will support your baby's sugar levels a little more closely in the first hours of life. Most GDM babies stabilize beautifully, feed well, and go home with their parents right on schedule.

You are not alone in this.
We are watching over both of you carefully, gently, and with so much compassion — making sure your baby transitions safely and peacefully into the world.

Shoulder Dystocia: What It Is and What You Need to Know

Shoulder dystocia is a birth situation that happens after the baby's head is delivered, when one of the shoulders becomes stuck behind the mother's pelvic bone. It is uncommon and usually resolved quickly but because it can be stressful in the moment, it helps to understand what it is, why it happens, and how your healthcare team responds.

Most importantly:

Shoulder dystocia is not anyone's fault.
Not yours, not the baby's, not the nurse's, not the provider's — it is an anatomical moment that can happen even in completely normal pregnancies.

Why Shoulder Dystocia Happens

While anyone can experience shoulder dystocia, certain factors slightly increase the chance:

- Larger baby (macrosomia)
- Gestational diabetes
- A baby with wider shoulders or chest
- Prolonged second stage (pushing)
- Assisted vaginal delivery (vacuum/forceps)
- Rapid delivery where the body follows too quickly

But shoulder dystocia still happens in **healthy, low-risk pregnancies** — so it is never a sign you did something wrong.

What It Looks Like From the Bedside

If shoulder dystocia occurs, we act **fast, coordinated, and calm**.

You may hear the provider say, "Shoulder dystocia or just Shoulder!," which activates a practiced response.

Your nurse and provider may:

- Bring your legs back into the **McRoberts** position (legs pulled all the way back, like the horse analogy I explained to you, only more exaggerated)
- Apply **suprapubic pressure** (firm pressure above your pubic bone)
- Ask you to stop pushing briefly
- Quickly change your position

From your view, things may feel urgent — but never chaotic.
We train for this constantly. Every move is purposeful and practiced.

What Happens for the Baby

Because the head is already delivered, the focus is on freeing the shoulder.

Most of the time, the baby delivers **within seconds to under a minute**.

Your baby may:

- Need brief stimulation to cry
- Need a quick assessment from NICU staff
- Have temporary arm weakness
- Have a small clavicle fracture (if it happens, it heals incredibly well)

These outcomes are usually **Short-lived** and resolve beautifully.

How We Care for You Afterward

After the birth, we will:

- Assess your bleeding
- Check your uterus frequently
- Evaluate for lacerations

- Explain everything clearly
- Offer emotional support

Many mothers process the event hours or even days later — and that's okay. We'll walk through it with you whenever you're ready.

Nurse's Reassurance

Shoulder dystocia can feel like a big moment — but you are surrounded by a team that trains for it regularly.

We know the maneuvers.
We know the sequence.
We know how to keep you and your baby safe.

Most shoulder dystocias resolve quickly with **healthy outcomes for both mom and baby**.

You are never alone — your nurse is at your side, your provider is guiding the delivery, and every person in the room has one shared goal:

A safe birth for you and your baby.

Nurse's Note

Always let your healthcare provider know if you experienced shoulder dystocia in a previous delivery. This information helps us prepare, plan positioning, and have the right hands in the room so we can respond quickly and safely.

From My Heart to Yours: A Note About Shoulder Dystocia

Know that I take shoulder dystocias — and the risks that come with them — *very* seriously in my practice. My first son, the 10 pound, 2 ounce, beautiful baby that he was, was a shoulder dystocia, and it left him with paralysis in his arm for three months. I wasn't a nurse at the time; I was just a young mother, terrified and devastated, not knowing what his future would look like. I was told that if he didn't regain movement within three months, he would need exploratory surgery to try to correct the injury.

So there my Randy and I were — driving to neurology and physical therapy **three times a week**, clinging to hope and doing everything we could to maintain his muscle tone and mobility. And then, almost three months to the day, I woke up to find him lying in his little bedside bassinet with his once-lifeless arm stretched high up into the air, as if saying, *"Hey Mom, I did it. Look, I'm going to be okay!"* And he has been more than o-kay ever since..

I still get chills every time I tell that story.

But for *you*, please know this:
A shoulder dystocia does **not** always mean injury. It is a risk, not a guarantee. There are good outcomes and bad outcomes and every situation is unique. What matters is that your health care team is trained, prepared, and ready to respond quickly and appropriately if it happens.

We will explain the risks honestly.
We will react with skill and urgency.
And we will do everything in our power to keep both you and your baby safe.

You are not alone — and your story is not written yet.

31

Preterm Labor: What It Is and What It Means for You and Your Baby

"The timing is unexpected. The courage is not."

Preterm labor is when your body begins preparing for birth **before 37 weeks of pregnancy**. It can be frightening to feel contractions or pressure earlier than expected, but I want you to know this:

You are not alone.
We respond quickly.
There is so much we can do to protect both you and your baby.

Preterm labor does **not** mean you did anything wrong. It is not a failure, not a sign you weren't careful enough and not something you could have prevented. Pregnancy is complex and sometimes the body moves ahead before we want it to — and that's exactly why we're here.

What Causes Preterm Labor?

Sometimes we can pinpoint a reason and sometimes we can't. Preterm labor can happen to anyone, even with a perfectly healthy pregnancy.

Common contributors include:

- Dehydration
- Infection (UTIs, kidney infections, vaginal infections)
- Stress or trauma
- Placental abruption
- Twins or multiples
- A short cervix or one that has had surgery
- Uterine defect
- Use of illicit drugs
- Polyhydramnios (too much amniotic fluid)
- High blood pressure or preeclampsia
- Diabetes
- Premature rupture of membranes (water breaking early)
- A history of preterm birth

But many women who experience preterm labor have **no risk factors at all**. This is why recognizing symptoms early is so important.

What Preterm Labor Feels Like

Every woman describes it differently, but the most common symptoms include:

Contractions

- Regular tightening
- Menstrual-like cramping
- Lower back pain that doesn't go away
- Pelvic or rectal pressure
- Contractions that continue even after resting or hydrating

Other Symptoms

- Increased vaginal discharge
- Fluid leaking (possible rupture of membranes)
- Spotting or bleeding
- A feeling that *"something isn't right"*

If you feel any of these before 37 weeks, call your provider immediately. You are **never** overreacting. We would always rather see you early than too late.

What Happens When You Come to the Hospital

If you come in with symptoms of preterm labor, your nurse and provider will take immediate steps to assess your situation. This usually includes:

Monitoring Your Contractions

You'll be placed on the monitor so we can see:

- How often you're contracting
- How long contractions last
- Whether they're consistent or irregular

Checking Baby's Well-Being

We'll assess your baby's heart rate pattern to make sure they're tolerating everything well and staying comfortably oxygenated.

Cervical Exam

Your cervix will be checked to see:

- Whether it's dilated
- Whether it's thinning (effacing)

- Whether it's changing over time

These changes help us determine whether you're in true preterm labor.

Ultrasound

Sometimes we need a deeper look — especially at:

- Cervical length
- Baby's position
- Amniotic fluid levels

Laboratory Tests

We may test for:

- **Urinary tract infection**
- **Dehydration/electrolyte imbalance**
- **Vaginal infections** (BV, yeast, trichomonas)
- **Ruptured membranes**
- **Fetal fibronectin** (a swab that helps predict your risk of delivering soon)

All of this gives us a clear picture of what your body is doing — and what your baby needs.

How We Treat Preterm Labor

Treatment depends on the cause and how far along you are. Options may include:

1. Hydration

Sometimes contractions are triggered by dehydration.
IV fluids can calm them down quickly and safely.

2. Medications to Stop or Slow Contractions (Tocolytics)

These medications don't *stop* labor permanently, but they buy us precious time — time to give steroids, prepare the NICU team, or transfer you to a higher-level facility if needed.

Common tocolytics include:

- **Nifedipine** (most common)
- **Terbutaline** (short-term use only) — may temporarily increase your heart rate

3. Steroids

If your baby might deliver soon, steroids help mature their:

- Lungs
- Gut
- Brain

These medications have saved *countless* premature babies and are one of the most important interventions in preterm labor.

4. Magnesium Sulfate

Given for **fetal neuroprotection** if delivery is expected before full gestation. The actual number of weeks depends on your particular provider and their practice. (See full Magnesium Sulfate section in the Preeclampsia Chapter)

5. Treating the Underlying Cause

Depending on what triggered the contractions, we may:

- Treat infections

- Rehydrate you
- Manage blood pressure or diabetes
- Monitor closely if your water has broken

6. Bed Rest or Activity Modification

Not always required but may be recommended depending on cervical changes, contraction patterns, and provider preference.

What This Means for Your Baby

Babies born preterm can need extra help transitioning after delivery, especially with:

- Breathing
- Feeding
- Maintaining temperature
- Keeping blood sugar stable

Depending on their gestational age, the **NICU team may be present** for your delivery.
This does **not** mean anything is wrong — it means we are ready.

Many babies born between **34–36 weeks** do wonderfully with only minimal support.

Babies born earlier may need:

- CPAP
- Oxygen support
- Feeding tubes
- Temperature regulation in an isolette
- Extra monitoring

But preterm babies are fighters — and they are cared for by specialists who know exactly what they need to thrive.

Betamethasone: What It Is and Why We Give It

Betamethasone — often called *"beta"* on the unit — is a steroid injection given to you when we think your baby may come early. It is one of the most powerful and effective tools we have to support premature babies.

Why We Give Betamethasone

It helps your baby's:

- Lungs mature
- Surfactant develop (the "coating" that keeps airways open)
- Brain and gut prepare for life outside the womb

Even **one dose** can significantly improve outcomes for babies born before **34–36 weeks**.

How It's Given

You'll receive:

- **Two injections**, 24 hours apart, some providers chose 12 if delivery looks imminent
- Usually in the hip, upper arm, or thigh
- A quick sting, but very tolerable
- Most hospitals aim to complete the full two-dose series if time allows

How Betamethasone Affects Blood Sugar (Important!)

Steroids naturally raise blood sugar — even in people who are not diabetic.
They cause your liver to release more glucose and temporarily make your body less responsive to insulin.

In Moms, This Means:

Your blood sugar can rise for **24–72 hours** after the injection.

If you have GDM, we will:

- Monitor your sugars more closely
- Adjust insulin if needed
- Encourage balanced meals

Even diet-controlled moms may see temporary spikes.
This is **normal** — and absolutely *not* your fault.

In Babies, This Means:

Your baby may experience a **temporary drop** in blood sugar after birth, so we:

- Check their sugars frequently
- Encourage early feeding
- Provide glucose gel if needed

These changes are **short-lived** and do *not* cause long-term issues.

Nurse's Reassurance

Betamethasone is one of the few medications in obstetrics that has **immediate, proven, lifesaving benefits** for premature infants.

If we recommend it, it is because we want your baby to have:

- Stronger lungs
- A safer transition
- A better outcome

And if your sugar rises — or your baby's drops — we know exactly how to manage it.
You will not be navigating any of this alone.

> **Nurse's Tip:** The little sting you feel from the needle during your betamethasone shot isn't usually the part that hurts the most – it's actually the *medicine* going in that causes the deeper burn. It's quick but I know it can be uncomfortable.
>
> Hang in there, mama. You are tougher than you think and you're doing this for your baby. This moment of discomfort is helping their tiny lungs grow stronger and that makes every second worth it. You've got this.

Your Emotions Matter

Preterm labor is scary. Full stop.

It brings uncertainty, fear, and a loss of control — and it is **okay** to feel that way.

Your nurse will:

- Explain every step
- Sit with you through the fear
- Calm the room
- Advocate fiercely for you and your baby

You did nothing to cause this.
You are doing everything right by seeking help.

Nurse's Reassurance

Preterm labor can feel unpredictable, but your care team is:

- Trained
- Prepared
- Experienced
- Ready

Many women who experience preterm labor go on to carry much longer and deliver healthy babies.
Every day your pregnancy continues is a **victory** and we will fight for every one of those days with you.

Surfactant: Your Baby's Lung Superpower

Surfactant is a slippery, foamy substance that lines the tiny air sacs inside your baby's lungs.
It's the "magic coating" that keeps the lungs open.

Without enough surfactant, the lungs can collapse between breaths — making breathing incredibly hard work.

Why Surfactant Is Crucial for Preemies

Surfactant doesn't fully develop until **34–36 weeks**.
If a baby is born early, this can lead to:

- Difficulty breathing
- Retractions
- Grunting
- Respiratory Distress Syndrome (RDS)

This is where medicine steps in.

How We Support Early Lungs

1. Betamethasone Before Birth

Helps the baby make more surfactant naturally — your two injections can make a huge difference.

2. Surfactant Replacement After Birth

If needed, the NICU team can give surfactant directly into your baby's lungs through a tiny breathing tube.

This:

- Opens the lungs
- Improves oxygen levels
- Reduces the work of breathing
- Dramatically improves outcomes

It is one of the greatest advances in neonatal medicine.

What You May See After Birth

If your baby is born premature, the NICU team will be ready the moment they arrive. Their role is to support your baby's transition with skill, gentleness, and constant communication.

Here's what the team may do right away:

- Dry and warm your baby to prevent heat loss
- Begin breathing support if your baby needs help ("CPAP" or gentle puffs of air)
- Monitor oxygen levels and breathing patterns
- Evaluate whether surfactant is needed for lung support
- Keep you updated every step of the way

It's completely normal for premature babies to:

- Need CPAP or soft nasal support
- Breathe fast or unevenly at first
- Use extra muscles to breathe (retractions)
- Look sleepy or tire easily
- Need help for a few hours, days, or longer depending on their gestational age

None of this means your baby is struggling — it means they are adjusting, and the NICU team is giving their tiny lungs all the help they need.

Nurse's Reassurance

Surfactant is one of the greatest protectors we have for premature babies — whether their lungs begin making it naturally or the NICU team gives it right after birth. If your baby arrives early, it does **not** mean they are weak. It means they need a little extra time, support, and gentle guidance as they adjust to life outside the womb.

Premature babies are some of the strongest fighters I've ever met. Their resilience is incredible and surfactant therapy is one of the tools that helps them do what they were born to do — grow, breathe, and thrive.

Your baby is never without help.
And **you will never be left out of the loop.**

Your team is here for both of you — every moment, every update, every heartbeat. 🤍

My Preterm Birth Story: A Reminder to Hold on to Hope

Before I ever became a nurse, I lived through a moment that changed me forever. My beloved dog, **Scout** — the dog my husband and I got when we were just teenagers — passed away after 13 beautiful years. I was devastated. Heartbroken. And my body reacted in a way I never expected: I went into **preterm labor**.

At just **29 weeks**, on New Year's Eve weekend, I found myself in the hospital getting **betamethasone shots** to help my baby's lungs and underwent an ultrasound. As if the contractions weren't scary enough, the ultrasound tech told me that **Brady's brain ventricles were enlarged**. Because of the holiday, I had to wait days for further evaluation.

I wasn't a nurse at the time — I had no medical knowledge, just the internet. So of course, I went straight to diagnosing him myself. The fear was overwhelming.

My preterm labor eventually subsided and I was sent home. Days later, I had another appointment confirming that yes, the ventricles were enlarged — and that we wouldn't know what that meant until he was born.

So I carried that fear all the way to **37 weeks**.
I delivered my sweet Brady **not knowing** if he would be okay.

But not only was he okay…
He was **absolutely perfect**.

Why I'm Telling You This

Because I know how terrified you may be right now — whether you're in preterm labor or an anomaly has been found on ultrasound. I know the late-night Googling, the fear, the "what-if" spiral.

But take it from someone who has lived it:

Please don't steal weeks of joy from yourself worrying about things you cannot control.

Have hope. Have faith. Things can be okay — beautifully, unexpectedly okay.

God works in mysterious ways.
And this story doesn't end here.

Full Circle: The Baby Named Scout

A couple of months ago, I had the honor of caring for the loveliest couple experiencing preterm labor with their long-awaited IVF pregnancy. They were terrified — she was only in the early third trimester. We stabilized her and weeks later she returned for her induction.

And wouldn't you know it…
I was her Labor Nurse.

I got to help bring their beautiful baby into the world — a baby they had prayed for, fought for, and feared for. And after all they had been through, after all *I* had been through years before…

They told me his name.
Not because they knew anything about my past.
Not because of my story.
Just because it was the name they chose.

His name was **Scout**.

I still get chills thinking about it.
Sometimes, God places you exactly where you're meant to be, with the exact people you're meant to care for — as a reminder that hope, healing, and full-circle moments are always possible.

32

Placental & Uterine Complications: What You Need to Know

"Complications don't define your birth.
The care you receive does."

The placenta is your baby's lifeline — it delivers oxygen, nutrients, and everything your little one needs to grow. Most pregnancies never experience placental problems, but when complications do occur, they can impact how we monitor you, how we manage your pregnancy, and sometimes how and when you deliver.

Below are the three major conditions you may hear about: **placenta previa**, **placenta accreta spectrum**, and **placental abruption**.

Placenta Previa

When the placenta covers the cervix

Normally, the placenta implants high on the uterine wall. Placenta previa happens when the placenta implants low and either touches or completely covers the cervix — the doorway your baby must pass through during birth.

Types of Previa

- **Complete previa:** Cervix fully covered
- **Partial previa:** Cervix partially covered
- **Marginal previa:** Placenta lies very close to the cervix
- **Low-lying placenta:** Within a few centimeters of the cervix

Symptoms

- Painless vaginal bleeding in the 2nd or 3rd trimester
- Bright red bleeding
- Bleeding that starts and stops

How We Manage It

- **No vaginal exams** (to prevent triggering bleeding)
- **Pelvic rest** (no intercourse, no tampons, no internal checks)
- **Regular ultrasounds** to track placenta movement
- **Possible hospitalization** if bleeding recurs or is heavy
- **C-section delivery** for complete or partial previa

Nurse's Reassurance

Placenta previa can sound alarming, but many low-lying placentas move upward as your uterus grows. If it remains a previa, we simply plan a safe, scheduled C-section — you won't be asked to labor or push. Safety and preparation guide every decision.

Placenta Accreta Spectrum (Accreta, Increta, Percreta)

When the placenta attaches too deeply

Placenta accreta occurs when the placenta grows firmly into the uterine wall, making it difficult (or impossible) to detach after birth. Without planning, this can cause serious bleeding — but with preparation, outcomes are overwhelmingly positive.

Levels of Invasion

- **Accreta:** Grows into the uterine lining
- **Increta:** Invades the uterine muscle
- **Percreta:** Grows through the uterus, sometimes into nearby organs

Risk Factors

- Prior C-sections (the biggest factor)
- Placenta previa
- Multiple uterine surgeries
- IVF
- Maternal age 35+

How It's Diagnosed

- Ultrasound (often the first clue)
- MRI for clearer visualization
- Referral to high-risk obstetrics (MFM)

How We Manage It

Placenta accreta deliveries are planned with extraordinary care:

- Delivery at a **high-risk obstetric center**
- **Scheduled C-section**, usually around 34–36 weeks
- A coordinated surgical team including OB, anesthesia, NICU, and sometimes urology
- A prepared blood bank
- **Planned hysterectomy** is often the safest approach after delivery

Nurse's Reassurance

Accreta is overwhelming to hear but these cases are **not** emergencies when planned appropriately. You will have a whole team designing every detail of your delivery well in advance. You will not be surprised, unprepared, or left alone — accreta care is one of the most coordinated, carefully managed situations in obstetrics.

Placental Abruption

When the placenta separates too early

Placental abruption occurs when the placenta partially or completely detaches from the uterine wall before birth. This disrupts oxygen and nutrient flow to the baby and can cause significant bleeding.

Abruption is **sudden, painful, and always treated as an emergency.**

Symptoms

- Severe abdominal pain
- A firm, rigid, or "boardlike" uterus
- Vaginal bleeding (light or heavy — both matter)
- Lower back pain
- Rapid, back-to-back contractions
- Baby showing distress on the monitor

Important: Bleeding may be **concealed** inside the uterus — meaning you may not see much blood even with a severe abruption.

Risk Factors

- High blood pressure
- Trauma (car accident, fall, impact)
- Smoking

- Drug use (especially cocaine)
- Previous abruption
- Multiple gestation
- Premature rupture of membranes

How We Manage It

Treatment depends on severity and gestational age:

Mild abruption:

- Close observation
- IV fluids
- Frequent vital signs
- Continuous fetal monitoring

Moderate to severe abruption OR any fetal distress:

- **Immediate delivery**, often a C-section
- Blood products if bleeding is significant
- Rapid, coordinated response by the entire team

Nurse's Reassurance

A placental abruption is one of the moments where the room shifts gears fast — but none of it is chaotic. Every person has a role. Every move is intentional. Your nurse will stay at your bedside, monitoring, explaining, supporting, and preparing you for what comes next. We move quickly **because it keeps you and your baby safe.**

Final Reassurance: You're Not Alone

Placental and uterine complications can feel frightening — but please remember:

You did not cause this.
You will be monitored closely.
You will never go through this alone.
Your team always has a plan.
Your nurse will be with you through every moment.

You don't need to know every medical term.
You don't need to understand every step.
You just need to tell us how you feel — and trust that we're watching over you both.

Uterine Rupture

Rare, serious, but carefully watched for

"Uterine rupture" is a phrase that understandably rattles people — but it deserves explanation, not fear.

A uterine rupture happens when a previous uterine scar (most commonly a C-section scar) opens during labor. It is rare but because it's serious, labor nurses and providers are highly trained to watch for the earliest signs.

This is especially monitored during:
TOLAC (Trial of Labor After Cesarean) or **VBAC** (Vaginal Birth After Cesarean).

What You Should Know

- Most women attempting a VBAC **do not** experience a rupture.
- VBAC success rates are high.
- Rupture rates remain very low.
- Continuous monitoring is used to keep you safe.

Your nurse will watch for subtle signs long before they become severe — things like sudden pain, fetal heart rate changes, or altered contraction patterns.

If a Rupture Happens

The team moves into immediate action:

- Stop Pitocin (if running)
- Prepare for an urgent C-section
- Stabilize you and your baby
- Communicate clearly with you and your support person

This is one of the most rehearsed emergency scenarios in obstetrics. You are surrounded by a team trained to respond within seconds.

Nurse's Reassurance

Uterine rupture may be rare, but vigilance is constant. You will never be left unmonitored, unsupported, or unheard. Whether you are attempting a VBAC or simply laboring with a uterine scar, your nurse is watching everything — not out of fear, but out of deep commitment to keeping you safe.

You are in good hands. Always.

Who Is at Risk for Uterine Rupture?

The biggest risk factor is a **previous cesarean birth** because it leaves a scar on the uterus. Most scars are strong and heal beautifully — but some types come with a higher risk than others.

Risk Is Higher With:

- Classical (vertical) uterine incision
- Multiple previous C-sections
- Short pregnancy spacing (< 18 months)
- Induction or augmentation during TOLAC

- A very thin lower uterine segment on ultrasound *(rarely checked routinely)*

Risk Is Lowest With:

- One prior **low-transverse incision** (the most common and safest type for VBAC)
- **Spontaneous labor** — when your body starts contractions on its own
- Minimal or no induction medications

Important: Hospitals that offer TOLAC/VBAC do so because they have the skills, staff, and OR readiness to manage it safely.

What We Look For During Labor

Uterine rupture almost never starts dramatically.
The **first signs usually appear on the fetal heart monitor**, which is why continuous monitoring is required during VBAC.

Here's what your nurse watches for:

1. Sudden Fetal Distress

- Recurrent late decelerations
- A prolonged deceleration
- **Sudden loss of fetal station** (baby moves *up* in the pelvis instead of down)

2. Severe Maternal Pain That Feels "Different"

- Pain between contractions
- Pain that doesn't match the contraction pattern
- A tearing or ripping sensation *(not always present)*

3. Maternal Vital Sign Changes

- Drop in blood pressure
- Increased heart rate
- Feeling faint, dizzy, or "not right"

4. Vaginal Bleeding

Can be light or heavy.

5. Loss of Uterine Tone

The uterus may stop contracting as strongly or regularly.

You may notice none of this — but your nurse will.
We read the monitor constantly during TOLAC.

How We Respond

If we suspect a uterine rupture, it becomes an obstetric emergency.
But please hear this: **it is a practiced emergency.**

Your team will move quickly *and* calmly. You may be taken immediately to the OR for a **stat C-section**.

Goals of Treatment:

- Deliver the baby safely
- Control bleeding
- Repair the uterus
- Stabilize both mom and baby

Your Response Team Usually Includes:

- Obstetrician

- Anesthesiologist
- Labor nurses
- OR nurses
- NICU staff (if needed)

You will not be alone — ever.

What Surgery Might Look Like

After baby is delivered, the surgeon will examine your uterus:

- Many uterine ruptures can be **repaired with stitches**.
- In rare cases, if bleeding is severe or the tear is extensive, a **life-saving hysterectomy** may be needed.

These decisions are made quickly, skillfully, and with **your safety as the top priority**.

Nurse's Reassurance: Uterine Rupture Is Rare — and Watched For Constantly

What I want you to truly feel:

Most VBACs are successful.
Most women will NOT experience uterine rupture.
Your team knows exactly what to look for.
Continuous monitoring is why we catch issues early.
You will never be ignored, minimized, or left unobserved.
If rupture occurs, we respond immediately and expertly.

We don't talk about uterine rupture to scare you. We talk about it to **empower you**, inform you, and make sure you feel prepared — not afraid.

VBAC is a safe and beautiful option for many women.
Understanding the risks simply helps you make the choices that feel best for your body, your pregnancy, and your birth story.

33

Special Deliveries: When Your Birth Journey Needs Something Extra

"Special deliveries aren't harder — they're just born with a little extra magic."

Every baby's arrival is unique and some pregnancies need a little extra planning, monitoring, and teamwork. These "special deliveries" don't make your birth risky — they simply mean your care is more *individualized.* And individualized care is what we do best.

As your nurse, I want you to know this:
You are not complicated.
You are not difficult.
You are not high-maintenance.
You simply need care tailored to *your* story — and we are honored to give you exactly that.

This chapter walks you through some of the most common situations that need a little extra attention: twins, TOLAC/VBAC, cerclage pregnancies, and more.

Twin (and Multiple) Gestation

Delivering twins is one of the most exhilarating experiences in all of Labor & Delivery — double heartbeats, double the teamwork, and double the joy. But it also means extra monitoring and very coordinated care.

How Twin Monitoring Works

We use **two fetal monitors** — one for each baby.

Sometimes they sit perfectly.
Sometimes they take turns doing acrobatics.
You may see me adjusting the monitors constantly — that's normal.

Twins love to hide behind each other and keeping two heartbeats separate on the screen can feel like tuning two radios at once.

Your Delivery Plan Depends On:

- Baby A's position
- Baby B's position
- Growth and weight of both babies
- How your pregnancy has progressed
- Your provider's experience
- Your hospital's resources

Vaginal Birth for Twins is absolutely possible

Especially if:

- Baby A is **head down**
- Baby B is head down **or** can be safely turned
- You and both babies are stable

Many providers deliver twins vaginally **in the operating room** — not because surgery is expected, but so that everything you need is already in place *if* Baby B suddenly needs help.

Cesarean Birth for Twins

Sometimes recommended if:

- Baby A is breech
- Large weight difference between babies
- Preterm instability
- Placenta previa
- Mono-mono twins (sharing one sac — extremely high monitoring needs)

Nurse's Reassurance

Twin deliveries have a special energy — the whole team is focused, coordinated, and fully prepared. You will never feel alone or unmonitored. We're watching carefully, adjusting constantly, and supporting you through every moment.

Nurse's Tip – The Twin Monitor Shuffle

If you're carrying twins, there will be moments where I'm adjusting those monitors every few minutes.

I promise:

- It's not because anything is wrong
- It's not because I'm trying to bother you
- It's not because the monitor isn't working

> It's simply because **twins love to hide behind each other.** They tag-team switching places, they roll, they wiggle, and sometimes they lie right on top of one another like stacked pancakes.
>
> *It feels like I'm tuning two radios at once while the babies do gymnastics inside you.*
>
> Thank you for your patience – every adjustment is done to keep both babies clearly and safely on the screen. Your comfort and your babies' safety are always my priorities.

TOLAC & VBAC

(Trial of Labor After Cesarean / Vaginal Birth After Cesarean)

Choosing a TOLAC means you're giving yourself the opportunity to labor after a previous cesarean with the hope of achieving a VBAC. Many women are excellent candidates and your chances of success are often higher than you think.

Who Qualifies for TOLAC/VBAC

You may be a strong candidate if you have:

- **A prior low-transverse uterine incision**
- **No history of uterine rupture**
- **No contraindication to vaginal birth**
- **A prior cesarean for a reason that is *not* guaranteed to repeat** (examples: breech baby, fetal distress, failed induction)

Why TOLAC Can Be Very Successful

Your body has done this before:

- Your cervix has dilated before
- Your uterus has contracted before
- Your pelvis has already proven itself
- Many second-time labors progress more efficiently

Your body remembers — even if your mind doesn't.

What We Monitor Closely

During a TOLAC, your nurse and provider will keep a close eye on:

- **Fetal heart tones**
- **Contraction pattern**
- **Signs of uterine rupture (rare)**
- **Progression of labor**

Continuous monitoring is required — not to restrict you but to keep you safe.

Benefits of VBAC

- **Shorter recovery time**
- **Less bleeding**
- **Lower risk of infection**
- **Avoiding repeat abdominal surgery**
- **More immediate mobility**
- **Faster return to normal activities**

VBAC is a safe and evidence-based option for many women.

Nurse's Reassurance

Choosing TOLAC does *not* mean choosing a risky or reckless path.
It means choosing a **monitored, supported, and informed** alternative to surgery.

You are not "trying something dangerous."
You are choosing a path your care team knows how to support.

And we will be with you through each contraction, each adjustment, and each decision.

A Note About Hospital Policies for TOLAC

Not every hospital offers TOLAC — and that's about *resources*, not judgment.

Some facilities do not have:

- 24/7 in-house anesthesia
- A dedicated OR team available at all times
- Staffing levels needed to quickly respond to emergencies

In these hospitals, they may recommend a scheduled repeat C-section because they want you somewhere equipped to support your goal safely.

Even in hospitals that **do** offer TOLAC, you may notice more cautious decision-making:

- Lower doses of Pitocin
- Avoidance of certain cervical-ripening agents
- Extra monitoring
- More frequent check-ins with the provider

This isn't hesitation — it's **evidence-based safety practice**.

Nurse's Reassurance

Your desire for a VBAC is *valid.*
Your goal is *respected.*
And it *deserves* to be supported — safely.

If TOLAC is important to you, talk to your provider early. Ask:

- "Does this hospital support VBAC?"
- "Does your practice support TOLAC?"
- "What are the induction policies for VBAC patients?"

The right environment — and the right team — make all the difference.

And we will help you find the safest, most supportive path to meet your baby.

PPROM: Preterm Premature Rupture of Membranes

(Your Water Breaking Before 37 Weeks)

PPROM happens when your water breaks early — **before 37 weeks and before labor has started on its own**. It can feel shocking, confusing, or scary, especially if you weren't expecting it. But I want you to know: we treat PPROM every single day and there is a clear, evidence-based plan for stabilizing you and protecting your baby.

You did **nothing wrong**.
Your body didn't "fail."
And you are not alone.

How You'll Know It's PPROM

Most people describe:

- A sudden gush of fluid
- A slow, continuous trickle
- Wet underwear that keeps re-wetting
- Fluid that doesn't smell like urine

If your water breaks early, you should come right in — even if you're not contracting.

What Happens When You Come to Labor & Delivery

As soon as you arrive, we start **stabilizing and assessing** both you and your baby. This includes:

1. Confirming Your Water Is Broken

We may do:

- A sterile speculum exam
- Testing the fluid
- Ultrasound to check fluid levels

(We avoid regular vaginal exams to reduce infection risk.)

2. Monitoring Baby

You'll be placed on continuous or intermittent fetal monitoring to see how your baby is tolerating everything.

3. Checking You for Infection

We monitor for:

- Fever
- Maternal vital signs
- Uterine tenderness
- Fetal tachycardia
- Abnormal discharge

4. Starting Antibiotics

You'll likely receive **latency antibiotics**, which help keep infection away and prolong pregnancy.

5. Steroids (Betamethasone)

If you're under 34–36 weeks, you'll likely receive steroid injections to:

- Mature baby's lungs
- Reduce NICU time
- Prevent complications

6. IV Fluids & Labs

We draw labs to check:

- Blood counts
- Inflammation markers
- Type & screen
- Infection markers

IV fluids help keep your body stable while we assess your next steps.

Nurse's Note: MFM & NEO Consults – Your Safety Net in PPROM

When you're diagnosed with PPROM, your care automatically becomes a *team effort* — and two of the most important specialists who step in are:

MFM (Maternal-Fetal Medicine)

High-risk pregnancy specialists who guide your medical plan, monitor complications, and help determine *when* and *how* you should deliver.

NEO (Neonatology)

Newborn specialists who prepare for your baby's needs if they arrive early. They explain what to expect in the NICU, breathing support, feeding plans, and what milestones your baby will need to reach before going home.

These consults aren't a sign that something is "wrong."
They're a sign that **you are being protected**.

MFM helps us keep your pregnancy going as long as safely possible.
NEO helps us prepare the safest transition for your baby — whether they're born tomorrow or weeks from now.

Both teams will talk with you directly, answer every question, and make sure you understand the plan. You're not fighting this battle alone — you have an entire village of experts standing behind you, watching you and your baby like hawks, advocating for the best possible outcome.

Their involvement is not scary — it's reassuring.
It means we are giving you *more* eyes, *more* expertise, and *more* support at exactly the moment you need it.

Why We Often Transfer You to Postpartum

Once you are stable — and **not in active labor** — most PPROM patients are moved from Labor & Delivery to Postpartum for ongoing monitoring.

This surprises a lot of people, but here's why:

1. PPROM is often a "wait and watch" condition.

Delivery may be days or even weeks away.

2. You don't need L&D-level monitoring 24/7.

Once baby looks good and you're not contracting, you're safe on the postpartum side. And you will appreciate the freedom.

3. Postpartum offers a quieter, calmer environment.

This is important because stress can increase contractions.

4. NICU is already involved behind the scenes.

Your baby's team is aware and prepared.

What Monitoring Looks Like on Postpartum

Your postpartum stay becomes a careful balance of **protecting you, reducing infection risk, and catching labor early**.

Expect:

- **Daily or twice-daily non-stress test (NSTs)** (monitoring baby's heart rate)
- **Vital-sign checks** to watch for infection
- **Regular assessment** for tightening, pain, bleeding, or new leakage
- **Temperature checks**
- **Monitoring your fluid loss/color** (how much you're leaking is important)
- **Ultrasounds as needed** to check fluid levels or fetal growth

You may stay on bedrest or modified activity depending on your provider.

When Delivery Happens

We deliver sooner if:

- Signs of infection develop
- Baby shows distress
- You reach a specific gestational age
- Labor starts on its own

- The cord or placenta becomes compromised

Many patients with PPROM **do not** deliver immediately — we often successfully prolong pregnancy to give baby more time to grow.

Nurse's Reassurance

PPROM can feel like your body betrayed you — but it didn't. This is something that happens unpredictably, even in perfectly healthy pregnancies.

You will be:

- Monitored closely
- Watched for infection constantly
- Supported emotionally
- Prepared for delivery when the time is right
- Surrounded by a team that knows PPROM inside and out

We stabilize you in L&D, then move you to postpartum to protect your pregnancy for as long as safely possible. The goal is simple:

Keep you safe.
Keep your baby safe.
Buy your little one as much time as possible.

You don't go through a single step of this alone.

AGA, LGA, and SGA: *What Size Is Your Delivery?*

During your ultrasound and sometimes after birth, you may hear your nurse or provider use terms like **AGA, LGA, or SGA** when describing your baby's size. These aren't labels of health — just clinical categories that compare your baby's weight to the average for their gestational age.

They help us tailor monitoring and feeding, but they do **not** define your baby's strength or wellness.

AGA - Appropriate for Gestational Age

This means your baby's weight falls **between the 10th and 90th percentile** for their gestational age.

Most newborns are AGA.

What this means:

- Baby grew as expected
- Typical feeding needs
- Standard newborn monitoring

SGA - Small for Gestational Age

SGA means your baby weighs **below the 10th percentile** for their gestational age.

Common reasons include:

- Genetics (small parents often make small babies!)
- Placental insufficiency
- High blood pressure disorders
- Smoking
- IUGR (intrauterine growth restriction)

SGA babies may need:

- More frequent blood sugar checks
- Help maintaining body temperature

- Extra feeding support

These babies are often **small but mighty** and with the right support, they grow beautifully.

LGA - Large for Gestational Age

LGA means your baby weighs **above the 90th percentile** for their gestational age.

Often associated with:

- Gestational diabetes
- Naturally larger families
- Post-dates pregnancy

LGA babies may need:

- Blood sugar monitoring (big babies burn through sugar faster)
- Extra help feeding if sleepy
- Monitoring during delivery for shoulder dystocia (most do great)

LGA babies are often the **adorable chunky rolls and cheeks** everyone swoons over!

Nurse's Reassurance

AGA, SGA, and LGA are **not judgments** — they are simply tools to guide the safest, most personalized care for your baby.

SGA babies need warmth, calories, and love.
LGA babies need sugar stability and gentle transitions.
AGA babies follow standard newborn pathways.

Every baby enters the world with their own story, their own pace, and their own beauty. And no matter what category they fall into, **we know exactly how to support them — and they are perfect exactly as they are.**

Macrosomia: What It Means When Your Baby Measures Big

Macrosomia simply means your baby is larger than average — usually weighing over **4,000–4,500 grams** (about **8 lb 13 oz to 9 lb 15 oz**) at birth. It's more common than people realize, and most big babies are born completely healthy.

A "big baby" isn't a diagnosis — it's a description.
And it does **not** mean anything is wrong with you or your baby.

Why Some Babies Grow Larger

There are several reasons a baby may measure big:

- Gestational diabetes (GDM)
- Genetics (big parents often have big babies!)
- Previous macrosomic baby
- Post-dates pregnancy
- Excess maternal weight gain
- Male babies tend to weigh slightly more

And sometimes there's **no medical reason at all** — it's simply how your baby was meant to grow.

How Macrosomia Affects Pregnancy and Birth

A bigger baby may influence how we plan your delivery. It doesn't guarantee complications — it just means we keep a closer eye on a few things.

During labor:

- Contractions may need to be strong and coordinated
- The pushing phase may take longer
- Position changes become extra important
- We stay alert and prepare for shoulder dystocia, just in case

Monitoring may include:

- Ultrasounds to estimate fetal weight (remember: these can be off by a pound!)
- Assessing baby's position
- Discussing induction options
- Having extra staff ready at delivery if baby is very large

How Big Babies Behave After Birth

Most macrosomic babies transition beautifully — pink, crying, and perfect. Others may have brief, expected adjustments like:

- Low blood sugar
- Trouble staying warm
- Sleepiness
- Difficulty latching at first

These babies are often considered **"sugar babies,"** and we support them with early feeding, glucose checks, and warmth.

The Connection Between Macrosomia & GDM

When a mom has gestational diabetes:

- Extra maternal glucose crosses to baby
- Baby produces more insulin

- Insulin acts as a growth hormone
- Baby stores more fat (especially in shoulders & abdomen)

This can slightly increase the risk of:

- Shoulder dystocia
- Low blood sugar after birth
- Larger fetal size, even with controlled GDM

But again — **most GDM babies do incredibly well** with early feeding and monitoring.

What Delivery Might Look Like

Your provider may discuss:

- Induction if baby is estimated to be very large
- Possible cesarean
- Active management during pushing
- Having extra personnel present

None of these recommendations mean anything is wrong — they are simply layers of safety.

And remember: **Ultrasound weight estimates can be off by more than a pound in either direction.**

Nurse's Note

Macrosomia (a larger-than-average baby) can increase the risk of shoulder dystocia during birth. This doesn't mean it *will* happen — it just means we're prepared. Your healthcare team stays two steps ahead so we can respond quickly and safely if needed.

Nurse's Reassurance

A big baby is still just **your baby** — perfect, loved, and wonderfully made. Macrosomia does not define your birth or your story.

With the right support, positioning, and teamwork, **many big babies are born vaginally with no issues at all.**

If we take extra precautions, it's simply to give you the safest, smoothest delivery possible.

You didn't cause this.
Your body isn't failing you.
Some babies are just meant to be big.

And as your nurse, I'll be right beside you — guiding the process, keeping you safe, and celebrating your little (big!) miracle the second they arrive.

Cerclage Pregnancies

A **cerclage** is a stitch placed in the cervix during pregnancy to help keep it closed when there's a risk of cervical insufficiency or early dilation.

Who Gets a Cerclage

A cerclage may be recommended for women who have:

- A previous preterm birth related to cervical change
- A short cervix seen on ultrasound
- A history of cervical trauma or surgery
- Early, painless dilation in a current pregnancy

It's a proactive way to support the pregnancy — not a sign that anything is "wrong."

What to Expect During Labor

If you come in contracting or are getting close to delivery, your provider will remove the cerclage stitch *before* your cervix dilates further.

This:

- Is usually quick
- Can feel crampy or uncomfortable
- Helps prevent cervical tearing

If removal is urgent or uncomfortable, pain relief options can be used to help you stay calm and comfortable.

If You Deliver Preterm

We monitor very closely for:

- Infection
- Cervical changes
- Contractions
- Baby's wellbeing

Cerclage removal does **not** prevent vaginal birth — it simply helps protect the cervix earlier in pregnancy.

Nurse's Reassurance

A cerclage doesn't diminish your ability to have a vaginal birth. Many women with cerclages deliver at term, go into labor normally, and never need another cerclage in future pregnancies.

You did nothing wrong — this is simply a tool we use to keep your pregnancy safe.

Nurse's Wisdom: The Cerclage Surprise

Believe it or not, some women who needed a **cerclage** during pregnancy — a stitch placed to keep the cervix from opening too soon — actually end up needing to be **induced** to get labor started. It's one of those ironic twists in obstetrics: we spend months trying to *stop* dilation, only to find that when it's finally time to have the baby, the cervix doesn't want to open at all.

The body can be unpredictable and every cervix has its own story. Just know this: whether your labor needs to be jump-started or your body takes over on its own, both paths are normal, safe, and supported every step of the way.

Other Special Circumstances You May Hear About

Some pregnancies require a bit more monitoring or collaboration among specialists. This isn't a reflection on your strength or health — it's just personalized care.

Intrahepatic Cholestasis of Pregnancy (ICP)

A liver condition causing **intense itching**, often on the hands and feet.

What we do:

- Check liver labs & bile acids
- Monitor the baby closely
- Discuss early delivery depending on severity

Oligohydramnios / Polyhydramnios

Low or high amniotic fluid levels.

This may lead to:

- More ultrasounds
- Closer fetal heart rate monitoring
- Positioning changes during labor
- Sometimes early induction

IUGR – Intrauterine Growth Restriction

Baby measuring smaller than expected.

Management includes:

- NSTs (nonstress tests)
- Frequent ultrasounds
- Doppler studies
- Early delivery if baby shows signs of stress

Advanced Maternal Age

Age 35+ may mean:

- More ultrasounds
- Additional screening options
- Slightly higher monitoring

Most AMA pregnancies are beautifully healthy.

Fetal Anomalies or Anticipated NICU Care

When a baby needs extra support at birth, we coordinate with:

- **Neonatology (NICU team)**
- **Maternal-Fetal Medicine (MFM)**
- **Anesthesia**
- **Specialty teams**, if needed

This coordination happens *weeks* before birth so that everything is ready and seamless.

Nurse's Note: You Are Never Alone in Special Circumstances

No matter what path your pregnancy takes, your care team works **around you**, not the other way around.

We anticipate.
We prepare.
We monitor.
We adjust.
We support.

Special circumstances don't make you "high risk" in spirit — they make your care **customized, thoughtful, and deeply intentional**.

You are safe.
You are supported.
And you are never navigating any of it alone.

34

Toys of the Trade: Tools That Help Us Help You

"We bring the tools. You bring the power."

In Labor & Delivery, you'll see us reach for certain tools, props, and devices that help position your body, support your movements, and maximize your comfort and progress. I lovingly call them our **"toys of the trade"** — the little helpers that make *big* differences during labor.

Some of these include:

- Peanut balls
- Birthing balls
- "Throne" or elevated back-of-bed positioning
- Warm blankets
- Side-lying releases
- Hands-and-knees maneuvering
- Squat bars
- Mirror (to help visualize progress and enhance pushing effectiveness)
- Stirrups (used appropriately during second stage)
- Birth stools (if your hospital supports them)

These tools come from years of obstetric practice, pelvic biomechanics, and nursing experience — but many of the techniques we use today have also been influenced by a brilliant, widely known education system:

Spinning Babies® – Giving Credit Where It's Due

Many of the modern physiologic positioning techniques used in L&D are influenced by the principles of **Spinning Babies®**, an approach created by **Gail Tully, CPM**.

Spinning Babies® emphasizes:

- Maternal positioning
- Balance of pelvic muscles and ligaments
- Creating space in the pelvis to help baby navigate the birth canal
- Simple, gentle techniques that support *fetal position* and *labor progress*

It is not a medical intervention — it's a **comfort-and-positioning philosophy** designed to work *with your body, not against it.*

Techniques Commonly Used From Spinning Babies® Concepts

- Side-lying Release
- Forward-Leaning Inversion (with support and approval)
- Open-Glottis pushing positions
- "Three Sisters of Balance" for pelvic alignment
- Dynamic labor positions to open the pelvic inlet and outlet

Not all techniques are used in every hospital — training, policy, and safety always guide practice — but the underlying philosophy is universal:

Balanced muscles + good positioning = smoother labor for mom and baby.

Nurse's Acknowledgment

Nurses have been using positional changes for decades, but the Spinning Babies® program beautifully organized and popularized many of the techniques we incorporate today.

We honor the work of **Gail Tully, CPM** and acknowledge her contributions to helping birthing families understand:

their bodies
their babies
and the power of movement during labor

Why These Techniques Matter in Your Labor

Movement and positioning aren't about "doing it right."
They're about:

- Comfort
- Progress
- Helping baby rotate and descend
- Supporting pelvic muscles and ligaments
- Optimizing contractions
- Reducing unnecessary interventions

Sometimes one *small* position change can transform an entire labor — and that's the magic of these "toys of the trade."

Nurse's Note

Changing your position throughout labor isn't just about comfort — it's about **progress**.

Every time we help you:

- roll,
- shift your hips,
- sit upright,
- lean forward,
- or try a new angle…

…we're encouraging your baby to find the best position to move down.

Staying in one spot too long can slow labor or make contractions feel less effective. That's why your nurse may adjust your position often, even when you're tired or have an epidural.

Trust that we're not trying to bother you — we're working with your body to keep labor moving safely and steadily for both you and your baby.

Movement is medicine in labor and we'll guide every step of it.

Words of Wisdom

If a position starts making you feel pressure or a bit uncomfortable, that's often a *good* sign.

It may mean:

- your baby is rotating
- your pelvis is opening
- progress is happening

Labor progress isn't always cozy — sometimes the positions that feel the strangest are the ones that help the most.

Trust your body. Trust the process.
You're doing exactly what you're meant to do.

Birthing Balls: How to Use Them Effectively

Birthing balls can be a powerful tool in labor — **when they're used the right way**.

When sitting on the ball, take a **wide, grounded position** with your legs out and your pelvis open. Many people find it most helpful to sit on the ball **facing the bed**, using the bed for support with your arms or upper body.

Try not to bounce on the ball.
Instead, gently **roll your hips in slow circles or a figure-eight motion**. This movement helps encourage your baby into a better position and promotes engagement.

If you bounce while your baby isn't well positioned, you may actually be bouncing your baby against your pelvic bone — which isn't helpful for positioning or progress.

Many moms describe sitting on the ball as uncomfortable — and there's a reason for that. It's often **effective**. The pressure helps bring your baby down onto the cervix, which can encourage dilation and progress in labor. That sensation doesn't mean something is wrong — it often means your body is doing exactly what it's meant to do.

This is one of those moments in labor where leaning into the work, rather than pulling away from it, can actually help things move forward.

You're not doing this wrong.
Your body is working hard — and **you've got this**.

35

Support People & Doulas: The Heart of Your Birth Team

"Your support team doesn't replace your strength — they amplify it."

Birth is not meant to be done alone. Whether you bring a partner, a parent, a best friend, or a doula, the people you choose to surround you during labor become part of your story — part of your strength, your comfort, and your calm. Their energy, their presence, and their words can shape the entire experience.

As your nurse, I see firsthand how powerful the right support can be. Labor is hard work: emotionally, mentally, and physically. Having someone who knows you, believes in you, and stays grounded with you can make every contraction feel a little more manageable.

Your support person does not need to know everything — they just need to **show up, stay present, and be centered on you.**

Why Support People Matter So Much

A good support person can:

- Remind you to breathe
- Massage your back or apply counterpressure
- Hold your hand during monitoring or epidural placement
- Encourage you when doubt creeps in
- Advocate for your wishes
- Keep the room calm and grounded
- Help with position changes
- Be your emotional anchor
- Celebrate your strength right alongside you

Support people don't replace the medical team — they **complement it.** They bring emotional comfort and personal connection that no nurse or provider can replicate.

There is something extraordinary about watching someone look at you with absolute belief in what you can do.

Doulas: Trained Support You Didn't Know You Needed

A **doula** is a trained labor-support professional whose role is to focus entirely on **your physical and emotional experience** during childbirth.

They do **not** perform medical tasks.
They **do** provide:

- Comfort techniques
- Breathing strategies
- Positioning guidance
- Continuous support

- Emotional grounding
- Advocacy
- Partner coaching
- Reassurance through every stage

Doulas stay with you continuously — something nurses wish we could do but realistically cannot.

Benefits of Having a Doula

Research shows doulas help reduce:

- Length of labor
- Need for pain medications
- Induction and augmentation
- C-section rates

They also increase:

- Birth satisfaction
- Sense of empowerment
- Confidence in labor

A doula works **with** your nurse and provider — a truly powerful team effort.

Nurse Shout-Out to Our Doula, Dania!

A special shout-out to our incredible **Doula Dania** — her soft-spoken, soul-hugging presence is a true asset to our unit. The way she supports our laboring moms with calm reassurance, steady encouragement, and unwavering compassion creates an atmosphere of safety and trust that is simply unmatched. You can feel the room shift when she enters — anxiety softens, breathing slows, and confidence grows. That kind of presence is a gift.

Doulas play a vital role in the birth experience by providing continuous emotional, physical, and informational support to birthing families. They help moms stay grounded through contractions, encourage movement and positioning, support breathing and coping techniques, and serve as steady advocates during vulnerable moments. Research consistently shows that doula support is associated with lower cesarean rates, shorter labors, decreased need for pain medication, and higher maternal satisfaction with the birth experience. For nurses, doulas are teammates — not replacements — enhancing the support we give at the bedside and strengthening the overall birth team.

Dania, your work matters more than you may ever know. You uplift our patients, support our staff, and embody everything that compassionate birth care should look like. Our moms are better because of you — and so is our unit.

Choosing the Right Person to Be With You

Your birth room is sacred.

Bring people who:

- Make you feel safe
- Bring calm energy
- Respect your choices
- Support **your** needs
- Stay emotionally steady
- Don't take over the space
- Don't project fear, stress, or negativity

Birth exposes every emotion — and you deserve people who can support you through all of them.

Nurse's Note: What Support Should Actually Look Like

Your support person should bring **calm, not chaos.**

Labor is not the place for arguments, criticism, tension, or emotional instability from others.

If someone in the room is upsetting you — even unintentionally — it can:

- slow labor,
- raise your stress hormones,
- and make everything harder.

If that happens, **tell me.**
Or give me the look — nurses are fluent in *that* look.

I can:

- Redirect conversation
- Step in as mediator
- Kindly remove someone for a break
- Advocate for your peace without drama

Your emotional safety matters just as much as your physical safety.

You Are Not Alone, Even If You Arrive Alone

Not every patient arrives with a partner or support team — and I see you.

I honor your strength.

I will never ask:

"Is someone coming?"
"Where's the father?"
"Are you expecting anyone else?"

Not because I don't care — but because I care deeply.

Those questions can unintentionally trigger:

- grief
- disappointment
- complicated emotions
- private stories
- wounds you shouldn't have to unpack in labor

You get to decide if or when you share that part of your life.

What matters is this:

You are supported right now.
You are not alone in this room.
I will hold steady with you through every moment.

Whether you arrive with a full birth team, one quiet friend, a doula, or entirely on your own — you are not alone. Your nurse steps in as whatever you need:

Encouragement.
Coach.
Calm presence.
Advocate.
Emotional anchor.

You are enough.
Your love for your baby is enough.
And your story is honored exactly as it is.

Final Thoughts

Your support team becomes part of your birth story forever.

Choose people who:

- Build you up
- Believe in you
- Bring steady, calming energy
- Support your choices
- Respect the sacredness of your space

And remember:

You and your nurse are a team, too.
We support you.
We advocate for you.
We protect your space.
We honor your experience.

Every step of the way.

36

Anxiety in Labor, Panic Attacks & Feeling Out of Control

*"Anxiety comes in waves — just like contractions.
And both pass."*

When Your Mind Needs Support as Much as Your Body

Most people talk about the physical intensity of labor — contractions, pain management, dilation, pushing. But fewer people talk openly about the **emotional intensity**, especially the anxiety that can show up unexpectedly.

Labor is powerful.
It is vulnerable.
It is unpredictable.

And even if you've prepared — taken classes, practiced breathing, visualized your birth — you may still find yourself feeling:

- Overwhelmed
- Panicky
- Out of control

- Scared
- Unable to focus
- Like everything is happening too fast
- Like your mind can't catch up with your body

You're not weak.
You're not failing.
You're not "bad at labor."

You're human.
And anxiety in labor is common, normal, and something we can absolutely help you with.

Why Anxiety Happens in Labor

Labor is an emotionally charged experience and your brain reacts to it in real time. Anxiety can be triggered by:

- Fear of pain
- Fear of the unknown
- Memories of previous trauma
- A difficult prior birth
- Fear of procedures
- Fear something will go wrong
- Feeling out of control
- Overstimulation (lights, noise, voices)
- Exhaustion
- Hormone surges
- Hyperventilation
- Rapid labors
- Pressure from yourself or others

Your body is doing one of the most intense things it will ever do.
Your nervous system is on high alert.

Anxiety is not a failure — it's your mind trying to keep up with what your body is experiencing. With gentle support, reassurance, and grounding, we help guide it back into safety.

Panic Attacks During Labor

Yes — panic attacks absolutely happen in labor.

A panic attack may feel like:

- Sudden fear
- Heart racing
- Rapid breathing
- Shaking
- Feeling like you can't get enough air
- Feeling like you might faint
- Feeling trapped
- Chest tightness
- Crying
- Feeling disconnected or "out of your body"
- Saying, "I can't do this."

None of this means you are doing anything wrong.
It means the **emotional intensity** is matching the **physical intensity** of labor.

Your nurse will help bring you back into your breath, your rhythm, and your body.

Signs You're Losing Control (And Why It's Okay)

Sometimes the first signs of emotional overwhelm are subtle:

- Feeling out of rhythm
- Struggling to cope between contractions

- Feeling overstimulated by touch or voices
- Wanting to run, escape, or change your mind
- Becoming loud, tearful, or restless
- Feeling too scared to ask for help

Here's the truth:
The moment you say **"I can't do this"** is often the exact moment your body is doing *exactly* what it needs to do.

Fear doesn't mean failure.
Fear often means **transition** — the most intense phase before pushing.

And you do **not** have to navigate any of this alone.

How Anxiety & Panic Can Cause Labor Dystocia

Labor dystocia = slow, stalled, or ineffective labor.
Anxiety and panic interfere with the body's normal labor hormones and muscle function through the **stress response**.

1. Stress Hormones Directly Suppress Oxytocin

Oxytocin is the hormone that drives contractions.

When someone is anxious or in panic:

- The body releases **catecholamines** (epinephrine & norepinephrine)
- These are **fight-or-flight hormones**
- They **block oxytocin**
- Result:
  Weaker contractions
  Slower cervical dilation
  Prolonged labor
  Increased need for Pitocin

This is why we often see labor **stall** during fear, arguments in the room, or emotional distress.

2. Pelvic Floor Tightening = Mechanical Obstruction

Fear causes:

- Involuntary **clenching of the pelvic floor**
- Increased **muscle tension**
- Guarding of the perineum and cervix

This leads to:

- Poor fetal descent
- Asynclitic or OP positioning
- Increased pushing time
- Shoulder dystocia risk
- Failed vacuum/forceps attempts
- Higher C-section rates for "failure to progress"

The body is literally trying to **protect itself instead of open.**

3. Hyperventilation & Oxygen Imbalance

During panic attacks:

- Rapid, shallow breathing
- Decreased CO_2 balance
- Reduced uterine & placental oxygen delivery

This can cause:

- Ineffective contractions
- Uterine fatigue

- Non-reassuring fetal tracings
- Increased operative delivery risk

4. Fear-Tension-Pain Cycle

This classic obstetric concept explains dystocia beautifully:

Fear → Muscle Tension → Increased Pain → More Fear → More Tension → Stalled Labor

Without intervention (support, breathing coaching, emotional safety), labor can **lock into dysfunction**.

5. Clinical Outcomes We See Linked to Anxiety

Patients with unmanaged anxiety or panic are statistically more likely to experience:

- Labor augmentation with Pitocin
- Epidural earlier than planned
- Prolonged second stage
- Operative vaginal delivery
- Unplanned cesarean
- Birth trauma & postpartum anxiety

What Breaks the Cycle

- Calm voice
- Breath coaching
- Dim lighting
- Reducing room traffic
- Emotional reassurance

- Continuous labor support (👀 doulas!)
- Grounding techniques
- Partner coaching
- Sometimes medication when appropriate

These **directly restore oxytocin dominance** and improve labor progress.

💖 Perfect Anxiety Storm Summary

Anxiety and panic activate the body's stress response, which suppresses oxytocin, tightens the pelvic floor, alters breathing patterns, and disrupts effective contractions. When the body perceives fear, it shifts from "let go" to "protect," increasing the risk for stalled labor, prolonged pushing, and operative delivery.

How to Cope When Anxiety Hits in Labor

Here are the real strategies we use at the bedside — the things that actually help when anxiety rises and labor feels overwhelming.

1. Breath Coaching

Your breath is your anchor — the one thing your mind can control even when your body feels intense.

We may guide you through:

- **Inhale for 4, exhale for 6**
- **Blowing out quickly** when you feel overwhelmed
- **Pursed-lip breathing**
- **Partner breathing with you**
- **Rhythmic breathing** synced to contractions

Breathing doesn't remove pain — **it restores control.**

2. Grounding Techniques

These bring your mind back into the present moment:

- Holding your nurse's or partner's hand
- Pressing both feet flat into the bed
- Making eye contact with someone calm
- Focusing on one spot in the room
- Naming things you see, hear, smell, feel

Grounding takes your brain out of the panic spiral and back into safety.

3. Changing Your Environment

You can ask for:

- Dimmed lights
- Quiet voices
- Fewer people in the room
- Music
- A warm blanket
- The door closed

Your birth space should feel like **your** space.

4. Position Changes

Movement interrupts anxiety patterns and shifts your mental focus.

Positions that help:

- Hands and knees
- Sitting upright
- Side-lying with a peanut ball
- Standing and swaying

- Leaning forward over the bed

A new position = a new mental reset.

5. Touch & Pressure

Depending on what calms you, we can try:

- Firm hip pressure
- Low-back counterpressure
- Light touch on the arms
- A reassuring hand on the shoulder
- Massage

Or **no touch at all** — your preference always comes first.

6. Clear, Calm Communication

Your nurse will:

- Slow down information
- Explain each step before it happens
- Ask before touching
- Give you choices
- Reassure you that you're safe

Knowledge reduces fear.
Clarity brings calm.

7. Reframing the Fear

Sometimes hearing the right words at the right moment changes everything.

You may hear:

- "You are safe."
- "This is intense, but you're not in danger."
- "Your body knows what to do."
- "I'm right here."
- "You're not alone."

Words can ground you.
Words can save you.
Words can help you reclaim control.

8. Pain Management Support

Anxiety skyrockets when pain becomes unmanageable. You are *always* allowed to ask for help.

Options include:

- Nitrous oxide
- IV medication
- Epidural
- Re-dosing an epidural that's fading
- Position changes for back labor

Pain control is emotional control.
This is **your birth**, not a test.

The Emotional Transition Stage

Transition (around 7–10 cm) is known for emotional overwhelm.

Common phrases during transition:

- "I can't do this."
- "I'm going to die."

- "Something is wrong."
- "I'm losing it."
- "Make it stop."

This is normal.
This is not failure.
This is labor reaching its most powerful point — often right before pushing.

Lean on your team.
Let us carry you through it.

After the Panic Passes

Once your anxiety settles:

- Your breathing softens
- Your voice quiets
- You may cry
- You may apologize
- You may feel embarrassed
- Or surprised at your own strength

Let me tell you the truth:

You're not dramatic.
You're not too much.
You're not "out of control."
You're laboring.

And you are doing beautifully.

Nurse's Note: Panic Is Common in Labor

If you feel panicky, overwhelmed, or scared, **tell me immediately.**

I can:

- Anchor your breath
- Adjust your environment
- Change your position
- Lower the room's stimulation
- Support you emotionally
- Help with pain control

You are *never* bothering us.
You are *never* alone.
We get through this together.

You Are Still in Control – Even When It Doesn't Feel Like It

Labor takes you to a primal place.
Your mind steps aside and your body takes over.

But you are not powerless.

You have:

A team that protects your safety
Choices and a voice
People guiding and supporting you
Strength you don't even realize you have

You may not control every detail of labor —
but you absolutely control **your needs, your voice, and your support.**

You are brave.
You are capable.
You are doing one of the hardest things a human has ever done.

And you are not doing it alone.

37

Birth Trauma & Emotional Safety in Labor

"You survived something big.
Be gentle with yourself."

Your Story Matters as Much as Your Safety

There is so much focus on the physical side of childbirth — dilation, contractions, epidurals, fetal monitoring — that sometimes the **emotional experience** gets pushed quietly into the background.

But labor is not just physical.

Labor is vulnerable.
Labor is intimate.
Labor is triggering.
Labor is raw.

And if you've experienced trauma in the past — sexual trauma, medical trauma, domestic violence, a previous traumatic birth, a loss, or a moment where you felt powerless — labor can bring those emotions back to the surface without warning.

I want you to know this, deep in your bones:

Your emotional safety is just as important as your physical safety.
Your past experiences deserve to be honored, not ignored.
You are allowed to speak up, set boundaries, and ask for exactly what you need.

In Labor & Delivery, you are not just a patient.
You are a whole person — with a history, a voice, and a story that matters.

What Birth Trauma Looks Like (It's More Common Than You Think)

Birth trauma can come from medical experiences such as:

- Feeling ignored or dismissed during a previous delivery
- A fast or chaotic labor that you didn't understand
- A baby needing resuscitation or NICU care
- Shoulder dystocia
- Emergency C-section or a Postpartum Hemorrhage
- A provider who didn't listen
- A moment where you felt powerless or unsafe

But trauma doesn't have to come from the delivery room.

It can come from:

- Sexual assault at any age
- Physical or emotional abuse
- Medical trauma or painful procedures
- A pregnancy loss or stillbirth
- Family conflict

- Feeling unsupported in your relationships
- A lifetime of not feeling heard

You don't need to "justify" trauma.
If your body remembers fear — **that is enough.**

Birth can reawaken those memories not because you are weak but because birth is **intense**, **exposed**, and **emotionally unfiltered.**

How Past Trauma Can Show Up During Labor

Your nervous system doesn't care that you're in a hospital — it only cares about safety.

Trauma may resurface as:

- Fear during vaginal exams
- Anxiety when privacy feels interrupted
- Panic during intense contractions
- Freezing or "checking out" (dissociation)
- Feeling overwhelmed by fast decisions
- Being triggered by certain tones or phrases
- Feeling like you're "not in control"
- Crying suddenly
- Feeling afraid to be touched without warning

None of these reactions mean:

You are weak
You are failing
You "can't handle" labor

These reactions mean:

Your nervous system is trying to protect you.

And with the right support, we can help you feel safe again.

How to Protect Your Emotional Safety During Birth

There are gentle, trauma-informed ways we can support you.
You are *allowed* to ask for them.
You *deserve* to ask for them.

1. Speak Up About Trauma–As Much or As Little as You Want

A simple sentence is enough:

- "I have a trauma history; please explain things before doing them."
- "Vaginal exams are hard for me; please go slow."
- "Please don't touch me without warning."
- "Certain positions make me feel vulnerable."
- "I prefer female providers when possible."

You do **not** owe anyone details.
You do **not** have to revisit your story in labor.
You only have to tell us what makes you feel safe.

And I promise — we will listen.

2. Ask for Consent-Based Language

You are allowed to ask your team to communicate in a way that centers your comfort and control.
You can request that your providers:

Tell you what they're about to do *before* they do it
Explain why something is needed
Move slowly during exams or procedures
Use calm, gentle, reassuring language
Allow you to decline anything that isn't urgent or emergent

Good providers do this routinely — but you are *always* empowered to advocate for your emotional needs.

3. Choose Support People Who Make You Feel Strong – Not Stressed

The birth room should feel safe, peaceful, and supportive.
Choose people who:

Speak gently
Calm you, not overwhelm you
Advocate for your needs
Keep tension out of the room
Bring comfort instead of chaos

Birth is not the place where you should be managing someone else's emotions.

4. Use Grounding Techniques Between Contractions

Grounding helps your brain shift from **fear → safety**.

You may find comfort in:

Slow breathing with someone counting for you
Holding your partner's or nurse's hand
Fixing your eyes on one object

Repeating a calming mantra ("I am safe," "My body knows what to do")
Dim lights, quiet voices, warm blankets

Small sensory changes can bring enormous relief to an overwhelmed nervous system.

5. Request Fewer Vaginal Exams If They Are Triggering

Unless medically necessary, vaginal exams can often be:

Spaced out
Replaced by visual or behavioral assessments
Done more gently and slowly
Performed by a preferred provider (if staffing allows)

You **always** have the right to ask for modifications.

6. Ask for a Quiet Room or Minimal Staff

Your birthing room is your sanctuary.
You can request:

Fewer people
A closed door
Dimmed lights
Minimal interruptions
Soft voices

Calm environments support calm nervous systems.

If Labor Becomes Overwhelming

Birth is unpredictable. Even the strongest, most prepared people can feel emotionally flooded.

If you start to feel fear, panic, or emotional overload, you can simply say:

- "I'm scared."
- "I don't feel okay."
- "This reminds me of something bad."
- "I feel out of control."

When you express this, We will immediately:

✓ Slow down
✓ Explain each step
✓ Ground you
✓ Quiet the room
✓ Adjust the environment
✓ Speak to you gently
✓ Make sure everyone treats you with dignity and respect

You do **not** have to hide your feelings or push through silently.

How Your Birth Team Helps Protect Your Emotional Safety

As your nurse, we will constantly asking ourselves:

How can I approach you gently?
Do you feel safe with the people in the room?
Do you need more privacy?
Do you need fewer exams or slower explanations?
Is your body language telling me you're overwhelmed?
Should the lights dim?
Do I need to pause and check in?
Is your partner supporting you well?

You deserve care that respects **your heart**, not just your cervix.

Nurse's Note: Your Emotional Safety Matters

Birth is emotional. If something feels triggering, overwhelming, or frightening, please tell us — even with just a look.

We will adjust immediately:

Softer language
Warmer tone
Slower steps
More explanation
Less stimulation
More grounding

Your past experiences matter.
Your comfort matters.
You matter.

When Birth Doesn't Go as Planned

Even when everything turns out physically okay, the *experience* itself can still be traumatic.

This includes:

- Emergency C-section
- Rapid, chaotic labor
- Shoulder dystocia
- NICU separation
- Postpartum hemorrhage
- Failed induction
- Feeling ignored or powerless

You are allowed to:

Grieve the birth you hoped for
Feel shaken, sad, angry, or numb
Seek counseling or support
Ask your providers to walk you through what happened

Birth trauma does **not** mean you failed.
It means you lived through something intense.

You Deserve a Healing Birth Experience

Your history does NOT make you difficult.
Your emotions do NOT make you dramatic.
Your triggers do NOT make you weak.

They make you human.
And in labor, **your humanity matters.**

I want you to feel:

Safe
Heard
Supported
Respected
In control
Empowered
Brave

And you are ALL of those things — no matter how your birth unfolds.

Your story matters.
Your emotions matter.
And you deserve a birth experience where your heart is cared for just as deeply as your body.

38

Postpartum Depression (PPD): When the Feelings Don't Match the Moment

"Asking for help isn't giving up — it's stepping toward healing."

Bringing a baby into the world is one of the most transformative experiences of your life — and with that transformation comes a tidal wave of hormones, exhaustion, adjustment, and emotion. Most people expect joy, gratitude, bonding, and instant connection.

But many women experience something entirely different.

Postpartum Depression (PPD) is **not weakness**, **not failure**, and **not your fault**. It is common, treatable, and nothing to be ashamed of. Your mind is recovering just as much as your body — and both deserve care.

You are not alone. You are not a bad mother. You are not broken.

"Baby Blues" vs. Postpartum Depression

Almost 70-80% of new mothers experience "baby blues" — a short-lived emotional shift in the first 2 weeks postpartum caused by hormonal changes (American Pregnancy Association, 2025).

Baby Blues:

Common symptoms:

- Crying for no clear reason
- Feeling overwhelmed
- Irritability
- Mood swings
- Feeling sensitive or easily triggered
- Trouble sleeping
- Anxiety

Baby blues usually:

✓ peak around days 3–5
✓ improve by week 2
✓ do *not* significantly impair functioning

Postpartum Depression (PPD):

PPD is more intense, longer lasting, and interferes with your ability to function or enjoy daily life.

It may start:

- within the first few weeks
- after the first 2 months
- or anytime in the first year

PPD is a medical condition — not an emotional failure.

Signs of Postpartum Depression

PPD can look very different from person to person. You might experience some or all of the following:

Emotional Symptoms

- Persistent sadness
- Feeling numb or disconnected
- Loss of interest in things you used to enjoy
- Crying constantly or feeling unable to cry
- Feeling hopeless or trapped
- Irritability or anger you can't control
- Guilt, shame, or believing you're "failing"

Cognitive Symptoms

- Feeling overwhelmed by simple tasks
- Difficulty concentrating
- Racing thoughts
- Feeling "out of it"

Physical Symptoms

- Changes in appetite
- Insomnia—even when the baby is sleeping
- Extreme fatigue
- Body aches

Thought-Based Symptoms

- Worrying you're not bonding with your baby
- Thinking your baby is better off without you
- Feeling like you're not meant to be a mother
- Scary thoughts you don't want (intrusive thoughts)

Intrusive thoughts do NOT mean you will act on them.
They are a symptom of anxiety and depression — and extremely common.

Postpartum Anxiety & OCD (Often Misdiagnosed as PPD)

Many women don't feel "sad." Instead, they feel:

- Constant worry
- Panic attacks
- Obsessive checking
- Fear of something happening to the baby
- Racing heart
- Trouble sleeping even when exhausted

Postpartum OCD can include unwanted intrusive thoughts that feel disturbing or frightening.

These conditions are real, treatable, and often appear alongside PPD.

What Causes PPD?

You are NOT to blame — this is biological, hormonal, and environmental.
PPD can be caused by:

Hormonal shifts
Lack of sleep
Blood loss or anemia
Stress
Breastfeeding challenges
Difficult birth
NICU separation
History of anxiety or depression
Trauma
Lack of support
Thyroid problems
Life changes

Your brain is recalibrating, your hormones are shifting, and your identity is expanding into motherhood. It's a lot.

How PPD Affects Bonding

One of the biggest fears mothers carry is:

"I don't feel bonded — does that mean I'm a bad mom?"

ABSOLUTELY NOT.

Bonding is not always instant.
It grows with time, rest, support, and recovery.
You can love your baby and still struggle.

Your worth as a mother is not measured by a moment — it's measured by your heart.

How We Treat PPD

PPD is **highly treatable**. Most women feel dramatically better with proper support.

1. Therapy

Talking with a perinatal therapist can help you process:

- fears
- intrusive thoughts
- identity shifts
- trauma
- relationship changes

2. Medication

Antidepressants are safe for breastfeeding and **often life-changing**.

SSRIs commonly used postpartum:

- Sertraline
- Escitalopram
- Fluoxetine

These can stabilize mood and bring back clarity.

3. Support

Help with meals, rest, chores, parenting.
Asking for help is not weakness — it's wisdom.

4. Sleep

Sleep is medicine.
A few protected hours can change everything.

5. Hormonal or thyroid evaluation

Sometimes your mood symptoms are biological and easily treatable.

You deserve care, not suffering.

When to Call Your Provider

Call your OB, midwife, or primary doctor if you experience:

- Depressive symptoms lasting more than 2 weeks
- Difficulty functioning
- Feeling detached from the baby

- Panic attacks
- Constant anxiety
- Intrusive thoughts you can't shake
- Feeling like you might accidentally harm the baby
- Feeling unable to care for yourself
- Feeling hopeless
- Thoughts of self-harm

You are never "bothering" us.
You are never overreacting.
You deserve help.

When to Seek IMMEDIATE Help

If you ever experience:

Thoughts of harming yourself
Thoughts of harming your baby
Feeling unsafe
Feeling like you might run away, disappear, or give up

Go to the ER, call 988, or contact your provider immediately.

You matter. Your life matters. You are needed.

Nurse's Note: You Are Not Failing

Postpartum Depression does not mean:

✗ You don't love your baby
✗ You're not grateful
✗ You're not a good mom
✗ You're weak

It means your body and brain are recovering from one of the most intense experiences of human life.

You deserve compassion.
You deserve rest.
You deserve treatment.
You deserve peace.

PPD is treatable. You will not feel this way forever.
Your joy is not gone — it's simply waiting for the fog to lift.

And we will help lift it with you.

39

Supporting a Teenager in the Childbirth Setting: Respecting Autonomy, Supporting Strength

"Support isn't about taking over. It's about lifting her up while she finds her own strength."

Caring for a teenager during pregnancy and birth is one of the most delicate, meaningful responsibilities in Labor & Delivery. Teen patients often arrive carrying layers of fear, uncertainty, and outside opinions — from family, friends, school, or life circumstances they never expected to navigate so young. But here's one truth I hold close as a bedside nurse:

A pregnant teenager is still a patient with full autonomy, full rights, and full humanity.

She is not "just a kid."
She is a mother in the making.
She deserves respect, privacy, and empowerment — not judgment.

Honoring Their Autonomy

Teenagers deserve the exact same informed consent process, explanations, and decision-making rights as an adult patient. That means:

- We speak *to her*, not around her
- We explain every procedure in clear, gentle language
- We ask her permission before touching her body
- We encourage questions and wait for her answers
- We give her space to think before deciding
- We remind her that *she* is the patient and *she* gets a say

Even when parents or guardians are present (and often supportive), this remains **her birth** and **her medical care**.

For many young mothers, labor is the first time an adult truly listens, respects, and empowers them — and that moment can stay with them forever.

Building Trust Through Kindness

Teen patients often need:

- More reassurance
- More repetition
- More time to process
- More emotional safety
- More gentle guidance

You would be amazed at the transformation when a scared teen hears:

"You're doing such a great job."
"You're stronger than you think."
"Your feelings make sense."
"I'm not going anywhere."
"You're not alone in this."

Birth is vulnerable for anyone — but for a teenager, it can feel like stepping into adulthood in a single night.

Your kindness becomes their anchor.

Involving Support People – While Centering the Teen

Support peoplc may include:

- Parents
- Grandparents
- A partner (teen or adult)
- A foster parent
- A guardian
- A trusted friend
- No one at all

Some families are loving and united.
Some are angry or disappointed.
Some are overwhelmed.
Some want to take control.
Some want to disappear.

As nurses, we navigate these dynamics by:

- Gently redirecting conversations to the teen
- Removing toxic influences when appropriate
- Keeping medical decisions focused on the patient
- Setting boundaries with visitors
- Ensuring the teen never feels shamed or overpowered

Many teens look at their nurse as the only adult in the room who isn't judging them. That responsibility matters.

Supporting Teens During Labor

Teenagers often need:

More explanation

What they feel
What they can expect
What's normal
What's safe

More coping guidance

Breathing
Positioning
Reassurance
Pain management support

More emotional validation

"Your fear is understandable."
"You're allowed to ask for help."
"You're doing everything right."

More privacy protections

Keeping the room calm
Asking who she wants present
Ensuring no one pressures or overwhelms her

Gentle reinforcement

Teen pregnancy doesn't erase capability.
Teen motherhood doesn't erase strength.
This birth is still hers — meaningful, powerful, and valid.

Pain Management for Teens

Many teenagers fear pain, medical procedures, or epidurals — often because they've never been in a hospital setting before. We can help by:

- Explaining pain options slowly
- Normalizing fear
- Reviewing choices without pressure
- Supporting their decisions even if they change
- Reassuring them that epidurals are safe
- Making sure they feel *in control*, not overwhelmed
- A calm conversation can transform their entire birth experience.

After Baby Is Born

Teen mothers may face unique emotional challenges:

- Fear of holding the baby "wrong"
- Worry about judgment
- Anxiety about parenting skills
- Difficulty with breastfeeding confidence
- Fear of disappointing family
- Grief for the girl they were before becoming a mother

They need:

- Encouragement
- Patience
- Validation
- Education without condescension
- Support without pressure
- Permission to learn
- Permission to struggle
- Permission to grow

Teen moms are every bit as capable of loving, nurturing, and bonding with their babies as any adult — they simply need support, not scrutiny.

Special Considerations in Teen Pregnancy

Teenage pregnancies may carry higher risk of:

- Preterm birth
- Low birth weight
- Anemia
- Hypertensive disorders
- Lack of prenatal care
- Social or environmental stressors

This is never the teen's fault.

It simply means we monitor more closely, educate more often, and support more deeply.

Nurse's Note: Teen Moms Need Safety, Not Judgment

Teenagers do not need:

✗ lectures
✗ shame
✗ assumptions
✗ someone "taking over"
✗ people speaking about them instead of to them

What they *do* need is people who:

✓ speaks respectfully
✓ protects their autonomy
✓ advocates for their choices
✓ shields them from harm or pressure
✓ treats them as the mother they are — not the stereotype people expect

Teen moms are some of the bravest patients I've ever cared for. They show resilience, tenderness, and courage far beyond their years.

Your job is not to fix them.
Your job is not to judge them.
Your job is to support them through one of the most important moments of their lives.

And I promise you — they will never forget how you made them feel.

The Truth About Teen Mothers

They are capable.
They are strong.
They are learning.
They are trying.
They deserve dignity.
They deserve support.
They deserve respect.
They deserve space to grow.

A teenager can still be an extraordinary mother.

And as their support people, you have the privilege of showing them just how extraordinary they already are.

Special Considerations in Teen Labor

Teen mothers may face unique challenges during labor and as the care team, we approach each of these with patience, gentleness, and respect.

1. Increased Anxiety

Many teens are scared to admit they're scared.
We normalize their feelings and provide grounding reassurance:

"You're safe. I'm right here. You're doing an amazing job."

2. Limited Prenatal Education

Some teens have had little or no childbirth education.
Our job is to *fill in the gaps* without a hint of judgment or condescension.

We explain slowly, clearly, and with kindness — never assuming they "should already know."

3. Trauma History

A trauma-informed approach is essential:

We will ask before touching
Explain what you're doing and why
Maintain privacy with intention
Normalize saying "stop," "slow down," or "I need a break"
Encourage their voice in every decision

Many teens have experienced trauma long before birth — and they deserve gentle hands and respectful care.

4. Social Pressure

Teen mothers often carry the weight of:

Judgment
Family dynamics
Stress

Unsolicited opinions
Fear of being dismissed

In the birth room, they deserve a space completely free of shame. We create a sanctuary where they can breathe, learn, and labor without criticism.

5. Support With Postpartum Adjustment

Teen parents may need additional support with:

Feeding education
Understanding baby cues
Recovery expectations
Holding, latching, diapering
Emotional reassurance
Guidance without lecturing

We don't "talk down." We empower.

Recognizing Their Bravery

Teen parents often show extraordinary resilience.
Birth can be a defining moment — not a setback, but a rise.

I've watched teenage mothers:

Labor with stunning strength
Advocate for themselves
Ask thoughtful questions
Protect their boundaries
Cry from fear, then keep going
Hold their baby with fierce love immediately

Age never limits capacity.
Strength rises in all forms.

Respect Is Non-Negotiable

Teen patients should never be spoken to:

Like they are children
Like they are a burden
With assumptions about their life
With judgment about their capability

Respect is the foundation — always.

Nurse's Voice for Her

A teenager in labor deserves the same dignity, autonomy, and steady support as any adult.

Speak gently.
Explain clearly.
Center **her** voice.

If family dynamics become tense, overwhelming, or emotionally unsafe, your nurse can step in as the buffer:

"I'm going to ask everyone to step out for a moment so she can regroup."

Use me. Signal me. Look at me.I will advocate for your emotional safety just as fiercely as your physical safety.

No one gets to make you feel small while you are doing something so incredibly big.

Nurse's Note: Teen Fathers Need a Voice Too

Teen fathers are often overlooked, underestimated, or dismissed — not because they don't care, but because they're young, scared, or unsure of their place in the room. But let me tell you something important:

Teen dads feel everything.
Fear.
Responsibility.
Pride.
Confusion.
Hope.
Pressure.
Love.

They may not always know how to show it, but they feel it deeply.

Many teen fathers:

- Want to be supportive but don't know how
- Feel intimidated by the hospital environment
- Fear being judged by staff or family
- Worry they'll "mess something up"
- Don't know whether they're allowed to speak up
- Are carrying their own trauma, stress, or lack of guidance
- Desperately want to belong in the birth space

As nurses, we can bring them into the experience instead of leaving them on the sidelines.

How We Can Support Teen Fathers

We can gently guide them through what's happening by:

- Showing them how to hold her hand during contractions
- Teaching them how to offer counterpressure
- Encouraging them to speak to her gently
- Praising their presence and involvement
- Explaining what they're seeing on the monitor

- Giving them small, meaningful jobs that build confidence
- Validating their feelings without judgment

A simple, "You're doing such a good job supporting her," can change the way a teen father sees himself — not as a boy in the room, but as a partner and a dad.

Why This Matters

Teen fathers often carry silent fears:

"Am I allowed to be here?"
"What if I'm not good enough for her or the baby?"
"What if her family doesn't want me here?"
"What if I disappoint everyone?"
"What if I don't know what I'm doing?"

Giving them a voice gives them confidence.
Giving them a role gives them purpose.
Giving them respect gives them pride.

And when a teen father feels supported, the entire birth atmosphere changes — calmer, more united, more hopeful.

A Message to Teen Fathers

If I could speak directly to every teen father I've cared for, I'd say this:

"You matter here.
Your presence matters.
Your support matters.
You don't have to have all the answers — just show up with love.
You're doing better than you think."

Teen moms are strong.
Teen dads are strong too.
And when both feel supported, respected, and included, they step into parenthood with confidence instead of fear.

Nurse's Reflection

I will tell you that some of the teenage moms I've taken care of have been among the **strongest** and most **resilient** patients I've ever seen. There is something uniquely powerful about the way they move through labor — a blend of instinct, determination, and raw courage that often leaves me in awe.

Many of them walk into birth carrying more on their shoulders than most adults ever will. They may be scared, overwhelmed, unsupported, or unsure of themselves — and yet, when it comes time to bring their baby into the world, they tap into a strength that is nothing short of extraordinary. I've seen teenage moms breathe through contractions with remarkable focus, advocate for themselves with quiet confidence, and push with a level of bravery that defies their age.

They remind me that motherhood doesn't wait for "the right time." It arrives with its own fierce wisdom and these young women rise to meet it with grit, grace, and a heart bigger than they even realize they possess.

I've learned not to underestimate them — ever. They are strong. They are capable. And they are some of the bravest people I've ever had the privilege to care for.

40

Teenage Pregnancy: Your Autonomy, Your Strength, Your Voice

"You didn't plan it, but you're rising to it."

A Message Just for You

If you're pregnant and you're a teenager, I want you to hear this clearly — from me, your nurse:

You are not "too young" to be respected.
You are not "too young" to make decisions.
You are not "too young" to be heard.

You are a patient with full rights.
You are a mother in the making.
You deserve dignity, privacy, and real support — not judgment.

You matter here.
Your voice matters here.
Your choices matter here.

Your Autonomy Matters

Even if you're the youngest one in the room, this is still your pregnancy and your birth. You get a say in everything that happens with your body and your baby.

When you're with me, I will always:

- talk to you, not over you
- explain things in clear, simple language
- ask your permission before touching you
- give you time to think before making decisions
- remind you that you're the patient — and you are allowed to speak up

Even if parents, guardians, or family are in the room, this is **your medical care**.
You deserve to understand what's happening and to be included every step of the way.

Sometimes, labor is the first time someone truly listens to you.
I promise to make sure you feel heard.

Building Trust With You

You might need:

- more reassurance
- more explanation
- more time to process
- more emotional safety

And that is completely okay.

You would be amazed how much your confidence grows when someone looks you in the eye and says:

"You're doing an amazing job."
"You're stronger than you think."
"You're allowed to feel scared."
"I'm right here. You're not alone."

Birth is vulnerable for anyone — but when you're young, it can feel like stepping into adulthood all at once.
Let me be your steady place.

Your Support People – and Your Space

Your support might be:

- a parent
- your partner
- a guardian or foster parent
- a friend
- or no one at all

Some people around you may be comforting.
Some may be stressed.
Some may be judgmental.
Some may try to take over.
Some may disappear.

But this room?
This room belongs to **you**.

I will:

- keep the focus on you
- redirect others when needed
- protect your space and privacy

- remove anyone who overwhelms or pressures you
- make sure your voice stays louder than theirs

You deserve a birth without shame or noise.
You deserve a nurse who has your back.

You Deserve Support During Labor

You deserve explanations that are gentle and clear:

- what you're feeling
- what's normal
- what's safe
- what's next

You deserve help with coping:

- breathing
- positioning
- pain management
- emotional reassurance

And you deserve validation:

"You're allowed to be scared."
"You're allowed to ask for help."
"You're doing everything right."

Teen pregnancy does not make you less capable.
You are still strong.
You are still smart.
You are still powerful.
This birth is still yours.

Pain Management: Your Choice, Not Anyone Else's

You might be afraid of pain, needles, or epidurals — especially if you've never been in a hospital before. That's normal.

I will help you by:

- explaining every option
- normalizing your fear
- supporting your decisions
- reminding you that epidurals are safe
- staying with you if you're scared
- going slowly so you don't feel overwhelmed

Pain management is not about being "tough."
It's about feeling in control. And your decision for pain management is entirely up to you to make. Do not let anyone else make you feel otherwise.

After Your Baby Is Born

Being a teen mom comes with feelings many people don't talk about:

- fear of doing something "wrong"
- worry about being judged
- anxiety about parenting
- feeling unsure about breastfeeding
- sadness over how life is changing
- pressure from family or partner

Let me tell you something:
You are allowed to learn.
You are allowed to struggle.
You are allowed to grow.

You don't need to know everything on Day One.
You just need someone to teach you with kindness — not criticism.

And that's what I'm here for.

Your Pregnancy Scorecard Is Not Your Fault

Teen pregnancies sometimes have higher risks, like:

- preterm labor
- low birth weight
- anemia
- blood pressure issues
- lack of early prenatal care

None of this is your fault.
It just means we watch you closely, care for you gently, and support you more intentionally.

You deserve safety — not blame.

Nurse's Note: You Deserve Respect – Always

You do **not** deserve:

✗ shame
✗ lectures
✗ assumptions
✗ people speaking about you instead of to you
✗ anyone taking over your decisions

You do deserve:

✓ respect
✓ autonomy

✓ compassion
✓ advocacy
✓ someone protecting your emotional and physical safety

You are not your situation.
You are not a stereotype.
You are not a problem to fix.

You are a young woman doing something unimaginably brave.

People may forget everything about your birth —
but you will never forget how your nurse made you feel.

I will do everything I can to make you feel safe, respected, and strong.

The Truth You Need to Hear

You are capable.
You are strong.
You are learning.
You are trying.
You deserve support.
You deserve dignity.
You deserve respect.

A teenager can still be an extraordinary mother.
And I want you to know this:

You already are.

41

Caring for You, Not Judging You
Substance Use Disorder in Pregnancy & Postpartum

"Compassion saves lives. Judgment destroys them."

If you are reading this and you have a history of substance use — or you're currently using — I want you to hear this first:

My job is to care for you. Not to judge you.

You are still a mother.
You are still worthy of respect, kindness, and safe, evidence-based care.
You are not "less than" because of what you've been through.

Many patients I've cared for have carried heavy stories long before they ever walked into Labor & Delivery — trauma, pain, abusive relationships, loss, mental health struggles, or years of trying to cope in the only ways they knew how.

No little girl dreams of growing up to fight addiction.
No one wakes up hoping they'll develop a substance use disorder.

So if this is part of your story, hear me clearly:

You are not alone.
You are not broken.
You are not beyond help.

Why I Need to Know About Your Substance Use (Past or Present)

One of the strongest, bravest things you can do is be honest with your nurse and provider about:

- What you use (prescription, non-prescription, street drugs, alcohol)
- How often you use it
- When you last used
- Whether you take treatment medications (methadone, Suboxone/buprenorphine, etc.)

This is not so we can judge you.
This is so we can keep **you** and **your baby** safe.

Substances can affect:

- Your blood pressure, heart rate, and breathing
- How you respond to pain or medications
- Your tolerance level
- How your baby transitions after birth
- Whether your baby may show withdrawal signs

If you don't tell us the truth, I might accidentally:

- Underdose your pain medication because I don't know you're tolerant
- Give you meds that interact dangerously
- Miss signs in your baby that need early treatment

But if you *do* tell me the truth, I can:

- Advocate for the right pain control
- Choose safer medications
- Monitor your baby correctly
- Prepare for extra support (lactation, pediatrics, social work)

Compassion Note: When you're honest with me, you're not "getting yourself in trouble." You're partnering with someone who wants you to feel safe.

"I Never Wanted to Go Down This Road..."

I believe you.

Addiction is not a moral failing.
It is a complex medical condition shaped by:

- Trauma
- Mental health
- Environment
- Genetics
- Coping limitations
- Survival strategies

Many moms cry and tell me:

"I hate that this is part of my story."
"I didn't want this life."
"I'm scared I ruined everything."

Here's the truth:

You can regret your past and still be a wonderful mother.
You can struggle and still deserve compassion.
You can fall down and rise again — and still be worthy of love.

In your delivery room, I don't see "an addict."

I see a mother.
I see a survivor.
I see someone doing her best in a hard world.

How Substance Use Changes Pain Management

If you use opioids — or are on medication-assisted treatment — you may have tolerance.

That means:

- Standard doses may not touch your pain
- You may need higher or different meds
- You may feel like no one believes how much it hurts

When I walk into your room, I am NOT thinking:

"She's drug-seeking."

I am thinking:

"She may need a different pain plan. I need to watch her closely and advocate."

Being vigilant means:

- Believing you when you say you're hurting
- Adjusting meds based on your tolerance
- Communicating frequently with anesthesia
- Using non-opioid techniques too: heat, position changes, breathing, water therapy, movement
- Protecting both safety AND comfort

You are not "drug-seeking." You are pain-seeking.
And you deserve relief.

> **Nurse Tip:** Please tell me if your pain feels unmanageable. I would rather you "bother" me ten times than suffer silently once.

How Substance Use Can Affect Your Baby

Depending on the substance, frequency, and timing, your baby may:

- Need extra monitoring
- Show withdrawal or withdrawal-like symptoms
- Have trouble feeding or sleeping
- Require a longer stay or NICU support

This does **not** mean you are a bad parent.
It means your baby needs a gentler transition.

What we may do:

- Keep lights low and sounds soft
- Use special scoring tools
- Encourage skin-to-skin
- Support feeding (breastfeeding may still be recommended!)
- Collaborate with pediatricians and neonatologists
- Involve social support when needed

Remember: You can love your baby fiercely AND have a history of substance use. Both can be true.

Will I Be Judged? Will I Lose My Baby?

This is one of the biggest fears I see in patients with a history of substance use — and it is a fear that lives deep, often long before they ever step foot into Labor & Delivery.

I want to speak to this clearly and honestly:

I cannot pretend that the system is perfect.
I cannot promise that social work or CPS will never be involved.
I cannot erase policies, reporting laws, or outside agencies.

But here is what I *can* promise you — with my whole heart and my professional integrity:

I will treat you with dignity while I do my job.
I will explain what I can, when I can, so you're never left in the dark.
I will speak to you with respect — always.
I will remember that you are a human being, not a diagnosis.
I will care for you and your baby with compassion, not judgment.

I may not control every part of the system, but I *do* control how I show up for you:

My tone.
My words.
My kindness.
My advocacy.
My presence.

And I take that responsibility seriously.

Compassion Note: You deserve to understand what's happening. You deserve to ask questions.You deserve to be talked to like a mother, not a problem.

How You Can Partner With Me

You do not have to walk into this alone.
You and I can work *together* — and when you let me in, I can protect you better.

Here's how we create a safe, honest team:

- **Tell me the truth** about your use — even if you feel ashamed.
- **Tell me if you're on methadone or Suboxone.**
- **Tell me what pain medications work for you and what doesn't.**
- **Tell me what you're afraid of:**
  - "I'm scared you'll judge me."
  - "I'm scared of losing my baby."
  - "I'm scared of withdrawal."
  - "I'm scared of relapsing."

Every fear you say out loud is something I can help you navigate.

If you tell me:

"I'm in recovery and I'm terrified of getting opioids."
→ We will make a plan *together.*

"I'm afraid I will relapse."
→ We can gather support before you even leave the hospital.

"I've been using and I don't know how to stop."
→ I can connect you with specialists who *want* to help, not punish.

Nurse Promise:

I will not be shocked by your story.
I have heard many stories.
I will not pull away from you.
I will lean *toward* you.

You Are Worth Showing Up For

I know that when you've been judged by society, family, partners, or previous providers, it can feel safer to shut down, hide the truth, or say nothing.

But your honesty gives me power — the power to:

- Keep you safe
- Keep your baby safe
- Treat your pain appropriately
- Avoid dangerous interactions
- Prepare for withdrawal if needed
- Advocate for the right postpartum supports
- Help you move toward recovery, if that's your goal

You deserve safe care.
You deserve real support.
You deserve someone who sees the *whole you*, not just the hard parts of your story.

And if no one has said this to you yet:

I see you.
I know you've survived things most people will never understand.
You are doing the best you can with what you've lived through.
My job is to care for you — not judge you.

And that is exactly what I will do.

To My Patients in Recovery

When you tell me you're in recovery, I want you to know that **"proud of you"** doesn't even come close to capturing what I feel for you. Walking away from a life that once held you — the habits, the coping, the escape, the numbness, the chaos — is one of the **hardest, bravest, most soul-shifting decisions a person can make**.

Choosing recovery means choosing discomfort, honesty, vulnerability, and growth every single day. It means facing your past instead of hiding from it. It means fighting for a future that is healthier, clearer, and rooted in love — especially love for the baby you're bringing into this world.

And I want you to hear this clearly:
You should be incredibly proud of yourself.
What you're doing takes strength that many people will never understand. You are rewriting your story. You are breaking cycles. You are choosing a path that demands courage over and over again — and you are showing up. That is extraordinary.

When you sit in front of me and say, "I'm in recovery," I don't see your past. I see your **resilience**, your **commitment**, your **hope**, and the incredible future you're building for yourself and your baby.

Keep going.
Keep fighting.
Keep choosing you.

And know that I see you — and I am truly, deeply proud of you.

42

Cultural Considerations & Translators: Honoring Every Voice in the Birth Room

"Birth looks different in every culture — respect is universal."

Every family who walks into Labor & Delivery brings their own culture, traditions, beliefs, values, and ways of understanding the world. Birth is deeply personal and for many families, it is also deeply cultural. As your nurse, one of the most sacred parts of my job is making sure you feel **seen, heard, respected, and understood** — no matter what language you speak or where your story began.

Communication in labor is not optional.
It is essential.
Your safety, comfort, and autonomy depend on it.

Language Access Is a Right – Not a Courtesy

If English is not your primary language — or even if you simply *feel more comfortable* in another language — you are entitled to a professional medical interpreter.

Not your partner.
Not your friend.
Not your child.
A *professional.*

Your hospital must provide access through:

- **Video interpretation**
- **Phone interpreter lines**
- **In-person interpreters** (when available)

You do **not** have to apologize.
You do **not** have to feel embarrassed.
You do **not** have to "try" English if it isn't what your heart thinks in.

And I will never let language become a barrier between you and your birth.

Cultural Sensitivity in Labor

Every culture has beliefs about:

- Touch
- Modesty and privacy
- Pain expression
- Who should be in the room
- Birth positions
- Feeding practices
- Postpartum rituals
- Decision-making
- Eye contact and communication styles

Your cultural identity **does not disappear** when you enter a hospital.

You don't leave your culture at the door — you bring it with you, and we honor it.

If something in our routine feels unfamiliar, uncomfortable, or contradictory to your beliefs, please tell me. I will adapt safely, respectfully, and creatively. There is almost always a way to meet your needs while keeping you safe.

Nurse's Note

Your cultural preferences matter — please share them with us.
Whether it's:

- Foods you prefer (or avoid)
- The temperature of your water
- Modesty preferences
- Prayer or spiritual routines
- Who you want involved
- Traditions after birth

These details help us support you in a familiar, comforting, respectful way. You deserve a birth experience that feels like **yours**, not someone else's.

Translators During Pushing – YES, Absolutely

One of the most important things I need you to know:

If you need a translator during pushing, we keep the translator on. I demand it!
If you need them during *every single contraction*, we keep them on.100%
If you need them continuously in the operating room, we keep them on. Without a doubt!

Birth is not the time for guessing or lip-reading.
You should never have to wonder what we are saying.
You should never be left out of your own birth due to language.

If that means:

- A phone interpreter listens for an hour,
- A video interpreter stays on for an entire delivery,
- They hear you cry, breathe, groan, or push…

That is **their job** — and they are honored to support you.

You deserve:

Full understanding
Full communication
Full autonomy

Even in your most intense moments.

Translators in the OR – 100% Yes

When you go to the operating room — for a C-section, an emergency, a repair, or any unexpected change — your emotions and your voice matter **more**, not less.

And I want you to know this clearly:

If you need a translator in the OR, we will keep the translator on.
If you want to understand every word while you are on the table, you deserve that.
If something feels wrong, confusing, or scary, I want to know immediately — and the translator makes that possible.

The OR can be overwhelming: bright lights, fast movement, unfamiliar equipment, new faces. When you add a language barrier to that environment, it can create fear, misunderstanding, or a sense of being alone inside your own procedure.

I will never allow that.

We keep the translator on because:

- You deserve to understand what's happening
- You deserve to be able to speak up
- You deserve to know why you're feeling what you're feeling
- You deserve to be able to tell me if something feels "off"
- You deserve to have your consent protected
- You deserve to stay connected to your own birth

If you feel a certain way, I want to know. Immediately. Clearly. In your own language.

The OR team may be focused on the technical work — the surgical field, your vital signs, your baby — but *your nurse is focused on you.* If the translator helps you communicate your fear, your discomfort, your pain, or even your confusion, then that translator is essential.

There is no such thing as "bothering" us.
There is no such thing as "too many questions."
There is no such thing as "the OR is too busy for interpretation."

Your voice does not get smaller just because the room is sterile.

You deserve to understand.
You deserve to be understood.
And I won't settle for anything less.

Protecting Your Dignity Through Communication

There is no scenario in labor where you should feel:

- Confused

- Ignored
- Talked over
- Talked around
- Rushed
- Left out
- Unsure of what someone is doing to your body

That is **not** the care you deserve.

With a translator, we can:

- Explain every step
- Walk you through emergencies
- Talk you through epidurals
- Coach you during pushing
- Clarify consent
- Answer all your questions
- Make sure you understand *your* options

This is how we protect your dignity, your voice, and your birth.

You deserve nothing less.

43

Adoption & Surrogacy — Paths of Love, Courage, and Selflessness

"Adoption is love chosen. Surrogacy is love given."

A Chapter for the Bravest Hearts

Not every family begins the same way. Some journeys start with biology, others with choice, others with miracles, others with unimaginable strength.
This chapter is for every parent whose path to birth looks different — for birth parents choosing adoption, for families welcoming through adoption, and for the remarkable women who choose to carry a baby for someone else through surrogacy.

These paths are not secondary.
They are not "less than."
They are not alternatives.

They are powerful, valid, love-filled ways of bringing a child into the world.

And every person involved deserves to be honored with tenderness, respect, and reverence.

Part I: Adoption – A Courageous Path of Love

A Choice Made From the Deepest Love

Choosing adoption is one of the most selfless decisions a parent can make. It is a choice rooted not in abandonment, but in **profound love**. It takes immense courage to look at your life, your circumstances, and your baby's future, and decide that the greatest act of love you can offer is to place them into the arms of another family.

If you are choosing adoption, I want you to hear this clearly:
You are not "giving your baby up." You are giving your baby a life you believe is best for them.
That decision comes from strength, not weakness.

The Emotional Journey of Adoption

Adoption brings a swirl of emotions — love, grief, pride, fear, relief, heartbreak, and hope — often all at once. There is no "right" way to feel. Your emotions are valid and deserve space.

Many birth parents silently wonder:

- *Will my baby be okay?*
- *Will they be loved?*
- *Am I doing the right thing?*
- *Will I be judged?*

These questions do not diminish your love — they **prove** it.

As Your Nurse, I Protect You

As your nurse, I want you to feel safe, respected, and supported through every moment of this process. Whether this is the most heartbreaking day of your life or a moment of peace, I will show up for **you**.

I will:

- honor your wishes
- protect your privacy
- advocate fiercely for your boundaries
- ensure you feel in control
- support your emotional needs
- sit with you if you need to cry
- speak up on your behalf if your voice shakes

You deserve dignity.
You deserve compassion.
You deserve a nurse who sees the depth of your love.

Your Choices Matter

Some birth parents want to hold their baby. Some want quiet moments alone. Some want to meet the adoptive family; others need space. Some want photos. Others don't.

Every choice is yours.
Every choice is right.

This is your story, and it will be cared for tenderly.

The Strength You Carry

One day, whether soon or years from now, you may understand just how brave you truly were. You put your baby's future first. You faced a decision most people will never have to face. And you walked through it with love.

You are strong.
You are loving.
You are worthy.

And your courage will be remembered.

Part II: Surrogacy – A Gift Beyond Measure

A Selfless Act of Pure Generosity

Surrogacy is one of the most extraordinary gifts a person can offer. To carry a baby for someone else — to give your body, your time, your health, your emotions to create a life for another family — is nothing short of remarkable.

If you are a surrogate, please know:
You are a hero in someone's story.
Your strength, compassion, and sacrifice are immeasurable.

The Surrogate's Journey

Surrogacy is beautiful but it is also emotionally complex. Surrogates often experience:

- Joy in giving life
- Deep responsibility
- Grief and gratitude woven together
- Physical demands of pregnancy
- A profound connection to the intended parents
- Emotional shifts during and after birth

No emotion you feel is wrong.
Your journey is unique and deserves to be honored.

As Your Nurse, I Safeguard Your Dignity

My promise to you as a surrogate is simple:
You will be treated with the utmost respect.

You deserve:

- a voice in your care
- emotional support
- clear communication
- physical comfort
- boundaries that are honored
- an advocate who sees *you*

You are not "just the surrogate."
You are a woman with a remarkable story — one that deserves tenderness and reverence.

A Moment That Changes Lives

When your labor ends and the intended parents meet their baby for the first time, the room becomes sacred. There is nothing like the joy on their faces — joy that you made possible. That moment belongs to all of you.

It is not a loss.
It is a victory.
A triumph of generosity.

A moment that proves how powerful the human heart can be.

A Shared Thread: Extraordinary Love

Adoption and surrogacy may look different but they share the same foundation:
love, sacrifice, courage, and the willingness to create a better future for a child.

Birth parents choosing adoption and surrogates choosing to carry for another family are connected by the same depth of heart — the willingness to put a child's wellbeing above their own comfort.

As your nurse, I want you to know:

I see your courage.
I respect your path.
I will protect your journey.
And I will honor your story with the tenderness it deserves.

44

Closing Chapter: From My Heart to Yours

"From one heartbeat to another, this book was my way of walking beside you."

As you reach the end of this book, I want you to pause and take a breath — not just because you've just absorbed a tremendous amount of knowledge, but because you've taken the time to invest in yourself and your birth experience. That says something **powerful** about who you are as a mother long before your baby ever takes their first breath.

Writing this book has been one of the greatest honors of my career. Every word, every explanation, every nurse's tip was written with one intention: to help you feel supported, educated, empowered, and safe. My wish is that you walk into your labor **not with fear, but with confidence** — knowing exactly what's happening, understanding your options, and feeling the strength inside yourself that maybe you haven't discovered yet.

I've been a Labor & Delivery nurse for a long time. I've stood at thousands of bedsides. I've held hands, held hearts, tied hair back, tucked legs into stirrups, wiped tears, coached pushes, celebrated victories, and sat in silence during the hardest moments a family can face. I've seen the entire spectrum of birth — **the beauty, the messiness, the miracles, and the moments** that feel like the world is standing still.

And through all of it, my greatest joy has never changed: **helping you feel cared for. Helping you feel seen. Helping you feel strong. Helping you feel like you're not doing this alone.**

If this book has given you even **one moment** of reassurance — **one moment** where you felt, *"Okay… I can do this"* — then **every hour** I spent writing it was worth it.

What I want most for you is simple:

I want you to walk into your birth feeling empowered.
I want you to feel respected and heard in every decision.
I want you to know you can speak up — and your voice matters.
I want you to feel safe, supported, and surrounded by people who care.
And I want you to look back on your experience and remember the strength you didn't even know you had.

When I think about my patients, I am reminded of one of my favorite sentiments, inspired by the timeless wisdom of Maya Angelou:

**"You may forget what I did, you may forget what I said,
but you will never forget how I made you feel."**

That is my purpose.
That is my calling.
That is why this book exists.

So wherever you are in your journey — preparing for labor, recovering postpartum, or holding your baby in your arms — remember this:

You are capable.
You are powerful.

You are made to do this.
You are worthy of a beautiful birth story.
And I am honored — truly honored, privileged, and it was my pleasure — to have walked even a small part of this path with you.

With all my heart,

Kim
Your Labor & Delivery Nurse

45

For the Families Who Need This: A Chapter of Compassion and Care

"There is no footprint too small to leave an everlasting mark."

This is a chapter I hope you never need—and yet, it is one of the most important ones I can offer. As an L&D nurse, I walk with families through some of the happiest moments of their lives. But I have also stood beside families during the darkest, most unimaginable moments—when a baby is born still or when a heartbeat that carried so much hope is no longer there.

This is the hardest part of my job. It changes you. It humbles you. It stays with you.

And if you are reading this because you are living through a loss, please hear this first:

You are not alone.
Your grief is real.
Your baby matters.
Your love is forever.
And this is not your fault.

That is the foundation of this chapter.

When Devastating News Is Given

No parent is ever prepared to hear the words:
"There is no heartbeat."

In that moment, time stops. Your world tilts. You may feel numb, sick, angry, confused—or nothing at all. Every reaction is normal. Every emotion is valid.

As nurses, we understand that this moment is sacred. It deserves:

slow, clear explanations
space for shock
room to breathe
the opportunity to ask questions or to say nothing at all

We will repeat ourselves as many times as you need.
We will sit quietly with you if silence is what you need.
We will stay with you through each step, so you never feel abandoned.

What Happens Medically

If your loss occurs in pregnancy or during labor, your care team will discuss what comes next with sensitivity and clarity.

1. Induction or Labor

In most cases, the safest option is to deliver your baby vaginally. This may feel overwhelming, but your body knows how to do this and we will help guide you through it gently.

Medications like Misoprostol or Pitocin may be used to start or support labor if you don't go into labor your own. Your comfort matters deeply—pain control (including an epidural) is absolutely available and appropriate.

2. No Rush, Unless Medically Necessary

You have time.
Time to process.
Time to breathe.
Time to gather support.
Time to hold your partner's hand.

There are very few instances where immediate action is required.

3. Your Care is Customized

We will tailor everything—your pain medicine, your environment, your pace—to what you need emotionally and physically.

The Birth of Your Baby

Your baby's birth still matters.
Your baby's story still matters.
And **you are still a parent**.

We protect this space as tenderly as we can.

What to Expect

Your labor may feel different because there is no fetal movement guiding the process. This is emotionally heavy and physically exhausting—but we are with you the entire way.

After delivery, you may choose:

to hold your baby
to bathe them
to dress them
to take photos

to create footprints or handprints
to have a naming ceremony
to invite family or keep it intimate
to spend minutes or hours
to let us hold your baby if you cannot

There is **no right way.**
There is **only your way**.

How Nurses Care for You

When loss enters the room, the way we care for you changes. It becomes slower. Softer. More intentional. We know that every word, every touch and every pause matters. In these moments, nursing is no longer about tasks or checklists — it is about walking with you through the unimaginable.

Here is how we care for you when your world has shifted:

1. We Protect Your Space

We dim the lights. We reduce noise. We soften our voices.

We place signs on the door so other staff enter quietly and respectfully. Your room becomes a protected sanctuary — a place where grief can be honored, not rushed.

2. We Move at Your Pace

Nothing is forced. Nothing is hurried.

If you need silence, we honor it.
If you need explanations, we give them gently.
If you need to pause and breathe, we sit with you.

We follow your cues, spoken or unspoken.
You lead; we walk beside you.

3. We Support Your Decisions – All of Them

This is your birth and your baby.

We ask:

Would you like to hold your baby?
Would you like us to prepare them for you?
Would you like photos or footprints?
Would you like to bathe or dress your baby?
Would you prefer privacy or support at your side?

There is no right or wrong answer.
There is only what's right for you in this moment.

4. We Care for Your Baby With Honor

If you need time before you're ready to hold your baby, we hold them for you.

We speak to them quietly.
We clean them gently.
We wrap them with tenderness.

We treat them like the precious child they are.

Every baby deserves to be honored.
Every baby deserves dignity.
Every baby is cared for as if they were our own.

5. We Help You Create Memories That Last

If you want them, we help you create things you can hold onto when your arms feel painfully empty:

tiny footprints
a handprint
photos
a lock of hair (if appropriate)
a memory box
a blanket
a hat
a card with your baby's name
written notes about the time you spent together

Some families treasure these items.
Some families aren't ready.
Either way — **we honor your choice.**

6. We See Your Tears and We Hold Space For Them

We don't rush your grief.
We don't "fix" your pain.
We don't fill silence with empty words.

We sit with you.
We listen.
We witness your love.

Sometimes the most powerful care we give is **our presence.**

7. We Care for Your Body As Tenderly As Your Heart

Even though your heart is breaking, your body has still been through labor and birth. We will:

manage your pain
monitor your bleeding
help you walk if you're weak
support you through milk suppression if needed
explain everything gently
ensure you're physically stable
protect your privacy and dignity

Your physical recovery matters, even in the midst of grief.

8. We Care for Your Partner and Support System Too

Loss affects the entire room. Partners often feel helpless, overwhelmed, or silent under the weight of their own grief.

We check on them.
We offer them water, food, a place to sit.
We answer their questions.
We remind them they matter too.

Everyone in that room needs care.

9. We Prepare You for What Happens Next

Not all families want to think ahead — but when you're ready, we talk you through:

The next steps....
funeral home or cremation options
what to expect in the days ahead
emotional resources
grief support
follow-up appointments

We give you information gently, in small pieces, never more than you can hold.

10. We Remember You

You may not realize this but we carry your family with us long after you leave the unit.

Your baby is remembered.
Your story stays with us.
Your strength leaves a mark on our hearts.

You are not just another patient.
Your baby is not forgotten.
Your experience becomes part of us.

Pain Management During a Loss

Pain is physical, but it is also emotional — and during a fetal loss, the emotional pain is already more than any heart should ever have to hold. I once had a patient ask me, "When should I get my epidural?" And I told her the truth, from one human to another:

"The moment you feel anything. Your heart is hurting enough. Any more pain would just be cruel."

In these moments, there is:

no prize for endurance
no reason to wait
no expectation to "tough it out"

Your body is doing the hardest thing it will ever be asked to do while your heart is breaking at the same time.

If you want an epidural, you can have it early.
If you want IV medication, you can have that too.
If you want to feel nothing physically, that is completely okay.

There is no right or wrong way to navigate this experience.
There is only **compassion** — for your body, for your heart, and for your grief.

Your comfort matters.
Your dignity matters.
And your nurse will advocate for whatever helps ease even one layer of pain in an already unthinkably painful moment.

You do not have to be strong.
You just have to be held.

And we will hold you through all of it.

Memory-Making and Hospital Support

Many hospitals offer:

cuddle cots (to allow more time with baby)
memory boxes
tiny hats, blankets, and clothing
photographs
certificates of remembrance
clay or ink footprints
little locks of hair (if appropriate)
the option of your baby not going to the morgue

These are small, priceless pieces of your baby's life story—**anchors of love** that families often cling to later.

You can decline any of these.
Or you can accept all of them.
You will be supported either way.

Your Emotions After Delivery

After delivery, emotions can feel overwhelming, unpredictable, or even distant. There is no single way you are *supposed* to feel.

You may experience:

- shock or disbelief
- denial or confusion
- sadness, anger, or guilt
- moments of relief
- waves of rage or frustration
- numbness or emotional quiet
- deep love
- profound grief
- or very little emotion at all

All of these responses are normal.

Grief does not move in a straight line. It comes in waves — some soft and quiet, others sudden and heavy. Some days you may feel okay. Other days, simply breathing may feel like enough.

Please allow yourself grace.
There is no timeline.
There is no right reaction.

Whatever you are feeling — or not feeling — is enough.
You are not doing this wrong.

Your Physical Recovery

Your body will recover just as it would after any birth — even when the outcome was not what you hoped or expected. Your body does not know the difference between joy and grief. It follows the same biological processes it was designed to follow.

You may experience:

Vaginal bleeding

Bleeding after birth is normal and expected. It may start heavier and gradually lighten over days to weeks. This is your uterus healing and shedding the lining that supported your pregnancy.

Cramping (afterpains)

You may feel cramps similar to strong menstrual cramps, especially during the first few days. These contractions help your uterus shrink back down and reduce bleeding.

Milk coming in

Your milk may come in a few days after birth, even if you are not breastfeeding. This can be physically uncomfortable and emotionally painful. Please know — we can help. There are gentle ways to support milk suppression and relieve discomfort, and you do not have to navigate this alone.

Fatigue

Your body has been through intense physical work. Healing takes energy, and exhaustion is common — both from birth itself and from the emotional toll your body is carrying.

Hormonal swings

After birth, hormone levels shift rapidly. You may experience mood changes, tearfulness, anxiety, or emotional numbness. These changes are physiological, not a reflection of weakness or coping ability.

Nurse Reassurance

Everything your body is doing right now is **normal**, even if it feels deeply unfair.

We will talk you through each change — gently and clearly. We will explain what's expected, what's temporary, and when to ask for help. You can ask questions as many times as you need. Nothing you're feeling is too small or too much.

Your body deserves care.
You deserve patience.
And you deserve support — every step of the way.

Partners and Support People

Partners and support people grieve in their own ways.

Some step into protector mode — focusing on logistics, decisions, and strength because it feels safer than feeling.
Some collapse, overwhelmed by shock, fear, or heartbreak they don't yet have words for.
Some go silent, unsure of how to speak without making things worse.
Some cry openly, allowing their grief to be seen.
Some look lost, standing beside the person they love while carrying their own unanswered pain.

There is no right or wrong way to grieve.

Partners often feel torn between their own emotions and the urge to stay strong for the birthing parent. Many feel pressure to "hold it together," even when they are breaking inside. Others feel invisible — unsure if their grief is allowed space when attention naturally centers on the patient.

But grief is not a competition.
Pain does not diminish because someone else is hurting too.

Partners and support people need care, reassurance, and permission to feel — just as much as the person giving birth. They may need space to talk, to cry, to sit in silence, or simply to be acknowledged.

Everyone deserves support.
No one should carry this pain alone.

If you are a partner or support person reading this: your feelings matter.
If you are the birthing parent: your partner may be grieving in ways that don't look like your own — and that doesn't mean they love you any less.

And if you are both in this space together, know this: healing does not mean forgetting. It means finding a way to breathe again, side by side, one moment at a time.

After You Leave the Hospital

This is often the hardest part.
The world moves on—but you don't.

Here are things that help many families:

follow-up appointments
grief counseling

support groups
faith-based support if meaningful to you
naming your baby
writing a letter
creating a memory box at home
planting a tree or flower
including your baby in family traditions
talking about your baby openly and often

There is no timeline for healing.
There is no "getting over it."
There is only learning to live with **love and loss intertwined.**

A Note From Your Nurse

This chapter is not written from a textbook.
It is written from years of **holding mothers as they shook**,
holding fathers as they cried,
and **holding babies whose lives, though brief, were immeasurably meaningful.**

The hardest part of my job is this.
And yet, it is the part I approach with the deepest honor.

If you are reading this because your world has shifted into grief, please know:

Your baby mattered.
Your baby is remembered.
And you will always be a parent.

We will walk with you in every moment we are allowed —
and your baby's story will stay with us long after you leave our unit.

You Are Not Alone

If this chapter is the only section of the book you needed,
I am wrapping you in compassion from a distance.
I am thinking of your baby.
I am holding space for your grief.

And I want you to remember this:

You loved your baby every moment of their life.
That love is eternal.
Nothing will ever take it from you.

46

The Rainbow After the Storm

"Your rainbow didn't come instead of your angel — they came because of them."

The term *rainbow baby* carries the weight of both sorrow and joy—a symbol of the beauty that can follow life's darkest storms. For families who have experienced the heart-wrenching loss of a baby, the arrival of a rainbow baby represents **hope, renewal, and a reminder that love does not end**, even after the most devastating of losses.

The Loss That Precedes the Rainbow

Before the rainbow, there is the storm.
The grief that comes with losing a child—whether through miscarriage, stillbirth, or fetal demise—creates a void that words can scarcely fill. It is a pain unlike any other, often isolating and profound.

As a nurse, I have seen firsthand the heavy hearts of parents who must navigate the unimaginable. Their grief is not only for the child they will never know, but for the **dreams, the hopes, and the plans** that will never be fulfilled.

But even in the depth of sorrow, there is a quiet knowing that this loss is *not* the end.
In time, many parents choose to try again, opening their hearts to the possibility of a new beginning—while never forgetting the one they lost.

And when that day comes—when they see those two pink lines or hear the heartbeat of a new baby—**a new chapter begins.**

A New Beginning

For parents who have experienced loss, pregnancy with a rainbow baby can be bittersweet.

There is **joy** but there is also **fear**.

Every kick, every movement, every ultrasound carries both hope and a tremor of worry. The echoes of loss linger in the background making every moment both precious and fragile.

It's important to acknowledge this truth:

A rainbow baby is *not* a replacement.
No child can ever take the place of the one lost.
Love for both children can coexist.

A rainbow baby does not erase grief—it simply **brings light into the darkness**. This child represents survival, resilience, and the heart's ability to love and heal again.

The Healing Power of the Rainbow

The arrival of a rainbow baby is one of the most beautiful, emotional, triumphant experiences a parent can have. It is a testament to their strength, perseverance, and their deep desire to love again.

This baby offers:

new memories
new hope
new joy
new healing

While the loss of a child is never forgotten, the rainbow baby gradually brings peace—softly filling shattered spaces with warmth and color.

The Role of the Nurse

As nurses, we are often the first to witness the emotional transformation of parents expecting a rainbow baby.

Our responsibility goes beyond tasks.
We support them not only during joyful moments but also during moments of fear, doubt, and anxiety.

Parents may:

- Need reassurance
- Need validation
- Need to talk about their previous loss
- Need extra emotional support

Providing a safe space for these conversations is just as important as caring for the physical aspects of pregnancy.

A rainbow baby pregnancy is unique.
Its emotional terrain is delicate.
And honoring that is part of our calling.

A New Chapter of Hope

The arrival of a rainbow baby is a celebration of **hope and healing**. It is a new beginning for families who have carried the heaviest grief.

To the families carrying these precious babies:

You are not defined by your loss.
You are defined by your love, your endurance, and your strength.
Your rainbow baby is a reflection of that resilience—bright, beautiful, and full of promise.

Their life honors both the past and the future.
Their presence is the soft light after the storm.

47

To the Mothers and Families I Have Cared for During Fetal Loss—

There are moments in nursing that shape us forever and caring for you in the midst of unimaginable heartbreak is one of them.

I want you to know:

It was an honor and a profound privilege to be by your side when the world felt unbearably heavy.

Many nurses come to work expecting to witness beginnings—first breaths, first cries, first chapters. But some days, we are called to witness **loss** instead.

Not everyone can step into that space, but I have always believed:

If I am there with you,
then I must show up fully—
with tenderness, steadiness, and whatever light I can offer in your darkest moment.

I hope I did that for you.
I hope I helped carry even a fraction of your grief.

Know this:

When I left that shift, I prayed for you.
I prayed for your strength.
And a piece of your story remains with me—quietly shaping the nurse I am today.

Your baby mattered.
Your love mattered.
And the depth of your sorrow reflects the depth of that love.

Whether you try again or choose a different future,
I hope peace finds you—softly, slowly, and in your own time.

Thank you for allowing me to walk with you through your most painful chapter.
I carry every one of you with me.

With all my heart,

Kim
Your Labor and Delivery Nurse

Acknowledgments

This book may have my name on the cover, but it carries the fingerprints of so many people who have shaped my life, my work, and my heart.

To my **Sons** — my very early teachers of Labor and Delivery. I hope, in some small way, you have watched this journey and learned that **hard work, perseverance, and grit matter**. I also hope you know that my happiness exist in you because without you, my existence would not matter.

To my Dad — you were a poor boy from the Atlantic City inlet who built a life for my brothers and I with grit, sacrifice, and an unshakable work ethic. Nothing was handed to you. You earned everything and in doing so, you showed us what it means to build something that lasts. You taught me to take chances, to stand on my own two feet, and to keep going when things got tough. You never promised it would be easy — only that it would be worth it.

End of the day, you did it "YOUR WAY", I did it "MINE". I hope you are as proud of me as I am of you.

To my heavenly Mother — you never got to see me become a nurse. That truth still stops me in my tracks. But you live inside of every patient I care for, every hand I hold, and every life I touch. Your love shaped my compassion long before I ever wore scrubs. When I walk into a delivery room, when I stand steady in an emergency, when I speak gently to a frightened mother — that is you moving through me and I carry you into every room with me. I hurried this book into the world so Dad could see me become an Author, holding the ache of knowing you never saw me become a nurse. But you never left. You just became something I carry instead of something I can see.

To **God** — for placing the passion for nursing inside of me, for trusting me to do His work through my hands, for protecting my patients, and for sustaining me when I was exhausted, overwhelmed, uncertain, or afraid. This calling is not mine alone — it is borrowed, guided, and protected by YOU. It is my purpose.

To **Lisa Lovett** — you were instrumental in my career in ways I can never fully repay. You helped secure both of my labor positions and placed me in the hearts of countless pregnant families. Because of you, I found my professional home. For that, I am truly grateful.

To **Lou Arpa** — my mentor and my boss during my first career in business — everything I learned about leadership, sales, strategy, and drive came from you. That knowledge now carries forward into the building of this brand. I carry your lessons with me daily.

And finally — to my **Husband**.

You are my **silent partner** in all of this. Everything I do in life is surrounded by you. We have lived an entire lifetime together — not always the easy kind — but through every struggle, every sacrifice, every uncertain moment, and every victory, **we stood side by side**. You are behind every late night, every idea, every page, every doubt, and every triumph in this book. This work carries my name — but **it exists because of your steady presence beside me throughout life and my entire career**. I wouldn't be who I am today without you.

REFERENCES

CHAPTER 1

Welcome to Labor and Delivery!

Larsen, D., & Maani, C. V. (2025). Nalbuphine. In *Statpearls [internet]*. StatPearls Publishing. https://www.ncbi.nlm.nih.gov/books/NBK534283/

CHAPTER 2

Your Birth Plan and Beyond

CHAPTER 3

Let's Get the Party Started!

American College of Obstetricians and Gynecologists. (2022). Gestational hypertension and preeclampsia. *ACOG PRACTICE BULLETIN, 135*(6). https://www.preeclampsia.org/frontend/assets/img/advocacy_resource/Gestational_Hypertension_and_Preeclampsia_ACOG_Practice_Bulletin,_Number_222_1605448006.pdf

Weller, M., Griffin, A., & Janssens, S. (2025). Introducing tranexamic acid into the protocol for management of post-partum haemorrhage: An observational study using repeated cross-sectional analysis. *Sexual & Reproductive Healthcare, 45*, 101110. https://doi.org/10.1016/j.srhc.2025.101110

CHAPTER 4

Understanding the Language of Labor and Delivery

ACOG clinical practice guideline no. 8: first and second stage labor management: correction. (2025). *Obstetrics & Gynecology, 145*(3), e126–e126. https://doi.org/10.1097/aog.0000000000005834

American College of Obstetricians and Gynecologists. (2022). Gestational hypertension and preeclampsia. *ACOG PRACTICE BULLETIN, 135*(6). https://www.preeclampsia.org/frontend/assets/img/advocacy_resource/Gestational_Hypertension_and_Preeclampsia_ACOG_Practice_Bulletin,_Number_222_1605448006.pdf

American College of Obstetricians and Gynecologists. (2018). Placenta accreta spectrum. *Obstetrics & Gynecology, 132*(6), 259–275. https://www.acog.org/-/media/project/acog/acogorg/clinical/files/obstetric-care-consensus/articles/2018/12/placenta-accreta-spectrum.pdf?rev=c00cd7ddadb54897bc450086708039db&hash=09EC778BDC6806E9B4149AE0C5417239

Cleveland Clinic. (2025). *Colostrum.* https://my.clevelandclinic.org/health/body/22434-colostrum

Davis, D. D., Roshan, A., & Varacallo, M. A. (2023). Shoulder dystocia. In *Statpearls [internet].* StatPearls Publishing. https://www.ncbi.nlm.nih.gov/books/NBK470427/

First and second stage labor management. (2024). *Obstetrics & Gynecology, 143*(1), 144–162 https://doi.org/10.1097/aog.0000000000005447

Jenkins SM, Van Hook JW. Induction of Labor. [Updated 2023 Feb 20]. In: StatPearls [Internet]. Treasure Island (FL): StatPearls Publishing; 2025 Jan-. Available from: https://www.ncbi.nlm.nih.gov/books/NBK459264/

Kauffmann, T., & Silberman, M. (2023). Fetal monitoring. In *Statpearls [internet].* StatPearls Publishing. https://www.ncbi.nlm.nih.gov/books/NBK589699/

Kunarathnam, V., Vadakekut, E. S., & Mahdy, H. (2025). Gestational diabetes. In *Statpearls [internet].* StatPearls Publishing. https://www.ncbi.nlm.nih.gov/books/NBK545196/

Pillarisetty, L. S., & Sharma, A. (2023). Pregnancy intrahepatic cholestasis. In *Statpearls [internet].* StatPearls Publishing. https://www.ncbi.nlm.nih.gov/books/NBK551503/

Raabe, V. N., & Shane, A. L. (2019). Group b streptococcus (streptococcus agalactiae). *Microbiology Spectrum, 7*(2). https://doi.org/10.1128/microbiolspec.gpp3-0007-2018

Sadiku, O. D., Aina, S. A., Odoemene, C. C., Ogunmoyin, T. E., Adedara, V. O., Olasimbo, O., Ashir, F. A., Adili, S. C., Kuteyi, A. O., Fakayode, O. O., Faletti, D. O., & Nogales Bernal, M. (2024). Approaches to the prevention and treatment of postpartum hemorrhage: A systematic review of past advances, recent developments, and best practices. *Cureus.* https://doi.org/10.7759/cureus.65096

Sharma, D. (2017). Golden hour of neonatal life: Need of the hour. *Maternal Health, Neonatology and Perinatology, 3*(1). https://doi.org/10.1186/s40748-017-0057-x

Simon, L. V., Shah, M., & Bragg, B. N. (2024). Apgar score. In *Statpearls [internet].* StatPearls Publishing. https://www.ncbi.nlm.nih.gov/books/NBK470569/

Togioka, B. M., & Tonismae, T. (2023). Uterine rupture. In *Statpearls [internet]*. StatPearls Publishing. https://www.ncbi.nlm.nih.gov/books/NBK559209/

Widström, A., Brimdyr, K., Svensson, K., Cadwell, K., & Nissen, E. (2019). Skin to skin contact the first hour after birth, underlying implications and clinical practice. *Acta Paediatrica*, *108*(7), 1192–1204. https://doi.org/10.1111/apa.14754

CHAPTER 5

Necessary Evils: The Things We Do That Don't Always Feel Good

American College of Obstetricians and Gynecologists. (2022). Gestational hypertension and preeclampsia. *ACOG PRACTICE BULLETIN*, *135*(6). https://www.preeclampsia.org/frontend/assets/img/advocacy_resource/Gestational_Hypertension_and_Preeclampsia_ACOG_Practice_Bulletin,_Number_222_1605448006.pdf

American College of Obstetricians & Gynecologists. (2025). *Routine tests during pregnancy*. Every Stage Health. Retrieved November 18, 2025, from https://www.acog.org/womens-health/faqs/routine-tests-during-pregnancy

Bauer, M. E., Arendt, K., Beilin, Y., Gernsheimer, T., Perez Botero, J., James, A. H., Yaghmour, E., Toledano, R. D., Turrentine, M., Houle, T., MacEachern, M., Madden, H., Rajasekhar, A., Segal, S., Wu, C., Cooper, J. P., Landau, R., & Leffert, L. (2021). The society for obstetric anesthesia and perinatology interdisciplinary consensus statement on neuraxial procedures in obstetric patients with thrombocytopenia. *Anesthesia & Analgesia*, *132*(6), 1531–1544. https://doi.org/10.1213/ane.0000000000005355

Fowler, J. R., & Simon, L. V. (2023). Chorioamnionitis. In *Statpearls [internet]*. StatPearls Publishing. https://www.ncbi.nlm.nih.gov/books/NBK532251/

Franklin, E., & Anjum, F. (2023). Incentive spirometer and inspiratory muscle training. In *Statpearls [internet]*. StatPearls Publishing. https://www.ncbi.nlm.nih.gov/books/NBK572114/

Hicks, M. A., & Tyagi, A. (2023). Magnesium sulfate. In *Statpearls [internet]*. StatPearls Publishing. https://www.ncbi.nlm.nih.gov/books/NBK554553/

Mohd Yassin, N., Kamarudin, M., Hamdan, M., & Tan, P. (2024). Self bladder emptying compared with foley catheter placement for planned cesarean delivery: A randomized controlled trial. *American Journal of Obstetrics & Gynecology MFM*, *6*(5), 101308. https://doi.org/10.1016/j.ajogmf.2024.101308

Pomajzl, A., & Siref, L. E. (2023). Postoperative urinary retention. In *Statpearls [internet]*. StatPearls Publishing. https://www.ncbi.nlm.nih.gov/books/NBK549844/

Sadiku, O. D., Aina, S. A., Odoemene, C. C., Ogunmoyin, T. E., Adedara, V. O., Olasimbo, O., Ashir, F. A., Adili, S. C., Kuteyi, A. O., Fakayode, O. O., Faletti, D. O., & Nogales Bernal, M. (2024). Approaches to the prevention and treatment of postpartum hemorrhage: A systematic review of past advances, recent developments, and best practices. *Cureus*. https://doi.org/10.7759/cureus.65096

Windermere, S., Sconzo, D., Askari, A., Filippidis, A., & Binello, E. (2024). Surgeon-led improvement in compliance with use of sequential compression devices in a neurosurgery patient population. *BMJ Open Quality*, *13*(3), e002807. https://doi.org/10.1136/bmjoq-2024-002807

CHAPTER 6

What's Going On Down There?

Ami, O., Maran, J.-C., Cohen, A., Hendler, I., Zabukovek, E., & Boyer, L. (2023). Childbirth simulation to assess cephalopelvic disproportion and chances for failed labor in a french population. *Scientific Reports*, *13*(1). https://doi.org/10.1038/s41598-023-28459-6

Cleveland Clinic. (2025). *Amniotic fluid.* https://my.clevelandclinic.org/health/body/23310-amniotic-fluid

Evbuomwan, O., & Chowdhury, Y. S. (2023). Physiology, cervical dilation. In *Statpearls [internet]*. StatPearls Publishing. https://www.ncbi.nlm.nih.gov/books/NBK557582/

Gomez, H. B., Hoffman, M., Caplan, R., Fawcett, M., & Sciscione, A. (2021). 177 incremental risk of chorioamnionitis associated with cervical examination. *American Journal of Obstetrics and Gynecology*, *224*(2), S119–S120. https://doi.org/10.1016/j.ajog.2020.12.199

Hutchison, J., Mahdy, H., Jenkins, S. M., & Hutchison, J. (2025). Normal labor: Physiology, evaluation, and management. In *Statpearls [internet]*. StatPearls Publishing. https://www.ncbi.nlm.nih.gov/books/NBK544290/

Kissler, K. J., Lowe, N. K., & Hernandez, T. L. (2020). An integrated review of uterine activity monitoring for evaluating labor dystocia. *Journal of Midwifery & Women's Health*, *65*(3), 323–334. https://doi.org/10.1111/jmwh.13119

CHAPTER 7

All Things Fluid

Cleveland Clinic. (2025). *Amniotic fluid.* https://my.clevelandclinic.org/health/body/23310-amniotic-fluid

Dayal S, Jenkins SM, Hong PL. Preterm and Term Prelabor Rupture of Membranes (PPROM and PROM) [Updated 2024 Oct 31]. In: StatPearls [Internet]. Treasure Island (FL): StatPearls Publishing; 2025 Jan-. Available from: https://www.ncbi.nlm.nih.gov/books/NBK532888/

Fowler, J. R., & Simon, L. V. (2023). Chorioamnionitis. In *Statpearls [internet].* StatPearls Publishing. https://www.ncbi.nlm.nih.gov/books/NBK532251/

Jenkins, S. M., & Hook, J. W. V. (2023). Induction of labor. In *Statpearls [internet].* StatPearls Publishing. https://www.ncbi.nlm.nih.gov/books/NBK459264/

Mahdy, H., & Eruo, F. U. (2023). Amniotomy. In *Statpearls [internet].* StatPearls Publishing. https://www.ncbi.nlm.nih.gov/books/NBK470167/

Sayad E, Silva-Carmona M. Meconium Aspiration. [Updated 2023 Apr 12]. In: StatPearls [Internet]. Treasure Island (FL): StatPearls Publishing; 2025 Jan-. Available from: https://www.ncbi.nlm.nih.gov/books/NBK557425/

Schmidt, P., Skelly, C. L., & Raines, D. A. (2022). Placental abruption. In *Statpearls [internet].* StatPearls Publishing. https://www.ncbi.nlm.nih.gov/books/NBK482335/

CHAPTER 8

Riding the Waves: Understanding Your Contractions

Broughton, K., Clark, A. G., & Ray, A. P. (2020). Nitrous oxide for labor analgesia: What we know to date. *Ochsner Journal, 20*(4), 419–421. https://doi.org/10.31486/toj.19.0102

Callahan, E. C., Lee, W., Aleshi, P., & George, R. B. (2023). Modern labor epidural analgesia: Implications for labor outcomes and maternal-fetal health. *American Journal of Obstetrics and Gynecology, 228*(5), S1260–S1269. https://doi.org/10.1016/j.ajog.2022.06.017

Ghanavatian S, Leslie SW, Derian A. Pudendal Nerve Block. [Updated 2024 Sep 2]. In: StatPearls [Internet]. Treasure Island (FL): StatPearls Publishing; 2025 Jan-. Available from: https://www.ncbi.nlm.nih.gov/books/NBK551518/

McEvoy, A., & Sabir, S. (2022). Physiology, pregnancy contractions. In *Statpearls [internet]*. StatPearls Publishing. https://www.ncbi.nlm.nih.gov/books/NBK532927/

Zuarez-Easton, S., Erez, O., Zafran, N., Carmeli, J., Garmi, G., & Salim, R. (2023). Pharmacologic and nonpharmacologic options for pain relief during labor: An expert review. *American Journal of Obstetrics and Gynecology, 228*(5), S1246–S1259. https://doi.org/10.1016/j.ajog.2023.03.003

CHAPTER 9

Your Epidural – What to Expect, What It Feels Like, and Why It's Okay to Want One

ACOG clinical practice guideline no. 8: first and second stage labor management: correction. (2025). *Obstetrics & Gynecology, 145*(3), e126–e126. https://doi.org/10.1097/aog.0000000000005834

Cai, L., Jiang, J.-J., Wang, T.-T., & Cao, S. (2023). Effects of combined spinal-epidural anesthesia on anxiety, labor analgesia and motor blocks in women during natural delivery. *World Journal of Psychiatry, 13*(11), 838–847. https://doi.org/10.5498/wjp.v13.i11.838

Callahan, E. C., Lee, W., Aleshi, P., & George, R. B. (2023). Modern labor epidural analgesia: Implications for labor outcomes and maternal-fetal health. *American Journal of Obstetrics and Gynecology, 228*(5), S1260–S1269. https://doi.org/10.1016/j.ajog.2022.06.017

Hofmeyr, G., Cyna, A. M., & Middleton, P. (2004). Prophylactic intravenous preloading for regional analgesia in labour. *Cochrane Database of Systematic Reviews.* https://doi.org/10.1002/14651858.cd000175.pub2

Linfield-Brown, G., Khullar, V., & Cardozo, L. (2025). Effect of epidural analgesia on postpartum bladder sensation. *European Journal of Obstetrics & Gynecology and Reproductive Biology, 308*, 96–98. Retrieved November 29, 2025, from https://doi.org/10.1016/j.ejogrb.2025.02.037

Plewa, M. C., Hall, W. A., & McAllister, R. K. (2025). Postdural puncture headache. In *Statpearls [internet]*. StatPearls Publishing. https://www.ncbi.nlm.nih.gov/books/NBK430925/

Tanaka, H., Kamiya, C., Katsuragi, S., Tanaka, K., Yoshimatsu, J., & Ikeda, T. (2018). Effect of epidural anesthesia in labor; pregnancy with cardiovascular disease. *Taiwanese Journal of Obstetrics and Gynecology, 57*(2), 190–193. https://doi.org/10.1016/j.tjog.2018.02.004

Tian, X., Niu, K., Cao, H., Zhan, G., Zhang, Y., Xu, F., Shangguan, W., & Gao, Y. (2021). Pruritus after continuous administration of epidural morphine for post-cesarean delivery analgesia: A case control study. *BMC Pregnancy and Childbirth, 21*(1). https://doi.org/10.1186/s12884-020-03522-6

Xu, C., Wang, X., Chi, X., Chen, Y., Chu, L., & Chen, X. (2023). Association of epidural analgesia during labor and early postpartum urinary incontinence among women delivered vaginally: A propensity score matched retrospective cohort study. *BMC Pregnancy and Childbirth, 23*(1). https://doi.org/10.1186/s12884-023-05952-4

CHAPTER 10

Epidural vs. IV Pain Medication

ACOG clinical practice guideline no. 8: first and second stage labor management: correction. (2025). *Obstetrics & Gynecology, 145*(3), e126–e126. https://doi.org/10.1097/aog.0000000000005834

Callahan, E. C., Lee, W., Aleshi, P., & George, R. B. (2023). Modern labor epidural analgesia: Implications for labor outcomes and maternal-fetal health. *American Journal of Obstetrics and Gynecology, 228*(5), S1260–S1269. https://doi.org/10.1016/j.ajog.2022.06.017

Zuarez-Easton, S., Erez, O., Zafran, N., Carmeli, J., Garmi, G., & Salim, R. (2023). Pharmacologic and nonpharmacologic options for pain relief during labor: An expert review. *American Journal of Obstetrics and Gynecology, 228*(5), S1246–S1259. https://doi.org/10.1016/j.ajog.2023.03.003

CHAPTER 11

Hello from the Inside!

American College of Obstetricians & Gynecologists. (2020, June 15). *Countdown to intern year, week 4: fetal heart tracings*. https://www.acog.org/community/districts-and-sections/district-iv/whats-new/countdown-to-intern-year-week-4-fetal-heart-tracings

Kauffmann, T., & Silberman, M. (2023). Fetal monitoring. In *Statpearls [internet]*. StatPearls Publishing. https://www.ncbi.nlm.nih.gov/books/NBK589699/

Jenkins, S. M., & Hook, J. W. V. (2023). Induction of labor. In *Statpearls [internet]*. StatPearls Publishing. https://www.ncbi.nlm.nih.gov/books/NBK459264/

Leathersich, S. J., Vogel, J. P., Tran, T., & Hofmeyr, G. (2018). Acute tocolysis for uterine tachysystole or suspected fetal distress. *Cochrane Database of Systematic Reviews, 2018*(7). https://doi.org/10.1002/14651858.cd009770.pub2

McEvoy, A., & Sabir, S. (2022). Physiology, pregnancy contractions. In *Statpearls [internet]*. StatPearls Publishing. https://www.ncbi.nlm.nih.gov/books/NBK532927/

MedCentral. (n.d.). *Terbutaline Subcutaneous*. https://www.medcentral.com/drugs/monograph/89203-382144/terbutaline-subcutaneous#cautions-3

Pfenniger, F., Leon, E., & Guirguis-Blake, J. (2013). What are the indications for intrapartum amnioinfusion? *Evidence-Based Practice, 16*(10), 7–8 https://doi.org/10.1097/01.ebp.0000540483.52742.b4

CHAPTER 12

How You Arrive: The Many Paths to Labor and Delivery

ACOG clinical practice guideline no. 8: first and second stage labor management: correction. (2025). *Obstetrics & Gynecology, 145*(3), e126–e126. https://doi.org/10.1097/aog.0000000000005834

Jenkins, S. M., & Hook, J. W. V. (2023). Induction of labor. In *Statpearls [internet]*. StatPearls Publishing. https://www.ncbi.nlm.nih.gov/books/NBK459264/

Mahdy, H., & Eruo, F. U. (2023). Amniotomy. In *Statpearls [internet]*. StatPearls Publishing. https://www.ncbi.nlm.nih.gov/books/NBK470167/

Pinas-Carrillo, A., & Chandraharan, E. (2025). Induction and augmentation of labor. In E. Chandraharan (Ed.), *The continuous textbook of women's medicine series: Obstetrics module* (Vol. 11, Labor and delivery). Global Academy of Medical Education and Training.

Uvnäs-Moberg, K. (2024). The physiology and pharmacology of oxytocin in labor and in the peripartum period. *American Journal of Obstetrics and Gynecology, 230*(3), S740–S758. https://doi.org/10.1016/j.ajog.2023.04.011

CHAPTER 13

Pitocin Is Not a Bad Word!

ACOG clinical practice guideline no. 8: first and second stage labor management: correction. (2025). *Obstetrics & Gynecology, 145*(3), e126–e126. https://doi.org/10.1097/aog.0000000000005834

American College of Obstetricians & Gynecologists. (2020, June 15). *Countdown to intern year, week 4: fetal heart tracings*. https://www.acog.org/community/districts-and-sections/district-iv/whats-new/countdown-to-intern-year-week-4-fetal-heart-tracings

Kauffmann, T., & Silberman, M. (2023). Fetal monitoring. In *Statpearls [internet]*. StatPearls Publishing. https://www.ncbi.nlm.nih.gov/books/NBK589699/

McAdow, M., Xu, X., Lipkind, H., Reddy, U. M., & Illuzzi, J. L. (2020). Association of oxytocin rest during labor induction of nulliparous women with mode of delivery. *Obstetrics & Gynecology*, *135*(3), 569–575. https://doi.org/10.1097/aog.0000000000003709

Osilla, E. V., Patel, P., & Sharma, S. (2025). Oxytocin. In *Statpearls [internet]*. StatPearls Publishing. https://www.ncbi.nlm.nih.gov/books/NBK507848/

Raees, S., Forgie, M., Mitchell, R., & Malloy, E. (2023). Calcium carbonate as a potential intervention to prevent labor dystocia: Narrative review of the literature. *Journal of Patient-Centered Research and Reviews*, *10*(3), 128–135. https://doi.org/10.17294/2330-0698.2010

CHAPTER 14

TRANSITION: The Hardest Part Before the Best Moment

Hutchison, J., Mahdy, H., Jenkins, S. M., & Hutchison, J. (2025). Normal labor: Physiology, evaluation, and management. In *Statpearls [internet]*. StatPearls Publishing. https://www.ncbi.nlm.nih.gov/books/NBK544290/

Young, E., Clarke, K.-A., Reed, R., & Hastie, C. (2025). Women's experiences of the transition phase of physiological labour during freebirth: A qualitative study. *Sexual & Reproductive Healthcare*, *45*, 101115. https://doi.org/10.1016/j.srhc.2025.101115

CHAPTER 15

The Final Stretch: Understanding the Pushing Stage

Bahl, R., Hotton, E., Crofts, J., & Draycott, T. (2024). Assisted vaginal birth in 21st century: Current practice and new innovations. *American Journal of Obstetrics and Gynecology*, *230*(3), S917–S931. https://doi.org/10.1016/j.ajog.2022.12.305

Simpson, K. (2006). When and how to push: Providing the most current information about second-stage labor to women during childbirth education. *Journal of Perinatal Education*, *15*(4), 6–9. https://doi.org/10.1624/105812406x151367

CHAPTER 16

THE ACT OF PUSHING: Working With Your Body to Bring Your Baby into the World

Bahl, R., Hotton, E., Crofts, J., & Draycott, T. (2024). Assisted vaginal birth in 21st century: Current practice and new innovations. *American Journal of Obstetrics and Gynecology*, *230*(3), S917–S931. https://doi.org/10.1016/j.ajog.2022.12.305

Barjon, K., Vadakekut, E. S., & Mahdy, H. (2024). Episiotomy. In *Statpearls [internet]*. StatPearls Publishing. https://www.ncbi.nlm.nih.gov/books/NBK546675/

Cahill, A. G., & Macones, G. A. (2024). Optimizing the length of the second stage and management of pushing. *American Journal of Obstetrics and Gynecology, 230*(3), S876–S878. https://doi.org/10.1016/j.ajog.2022.07.017

Davis, D. D., Roshan, A., & Varacallo, M. A. (2023). Shoulder dystocia. In *Statpearls [internet]*. StatPearls Publishing. https://www.ncbi.nlm.nih.gov/books/NBK470427/

Kauffmann, T., & Silberman, M. (2023). Fetal monitoring. In *Statpearls [internet]*. StatPearls Publishing. https://www.ncbi.nlm.nih.gov/books/NBK589699/

Lemos, A., Amorim, M., Dornelas de Andrade, A., de Souza, A. I., Cabral Filho, J., & Correia, J. B. (2017). Pushing/bearing down methods for the second stage of labour. *Cochrane Database of Systematic Reviews, 2017*(3). https://doi.org/10.1002/14651858.cd009124.pub3

Simpson, K. (2006). When and how to push: Providing the most current information about second-stage labor to women during childbirth education. *Journal of Perinatal Education, 15*(4), 6–9. https://doi.org/10.1624/105812406x151367

Yao, J., Roth, H., Anderson, D., Lu, H., Li, X., & Baird, K. (2022). Benefits and risks of spontaneous pushing versus directed pushing during the second stage of labour among women without epidural analgesia: A systematic review and meta-analysis. *International Journal of Nursing Studies, 134*, 104324. https://doi.org/10.1016/j.ijnurstu.2022.104324

CHAPTER 17

C-Sections: Planned, Unplanned, and Always Powerful

Sung, S., Mikes, B. A., Martingano, D. J., & Mahdy, H. (2024). Cesarean delivery. In *Statpearls [internet]*. StatPearls Publishing. https://www.ncbi.nlm.nih.gov/books/NBK546707/

Wilson, R., Caughey, A. B., Wood, S. L., Macones, G. A., Wrench, I. J., Huang, J., Norman, M., Pettersson, K., Fawcett, W. J., Shalabi, M. M., Metcalfe, A., Gramlich, L., & Nelson, G. (2018). Guidelines for antenatal and preoperative care in cesarean delivery: Enhanced recovery after surgery society recommendations (part 1). *American Journal of Obstetrics and Gynecology, 219*(6), 523.e1–523.e15. https://doi.org/10.1016/j.ajog.2018.09.015 https://www.rxlist.com>alpha_z

CHAPTER 18

The Placenta, Cord, and Delivering the Placenta

Cleveland Clinic. (2025). *Nucal Cord.* https://my.clevelandclinic.org/health/diseases/nuchal-cord

Gaikwad, V., Yalla, S., & Salvi, P. (2023). True knot of the umbilical cord and associated adverse perinatal outcomes: A case series. *Cureus.* https://doi.org/10.7759/cureus.35377

Herrick, E. J., & Bordoni, B. (2023). Embryology, placenta. In *Statpearls [internet].* StatPearls Publishing. https://www.ncbi.nlm.nih.gov/books/NBK551634/

Johnson, S., Pastuschek, J., Rödel, J., Markert, U., & Groten, T. (2018). Placenta – worth trying? human maternal placentophagy: Possible benefit and potential risks. *Geburtshilfe und Frauenheilkunde, 78*(09), 846–852. https://doi.org/10.1055/a-0674-6275

Karimi, N., Molaee, G., Tarkesh Esfahani, N., & Montazeri, A. (2022). Placental cord drainage and its outcomes at third stage of labor: A randomized controlled trial. *BMC Pregnancy and Childbirth, 22*(1). https://doi.org/10.1186/s12884-022-04877-8

Schaffer, L. (2024, September 12). *Nucal cord.* UptoDate. Retrieved November 30, 2025, from https://www.uptodate.com/contents/nuchal-cord/print

Sung, S., Mikes, B. A., Martingano, D. J., & Mahdy, H. (2024). Cesarean delivery. In *Statpearls [internet].* StatPearls Publishing. https://www.ncbi.nlm.nih.gov/books/NBK546707/

CHAPTER 19

The First Moments After Birth

Background. (2014). In *Guideline: Delayed umbilical cord clamping for improved maternal and infant health and nutrition outcomes.* World Health Organization. https://www.ncbi.nlm.nih.gov/books/NBK310514/

Sakharkar, S., Tiwari, D., Pansare, A., & Kabra, N. (2023). Neonatal resuscitation program algorithm with timeline- a concise flow chart for delivery room resuscitation. *Resuscitation Plus, 15,* 100445. https://doi.org/10.1016/j.resplu.2023.100445

Simon, L. V., Shah, M., & Bragg, B. N. (2024). Apgar score. In *Statpearls [internet].* StatPearls Publishing. https://www.ncbi.nlm.nih.gov/books/NBK470569/

Widström, A., Brimdyr, K., Svensson, K., Cadwell, K., & Nissen, E. (2019). Skin-to-skin contact the first hour after birth, underlying implications and clinical practice. *Acta Paediatrica, 108*(7), 1192–1204. https://doi.org/10.1111/apa.14754

CHAPTER 20

NICU Admission - What It Means for Baby and Mom

Alhamawi, N. J., Alharbi, H. A., & Alqahtani, M. H. (2024). Reasons and factors affecting the neonatal intensive care unit (nicu) length of stay of full-term newborns: A systematic review. *Cureus*. https://doi.org/10.7759/cureus.73892

Sakharkar, S., Tiwari, D., Pansare, A., & Kabra, N. (2023). Neonatal resuscitation program algorithm with timeline- a concise flow chart for delivery room resuscitation. *Resuscitation Plus, 15*, 100445. https://doi.org/10.1016/j.resplu.2023.100445

CHAPTER 21

Immediate Postpartum Recovery - Vaginal and C-Section Births

American Pregnancy Association. (2025). *Baby Blues*. https://americanpregnancy.org/healthy-pregnancy/first-year-of-life/baby-blues/

Berens, P. (2025, July 11). *Overview of the postpartum period: normal physiology and routine maternal care*. UptoDate. Retrieved from November 30, 2025, from https://www.uptodate.com/contents/overview-of-the-postpartum-period-normal-physiology-and-routine-maternal-care

Bienstock, J. L., Eke, A. C., & Hueppchen, N. A. (2021). Postpartum hemorrhage. *New England Journal of Medicine, 384*(17), 1635–1645. https://doi.org/10.1056/nejmra1513247

Binyamin, Y., Orbach-Zinger, S., & Heesen, M. (2025). Current strategies for the diagnosis and management of postpartum hemorrhage: A focused review of four cochrane systematic reviews from 2024 and 2025. *International Journal of Obstetric Anesthesia, 63*, 104692. https://doi.org/10.1016/j.ijoa.2025.104692

Carlson, K., Mughal, S., Azhar, Y., & Siddiqui, W. (2025). Perinatal depression. In *Statpearls [internet]*. StatPearls Publishing. https://www.ncbi.nlm.nih.gov/books/NBK519070/

Chauhan, G., & Tadi, P. (2022). Physiology, postpartum changes. In *Statpearls [internet]*. StatPearls Publishing. https://www.ncbi.nlm.nih.gov/books/NBK555904/

Cleveland Clinic. (2025). *Lochia*. https://my.clevelandclinic.org/health/body/22485-lochia

Lopez-Gonzalez, D. M., & Kopparapu, A. K. (2022). Postpartum Care of the new mother. In *Statpearls [internet]*. StatPearls Publishing. https://www.ncbi.nlm.nih.gov/books/NBK565875/

Osilla, E. V., Patel, P., & Sharma, S. (2025). Oxytocin. In *Statpearls [internet]*. StatPearls Publishing. https://www.ncbi.nlm.nih.gov/books/NBK507848/

Oxytocin. (2025). In *Drugs and lactation database (lactmed®) [internet]*. National Institute of Child Health and Human Development. https://www.ncbi.nlm.nih.gov/books/NBK501490/

World Health Organization. (2022). Executive summary. In *Who recommendations on maternal and newborn care for a positive postnatal experience [internet]*. https://www.ncbi.nlm.nih.gov/books/NBK579653/

Chapter 22

Vaginal Birth Recovery

Berkowitz, L. R. (2025, August 11). *Postpartum perineal care and management of complications*. UptoDate. Retrieved November 30, 2025, from https://www.uptodate.com/contents/postpartum-perineal-care-and-management-of-complications

Lopez-Gonzalez, D. M., & Kopparapu, A. K. (2022). Postpartum Care of the new mother. In *Statpearls [internet]*. StatPearls Publishing. https://www.ncbi.nlm.nih.gov/books/NBK565875/

Roman, A. S. (2025, October 14). *Management of hematomas incurred as a result of obstetric delivery*. UptoDate. . Retrieved November 30, 2025, from https://www.uptodate.com/contents/management-of-hematomas-incurred-as-a-result-of-obstetric-delivery

Chapter 23

C-Section Birth Recovery

Berghella, V. (2025, March 24). *Cesarean birth: postoperative care, complications, and long-term sequelae*. UptoDate. Retrieved November 30, 2025, from https://www.uptodate.com/contents/cesarean-birth-postoperative-care-complications-and-long-term-sequelae?search=antiemetics%20after%20post%20cesarean&source=search_result&selectedTitle=1~150&usage_type=default&display_rank=1

Carvalho, B. (2025, October). *Post-cesarean delivery analgesia*. UptoDate. Retrieved November 30, 2025, from https://www.uptodate.com/contents/post-cesarean-delivery-analgesia

Hailu, S., Mekonen, S., & Shiferaw, A. (2022). Prevention and management of postoperative nausea and vomiting after cesarean section: A systematic literature review. *Annals of Medicine & Surgery, 75*. https://doi.org/10.1016/j.amsu.2022.103433

Lopez-Gonzalez, D. M., & Kopparapu, A. K. (2022). Postpartum Care of the new mother. In *Statpearls [internet]*. StatPearls Publishing. https://www.ncbi.nlm.nih.gov/books/NBK565875/

Singh, P. M., Sultan, P., O'Carroll, J., Blake, L., Carvalho, B., Singh, N. P., & Monks, D. T. (2023). Pharmacological agents for prevention of pruritus in women undergoing caesarean delivery with neuraxial morphine: A systematic review and bayesian network meta-analysis. *British Journal of Anaesthesia, 131*(3), 556–571. https://doi.org/10.1016/j.bja.2023.05.028

Sung, S., Mikes, B. A., Martingano, D. J., & Mahdy, H. (2024). Cesarean delivery. In *Statpearls [internet]*. StatPearls Publishing. https://www.ncbi.nlm.nih.gov/books/NBK546707/

Tian, X., Niu, K., Cao, H., Zhan, G., Zhang, Y., Xu, F., Shangguan, W., & Gao, Y. (2021). Pruritus after continuous administration of epidural morphine for post-cesarean delivery analgesia: A case control study. *BMC Pregnancy and Childbirth, 21*(1). https://doi.org/10.1186/s12884-020-03522-6

CHAPTER 24

Your First Moments Together

Babakazo, P., Bosonkie, M., Mafuta, E., Mvuama, N., & Mapatano, M.-A. (2022). Common breastfeeding problems experienced by lactating mothers during the first six months in Kinshasa. *PLOS ONE, 17*(10), e0275477. https://doi.org/10.1371/journal.pone.0275477

Blackmon, M. M., Nguyen, H., Vadakekut, E. S., & Mukherji, P. (2024). Acute mastitis. In *Statpearls [internet]*. StatPearls Publishing. https://www.ncbi.nlm.nih.gov/books/NBK557782/

Cleveland Clinic. (2025). *Colostrum*. https://my.clevelandclinic.org/health/body/22434-colostrum

Shorey, S., He, H.-G., & Morelius, E. (2016). Skin-to-skin contact by fathers and the impact on infant and paternal outcomes: An integrative review. *Midwifery, 40*, 207–217. https://doi.org/10.1016/j.midw.2016.07.007

United States Department of Agriculture - WIC Breastfeeding Support. (n.d.). *Pumping and hand expression basics*. USDA WIC breastfeeding support. https://wicbreastfeeding.fns.usda.gov/pumping-and-hand-expression-basics

Widström, A., Brimdyr, K., Svensson, K., Cadwell, K., & Nissen, E. (2019). Skin-to-skin contact the first hour after birth, underlying implications and clinical practice. *Acta Paediatrica, 108*(7), 1192–1204. https://doi.org/10.1111/apa.14754

CHAPTER 25

Baby Care in Recovery

Conis, E. (2011). "Do we really need hepatitis b on the second day of life?" vaccination mandates and shifting representations of hepatitis b. *Journal of Medical Humanities, 32*(2), 155–166. https://doi.org/10.1007/s10912-010-9132-2

McKee-Garrett, T. M. (2025, October 8). *Overview of the routine management of the healthy newborn infant.* UptoDate. Retrieved November 30, 2025, from https://www.uptodate.com/contents/overview-of-the-routine-management-of-the-healthy-newborn-infant

Mitanchez, D. (2015). What neonatal complications should the pediatrician be aware of in case of maternal gestational diabetes? *World Journal of Diabetes, 6*(5), 734. https://doi.org/10.4239/wjd.v6.i5.734

MotherToBaby | Fact Sheets [Internet]. Brentwood (TN): Organization of Teratology Information Specialists (OTIS); 1994-. Gestational Diabetes. 2025 Mar. Available from: https://www.ncbi.nlm.nih.gov/books/NBK582729/

Pulsifer, A., Puopolo, K. M., Skerritt, L., Dhudasia, M. B., Pyle, B., Schumacher, A., & Mukhopadhyay, S. (2021). Improving compliance with revised newborn hepatitis b vaccination policy. *Hospital Pediatrics, 11*(12), 1354–1363. https://doi.org/10.1542/hpeds.2021-005969

Warees, W. M., Anand, S., Leslie, S. W., & Rodriguez, A. M. (2024). Circumcision. In *Statpearls [internet].* StatPearls Publishing. https://www.ncbi.nlm.nih.gov/books/NBK535436/

CHAPTER 26

Transition from Immediate Recovery to Postpartum: The Hand-Off of Care

Berkowitz, L. R. (2025, August 11). *Postpartum perineal care and management of complications.* UptoDate. Retrieved November 30, 2025 from https://www.uptodate.com/contents/postpartum-perineal-care-and-management-of-complications

CHAPTER 27
Common Infections in Labor & Delivery: What They Are & How We Treat Them

Abu Esba, L., Al Mardawi, G., Al Mardawi, E., Almadhi, F., & Ardah, H. I. (2023). Misoprostol-induced fever and unnecessary antibiotic prescribing: A retrospective study. *Infectious Diseases and Therapy*, *12*(9), 2259–2268. https://doi.org/10.1007/s40121-023-00865-3

Asafo-Agyei, K. O., & Samant, H. (2025). Pregnancy and viral hepatitis. In *Statpearls [internet]*. StatPearls Publishing. https://www.ncbi.nlm.nih.gov/books/NBK556026/

Belyayeva, M., Leslie, S. W., & Jeong, J. M. (2024). Acute pyelonephritis. In *Statpearls [internet]*. StatPearls Publishing. https://www.ncbi.nlm.nih.gov/books/NBK519537/

Dombrowski, J. C. (2021). Chlamydia and gonorrhea. *Annals of Internal Medicine*, *174*(10), ITC145–ITC160. https://doi.org/10.7326/aitc202110190

Fowler, J. R., & Simon, L. V. (2023). Chorioamnionitis. In *Statpearls [internet]*. StatPearls Publishing. https://www.ncbi.nlm.nih.gov/books/NBK532251/

Gigi, R. S., Buitrago-Garcia, D., Taghavi, K., Dunaiski, C.-M., van de Wijgert, J. M., Peters, R. H., & Low, N. (2023). Vulvovaginal yeast infections during pregnancy and perinatal outcomes: Systematic review and meta-analysis. *BMC Women's Health*, *23*(1). https://doi.org/10.1186/s12905-023-02258-7

Habak, P. J., Carlson, K., & Jr, R. P. G. (2024). Urinary tract infection in pregnancy. In *Statpearls [internet]*. StatPearls Publishing. https://www.ncbi.nlm.nih.gov/books/NBK537047/

Hammad, W., & Konje, J. C. (2021). Herpes simplex virus infection in pregnancy – an update. *European Journal of Obstetrics & Gynecology and Reproductive Biology*, *259*, 38–45. https://doi.org/10.1016/j.ejogrb.2021.01.055

Irshad, U., Mahdy, H., & Tonismae, T. (2023). Hiv in pregnancy. In *Statpearls [internet]*. StatPearls Publishing. https://www.ncbi.nlm.nih.gov/books/NBK558972/

Ng, B., Chuah, J., Cheah, F., Mohamed Ismail, N., Tan, G., Wong, K., & Lim, P. (2023). Maternal and fetal outcomes of pregnant women with bacterial vaginosis. *Frontiers in Surgery*, *10*. https://doi.org/10.3389/fsurg.2023.1084867

Raabe, V. N., & Shane, A. L. (2019). Group b streptococcus (streptococcus agalactiae). *Microbiology Spectrum*, *7*(2). https://doi.org/10.1128/microbiolspec.gpp3-0007-2018

Zamstein, O., Wainstock, T., & Sheiner, E. (2023). Intrapartum maternal fever and long-term infectious morbidity of the offspring. *Journal of Clinical Medicine, 12*(9), 3329. https://doi.org/10.3390/jcm12093329

CHAPTER 28

Hypertensive Disorders including Pre-Eclampsia and her Ugly Sisters: What You Need to Know

August, P. (2025, March 6). *Treatment of hypertension in pregnant and postpartum patients.* UptoDate. https://www.uptodate.com/contents/treatment-of-hypertension-in-pregnant-and-postpartum-patients?search=severe%20hypertension%20treatment&source=search_result&selectedTitle=5~150&usage_type=default&display_rank=5

Bienstock, J. L., Eke, A. C., & Hueppchen, N. A. (2021). Postpartum hemorrhage. *New England Journal of Medicine, 384*(17), 1635–1645. https://doi.org/10.1056/nejmra1513247

Binyamin, Y., Orbach-Zinger, S., & Heesen, M. (2025). Current strategies for the diagnosis and management of postpartum hemorrhage: A focused review of four cochrane systematic reviews from 2024 and 2025. *International Journal of Obstetric Anesthesia, 63*, 104692. https://doi.org/10.1016/j.ijoa.2025.104692

Eppes, C., Mundy, K., Rhodes, M., Handy, W., Davidson, C. M., Leke, E. B., & Lundeen, S. (2024). Postpartum hemorrhage. *American Journal of Obstetrics and Gynecology, 220*(1). https://doi.org/10.1016/j.ajog.2018.11.267

Hicks, M. A., & Tyagi, A. (2023). Magnesium sulfate. In *Statpearls [internet]*. StatPearls Publishing. https://www.ncbi.nlm.nih.gov/books/NBK554553/

Khalid, F., Mahendraker, N., & Tonismae, T. (2023). Hellp syndrome. In *Statpearls [internet]*. StatPearls Publishing. https://www.ncbi.nlm.nih.gov/books/NBK560615/

Luger, R. K., & Kight, B. P. (2022). Hypertension in pregnancy. In *Statpearls [internet]*. StatPearls Publishing. https://www.ncbi.nlm.nih.gov/books/NBK430839/

Onishi, K., Seagraves, E., Baraki, D., Donaldson, T., Barake, C., Abuhamad, A., Huang, J. C., & Kawakita, T. (2023). Comparison of adverse maternal outcomes between early- and late-onset superimposed preeclampsia. *American Journal of Perinatology, 41*(S 01), e2010–e2016. https://doi.org/10.1055/a-2096-3403

Norwitz, E. R. (2025, October). *Preeclampsia: intrapartum and postpartum management and long-term prognosis.* UptoDate. Retrieved December 1, 2025, from https://www.uptodate.com/contents/preeclampsia-intrapartum-and-postpartum-management-and-long-term-prognosis?search=magnesium%20sulfate%20and%20newborns&source=search_result&selectedTitle=7~150&usage_type=default&display_rank=6

Yang, H., Sun, G., Cheng, Y., Cao, D., & Zhao, Y. (2022). Bakri balloon tamponade to treat postpartum hemorrhage. *Chinese Medical Journal, 135*(18), 2258–2260. https://doi.org/10.1097/cm9.0000000000002387

CHAPTER 29
POSTPARTUM HEMORRHAGE (PPH): WHAT IT IS, WHY IT HAPPENS, AND HOW WE RESPOND

Abu Esba, L., Al Mardawi, G., Al Mardawi, E., Almadhi, F., & Ardah, H. I. (2023). Misoprostol-induced fever and unnecessary antibiotic prescribing: A retrospective study. *Infectious Diseases and Therapy, 12*(9), 2259–2268. https://doi.org/10.1007/s40121-023-00865-3

Bienstock, J. L., Eke, A. C., & Hueppchen, N. A. (2021). Postpartum hemorrhage. *New England Journal of Medicine, 384*(17), 1635–1645. https://doi.org/10.1056/nejmra1513247

Binyamin, Y., Orbach-Zinger, S., & Heesen, M. (2025). Current strategies for the diagnosis and management of postpartum hemorrhage: A focused review of four cochrane systematic reviews from 2024 and 2025. *International Journal of Obstetric Anesthesia, 63*, 104692. https://doi.org/10.1016/j.ijoa.2025.104692

Brown, M., Hong, M., & Lindquist, J. (2021). Uterine artery embolization for primary postpartum hemorrhage. *Techniques in Vascular and Interventional Radiology, 24*(1), 100727. https://doi.org/10.1016/j.tvir.2021.100727

Clark, M., & MacDougall, D. (2022). Vacuum-induced uterine tamponade for postpartum hemorrhage. In Canadian Agency for Drugs and Technologies in Health. https://www.ncbi.nlm.nih.gov/books/NBK596675/

Cooper, D. B., & Menefee, G. W. (2023). Dilation and curettage. In *Statpearls [internet]*. StatPearls Publishing. https://www.ncbi.nlm.nih.gov/books/NBK568791/

Eppes, C., Mundy, K., Rhodes, M., Handy, W., Davidson, C. M., Leke, E. B., & Lundeen, S. (2024). Postpartum hemorrhage. *American Journal of Obstetrics and Gynecology, 220*(1). https://doi.org/10.1016/j.ajog.2018.11.267

Kallianidis, A. F., Rijntjes, D., Brobbel, C., Dekkers, O. M., Bloemenkamp, K. M., & van den Akker, T. (2022). Incidence, indications, risk factors, and outcomes of emergency peripartum hysterectomy worldwide. *Obstetrics & Gynecology, 141*(1), 35–48. https://doi.org/10.1097/aog.0000000000005022

Rajaretnam, N., Okoye, E., & Burns, B. (2023). Laparotomy. In *Statpearls [internet]*. StatPearls Publishing. https://www.ncbi.nlm.nih.gov/books/NBK525961/

Roberts, I., Brenner, A., & Shakur-Still, H. (2023). Tranexamic acid for bleeding: Much more than a treatment for postpartum hemorrhage. *American Journal of Obstetrics & Gynecology MFM*, *5*(2), 100722. https://doi.org/10.1016/j.ajogmf.2022.100722

Sadiku, O. D., Aina, S. A., Odoemene, C. C., Ogunmoyin, T. E., Adedara, V. O., Olasimbo, O., Ashir, F. A., Adili, S. C., Kuteyi, A. O., Fakayode, O. O., Faletti, D. O., & Nogales Bernal, M. (2024). Approaches to the prevention and treatment of postpartum hemorrhage: A systematic review of past advances, recent developments, and best practices. *Cureus*. https://doi.org/10.7759/cureus.65096

Wei, C., Chang, X., Dong, J., & Zhou, Q. (2020). Remifentanil for carboprost-induced adverse reactions during cesarean delivery under combined spinal-epidural anesthesia. *Frontiers in Pharmacology*, *11*. https://doi.org/10.3389/fphar.2020.00980

Wormer, K. C., Jamil, R. T., & Bryant, S. B. (2024). Postpartum hemorrhage. In *Statpearls [internet]*. StatPearls Publishing. https://www.ncbi.nlm.nih.gov/books/NBK499988/

Yang, H., Sun, G., Cheng, Y., Cao, D., & Zhao, Y. (2022). Bakri balloon tamponade to treat postpartum hemorrhage. *Chinese Medical Journal*, *135*(18), 2258–2260. https://doi.org/10.1097/cm9.0000000000002387

CHAPTER 30

Other Pregnancy Complications

Davis, D. D., Roshan, A., & Varacallo, M. A. (2023). Shoulder dystocia. In *Statpearls [internet]*. StatPearls Publishing. https://www.ncbi.nlm.nih.gov/books/NBK470427/

Durnwald, C. (2025, September 19). *Patient education: gestational diabetes (beyond the basics)*. UptoDate. Retrieved December 8, 2025, from https://www.uptodate.com/contents/gestational-diabetes-beyond-the-basics

Kunarathnam, V., Vadakekut, E. S., & Mahdy, H. (2025). Gestational diabetes. In *Statpearls [internet]*. StatPearls Publishing. https://www.ncbi.nlm.nih.gov/books/NBK545196/

CHAPTER 31

Preterm Labor: What It Is and What It Means for You and Your Baby

American College of Obstetricians and Gynecologists. (2010). *Magnesium sulfate before anticipated preterm birth for neuroprotection*. ACOG clinical. https://www.acog.org/clinical/clinical-guidance/committee-opinion/articles/2010/03/magnesium-sulfate-before-anticipated-preterm-birth-for-neuroprotection

Chawla, S., Wyckoff, M. H., Lakshminrusimha, S., Rysavy, M. A., Patel, R., Chowdhury, D., Das, A., Greenberg, R. G., Natarajan, G., Shankaran, S., Bell, E. F., Ambalavanan, N., Younge, N. E., Laptook, A. R., Pavlek, L. R., Backes, C. H., Van Meurs, K. P., Werner, E. F., Carlo, W. A.,...Shankaran, S. (2025). Short duration of antenatal corticosteroid exposure and outcomes in extremely preterm infants. *JAMA Network Open*, *8*(2), e2461312. https://doi.org/10.1001/jamanetworkopen.2024.61312

Funai, E. F. (2024, May 31). *Patient education: preterm labor (beyond the basics).* UptoDate. Retrieved December 8, 2025, from https://www.uptodate.com/contents/preterm-labor-beyond-the-basics/print

Jenkins, S. M., & Mikes, B. A. (2025). Preterm labor. In *Statpearls [internet].* StatPearls Publishing. https://www.ncbi.nlm.nih.gov/books/NBK536939/

Khawar, H., & Marwaha, K. (2023). Surfactant. In *Statpearls [internet].* StatPearls Publishing. https://www.ncbi.nlm.nih.gov/books/NBK546600/

Lim, H., Yu, S., Lee, H., Hwang, S., Kim, D., Park, J., & Lee, L. P. (2025). Understanding the impact of antenatal corticosteroids via placenta and fetal lung microphysiological analysis platform (map) on a chip. *Trends in Biotechnology*, *43*(10), 2665–2679. https://doi.org/10.1016/j.tibtech.2025.06.006

MedCentral. (n.d.). *Terbutaline Subcutaneous.* https://www.medcentral.com/drugs/monograph/89203-382144/terbutaline-subcutaneous#cautions-3

Saldaña-García, N., Espinosa-Fernández, M., Martínez-Pajares, J., Tapia-Moreno, E., Moreno-Samos, M., Cuenca-Marín, C., Rius-Díaz, F., & Sánchez-Tamayo, T. (2022). Antenatal betamethasone every 12 hours in imminent preterm labour. *Journal of Clinical Medicine, 11*(5), 1227. https://doi.org/10.3390/jcm11051227

Songthamwat, S., Na Nan, C., & Songthamwat, M. (2018). Effectiveness of nifedipine in threatened preterm labor: A randomized trial. *International Journal of Women's Health, Volume 10*, 317–323. https://doi.org/10.2147/ijwh.s159062

CHAPTER 32

Placental & Uterine Complications: What You Need to Know

American College of Obstetricians and Gynecologists. (2018). Placenta accreta spectrum. *Obstetrics & Gynecology*, *132*(6), 259–275. https://www.acog.org/-/media/project/acog/acogorg/clinical/files/obstetric-care-consensus/articles/2018/12/placenta-accreta-spectrum.pdf?rev=c00cd7ddadb54897bc450086708039db&hash=09EC778BDC6806E9B4149AE0C5417239

Anderson-Bagga, F. M., & Sze, A. (2023). Placenta previa. In *Statpearls [internet]*. StatPearls Publishing. https://www.ncbi.nlm.nih.gov/books/NBK539818/

Schmidt, P., Skelly, C. L., & Raines, D. A. (2022). Placental abruption. In *Statpearls [internet]*. StatPearls Publishing. https://www.ncbi.nlm.nih.gov/books/NBK482335/

Togioka, B. M., & Tonismae, T. (2023). Uterine rupture. In *Statpearls [internet]*. StatPearls Publishing. https://www.ncbi.nlm.nih.gov/books/NBK559209/

CHAPTER 33

Special Deliveries: When Your Birth Journey Needs Something Extra

Akanmode, A. M., & Mahdy, H. (2025). Macrosomia. In *Statpearls [internet]*. StatPearls Publishing. https://www.ncbi.nlm.nih.gov/books/NBK557577/

Bieber, K. B., & Olson, S. M. (2023). Cervical cerclage. In *Statpearls [internet]*. StatPearls Publishing. https://www.ncbi.nlm.nih.gov/books/NBK560523/

Chew, L. C., Osuchukwu, O. O., Reed, D. J., & Verma, R. P. (2024). Fetal growth restriction. In *Statpearls [internet]*. StatPearls Publishing. https://www.ncbi.nlm.nih.gov/books/NBK562268/

Cleveland Clinic. (2025). *Amniotic fluid*. https://my.clevelandclinic.org/health/body/23310-amniotic-fluid

Dalvi, S. (2025). Fetal anomalies: An obstetrician's overview. *The Journal of Obstetrics and Gynecology of India*, *75*(4), 275–281. https://doi.org/10.1007/s13224-025-02211-8

Dayal, S., Jenkins, S. M., & Hong, P. L. (2024). Preterm and term prelabor rupture of membranes (pprom and prom). In *Statpearls [internet]*. StatPearls Publishing. https://www.ncbi.nlm.nih.gov/books/NBK532888/

Fenton, T. R., Merlino Barr, S., Elmrayed, S., & Alshaikh, B. (2024). Expected and desirable preterm and small infant growth patterns. *Advances in Nutrition*, *15*(6), 100220. https://doi.org/10.1016/j.advnut.2024.100220

Glick, I., Kadish, E., & Rottenstreich, M. (2021). Management of pregnancy in women of advanced maternal age: Improving outcomes for mother and baby. *International Journal of Women's Health*, *Volume 13*, 751–759. https://doi.org/10.2147/ijwh.s283216

Habak, P. J., Khaparde, G., & Vadakekut, E. S. (2025). Vaginal birth after cesarean delivery. In *Statpearls [internet]*. StatPearls Publishing. https://www.ncbi.nlm.nih.gov/books/NBK507844/

Pillarisetty, L. S., & Sharma, A. (2023). Pregnancy intrahepatic cholestasis. In *Statpearls [internet]*. StatPearls Publishing. https://www.ncbi.nlm.nih.gov/books/NBK551503/

CHAPTER 34

Toys of the Trade: Tools That Help Us Help You

Mazzeo Melchionda, M., Aloi, T., Bruno, F., De Lazzari, A., Mauri, P., & Esposito, G. (2025). Spinning babies® approach: A way to promote fetal head rotation during labor? *European Journal of Midwifery, 9*(September), 1–4. https://doi.org/10.18332/ejm/206972

CHAPTER 35

Support People & Doulas: The Heart of Your Birth Team

CHAPTER 36

Anxiety in Labor, Panic Attacks & Feeling Out of Control

Hishikawa, K., Kusaka, T., Fukuda, T., Kohata, Y., & Inoue, H. (2019). Anxiety or nervousness disturbs the progress of birth based on human behavioral evolutionary biology. *The Journal of Perinatal Education, 28*(4), 218–223. https://doi.org/10.1891/1058-1243.28.4.218

Kundarti, F., Kiswati, & Komalyna, I. (2024). Mindfulness based intervention reduce anxiety in labor. *Gaceta Sanitaria, 38*, 102359. https://doi.org/10.1016/j.gaceta.2024.102359

CHAPTER 37

Birth Trauma & Emotional Safety in Labor

Fugate, S., Conklin, A., & Maines, J. (2025). Birth trauma. In *Statpearls [internet]*. StatPearls Publishing. https://www.ncbi.nlm.nih.gov/books/NBK539831/

CHAPTER 38

Postpartum Depression (PPD): When the Feelings Don't Match the Moment

American Pregnancy Association. (2025). *Baby Blues*. https://americanpregnancy.org/healthy-pregnancy/first-year-of-life/baby-blues/

Carlson, K., Mughal, S., Azhar, Y., & Siddiqui, W. (2025). Perinatal depression. In *Statpearls [internet]*. StatPearls Publishing. https://www.ncbi.nlm.nih.gov/books/NBK519070/

CHAPTER 39

Supporting a Teenager in the Childbirth Setting: Respecting Autonomy, Supporting Strength

Cox, J. E. (2024, November 26). *Pregnancy in adolescents*. UptoDate. Retrieved December 8, 2025, from https://www.uptodate.com/contents/pregnancy-in-adolescents?search=teenage%20pregnancy%20risk%20factors&source=search_result&selectedTitle=1~25&usage_type=default&display_rank=1

Harding, J. F., Zief, S., Farb, A., & Margolis, A. (2020). Supporting expectant and parenting teens: New evidence to inform future programming and research. *Maternal and Child Health Journal, 24*(S2), 67–75. Retrieved March 23, 2025, from https://doi.org/10.1007/s10995-020-02996-2

CHAPTER 40

Teenage Pregnancy: Your Autonomy, Your Strength, Your Voice

Cox, J. E. (2024, November 26). *Pregnancy in adolescents*. UptoDate. Retrieved December 8, 2025, from https://www.uptodate.com/contents/pregnancy-in-adolescents?search=teenage%20pregnancy%20risk%20factors&source=search_result&selectedTitle=1~25&usage_type=default&display_rank=1

CHAPTER 41

Caring for You, Not Judging You

Substance Use Disorder in Pregnancy & Postpartum

Lim, G., Carvalho, B., George, R. B., Bateman, B. T., Brummett, C. M., Ip, V. H., Landau, R., Osmundson, S., Raymond, B., Richebe, P., Soens, M., & Terplan, M. (2025). Consensus statement on pain management for pregnant patients with opioid use disorder from the society for obstetric anesthesia and perinatology, society for maternal-fetal medicine, and american society of regional anesthesia and pain medicine. *American Journal of Obstetrics and Gynecology, 233*(4), B1–B29.

Prince, M. K., Daley, S. F., & Ayers, D. (2023). Substance use in pregnancy. In *Statpearls [internet]*. StatPearls Publishing. https://www.ncbi.nlm.nih.gov/books/NBK542330/

www.ingramcontent.com/pod-product-compliance
Ingram Content Group UK Ltd.
Pitfield, Milton Keynes, MK11 3LW, UK
UKHW020128290926
15471UKWH00003B/359

9 798994 317303